Clinical Conundrums to Practice Diagnostic Reasoning

Smitha Bhat

Clinical Conundrums to Practice Diagnostic Reasoning

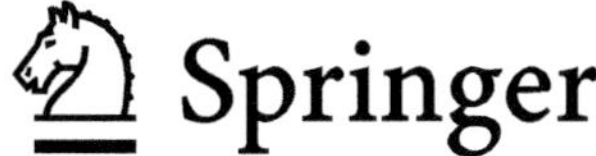

Smitha Bhat
Department of Medicine
Father Muller Medical College
Mangaluru, Karnataka, India

ISBN 978-981-95-0635-4 ISBN 978-981-95-0636-1 (eBook)
https://doi.org/10.1007/978-981-95-0636-1

This Springer imprint is published by the registered company Springer Nature Singapore Pte Ltd.
The registered company address is: 152 Beach Road, #21-01/04 Gateway East, Singapore 189721, Singapore

To

Dr. Sandeep Gopal—the wind beneath my wings...

Foreword by Swati Srivastava

It is truly a great honor to write the foreword for *Clinical Conundrums to Practice Diagnostic Reasoning*.

To develop strong diagnostic reasoning skills, one must engage in deliberate practice by working through clinical conundrums, whether real or simulated, while articulating the reasoning process. Comparing one's approaches with expert insights helps identify cognitive errors and knowledge gaps. Clinical problem-solving abilities vary significantly among clinicians and are dependent not only on their level of expertise within a specific domain, but also their ability to correlate and integrate information from various sources.

Dr. Smitha Bhat has taken up the task of creating and discussing cases that stimulate the diagnostic reasoning process. Dr. Smitha Bhat is a Professor of Medicine at Father Muller Medical College, Mangalore. She is passionate about teaching and assessment and is a noted medical educationist. Her special interests are bedside teaching and assessment—especially workplace-based assessment. She includes a number of innovations in her interaction with students: open book exams, clinical puzzles to encourage diagnostic reasoning, and gamification. Dr. Smitha's contribution to teaching has been recognized by various universities: She is a member of the Board of Studies of the Rajiv Gandhi University of Health Sciences, a former member of the Faculty of Medicine for Sri Devaraj Urs University, and of the Board of Studies for JSS university Mysore, and a member of the Staff Development Council for Nitte University, Mangalore. She is an undergraduate and postgraduate examiner, examiner for the National Board of examinations, and for MRCP PACES. She has co-authored a book *Linker Case Primer: Integrated Teaching in CBME* curriculum.

Considering the clinical utility and significance of clinical practice diagnostic reasoning, I am sure this book will be a learning experience for medical students, postgraduate residents, and internists. I compliment Dr. Smitha for having written this fascinating book.

Swati Srivastava

Governor, American College
of Physicians, India Chapter
Jaipur, Rajasthan, India
Fellow In Diabetes Management
(CMC VELLORE)
Vellore, India
Senior Professor & Unit Head,
SMS Medical College
Jaipur, Rajasthan, India
Past National Chair: Medical Student
Committee, ACP, India Chapter
Jaipur, Rajasthan, India
Member AACE Diabetes and Thyroid
Disease State Network 2020-2021
Jaipur, Rajasthan, India
Vice-Chairman: RSSDI Rajasthan
District Coordinator Committee
Jaipur, Rajasthan, India
Governing Body Member, Rajasthan RSSDI
Jaipur, Rajasthan, India
Joint Secretary: Rajasthan API
Jaipur, Rajasthan, India
Organising Secretary: IPF
Jaipur, Rajasthan, India
Member Executive Committee: Raj RSSDI
Jaipur, Rajasthan, India

Foreword Anuj Maheshwari

Dr. Smitha Bhat is a Professor of Medicine and consultant physician at Father Muller Medical College, Mangalore. She is a reputed speaker at numerous national conferences and fora. Dr. Smitha has authored this book that focuses on diagnostic reasoning—to stimulate analytical skills and critical thinking—something she is passionate about.

Diagnostic reasoning is the skill that distinguishes exceptional clinicians from merely competent practitioners. This volume, *Clinical Conundrums to Practice Diagnostic Reasoning*, uses the powerful instrument of storytelling to guide readers through the intricacies of integrating history, physical examination findings, and lab investigations to reach a diagnosis. By presenting clinical scenarios that deliberately introduce diagnostic ambiguity, the author encourages the reader to think, reflect, and analyze.

Each chapter begins with a story. The tales are sometimes funny and sometimes sad, and are based on characters one can identify with. They underscore the fundamental principle that behind every complex medical presentation lies a unique human experience. The story is followed by the analytical approach to reach the diagnosis, and then a brief summary of the aetiopathogenesis, signs, symptoms, and treatment of the disease.

For medical students, postgraduate residents, and internists committed to continuous professional development, this volume represents an indispensable resource.

It challenges readers to move beyond easy answers, encouraging a more analytical and nuanced approach to clinical problem-solving.

I recommend that this book be added to the arsenal of anyone who is interested in the fascinating ever-changing field of internal medicine.

Anuj Maheshwari

Professor, General Medicine, Hind Institute of Medical Sciences
Ataria, Sitapur, UP, India
Immediate Past Governor, American College of Physicians, India Chapter
Jaipur, Rajasthan, India
President Elect Research Society for Study of Diabetes in India
New Delhi, Delhi, India
President, Asian Pacific Society of Hypertension
Lucknow, India
Secretary General of Indian Society of Hypertension
Lucknow, India
Vice President, International Society of Medical Nutrition
Lucknow, India

Acknowledgments

From the germ of the idea in the brain to getting it on paper—it's been a long journey, and I wouldn't have been able to complete it without the support of my family, friends, and colleagues.

I'm grateful to my parents—Professor S. V. Bhat and Mrs. Anitha Bhat, for starting me on the path of learning and teaching, and to my husband Dr. Sandeep Gopal and our son Pramath, for being the center and strength of my life.

I'm fortunate to work and teach in Father Muller Medical College, Mangalore, and I acknowledge the support of the Directors of Father Muller Charitable institutions—Rev. Fr Baptist Menezes, Rev. Fr Patrick Rodrigues, Rev. Fr Richard Aloysius Coelho, and Rev. Fr Faustine Lucas Lobo. I am thankful to the administrators of Father Muller Medical College and Father Muller Hospital—Rev. Fr Lawrence D'Souza, Rev. Fr Denis D'Sa, Rev. Fr Stany Tauro, Rev. Fr Rudolph Ravi D'Sa, Rev. Fr Ajith B. Menezes, Rev. Fr George Jeevan Sequeira, and Rev. Fr. Michael Santhumayor. I am grateful to the Deans of Father Muller Medical College—Dr. Sanjeev Rai, Dr. J P Alva, and Dr. Antony Sylvan D Souza and Chief of Research Dr. Ramesh Bhat, for their constant motivation to excel. I am especially grateful to the heads of the Department of Medicine—Dr. K S Bhat, Dr. B M Venkatesh, Dr. Arunachalam, and Dr. Roshan, and my colleagues—passionate and committed internists—for their interest and encouragement when I was developing the puzzles.

This book was written to share my love for the subject of internal medicine with my students—it is their interest and enthusiasm that motivated me to write. I acknowledge the contribution of Dr. Vimala Colaco, Associate Professor of Neurology, FMMC, who has contributed images and her expertise to many of the chapters on neurology.

I am very thankful to the immediate past governor and governor of the American College of Physicians, India Chapter, Dr. Anuj Maheshwari and Dr. Swati Srivastava, for writing the foreword, and for their support at every step of my journey. Many fellow physicians have played a role in the blossoming of my career as physician, teacher, and writer—Dr. Mukhyaprana Prabhu, Dr. Bijay Patni, Dr. Narsingh Verma, Dr. Akash Singh, Dr. Ashutosh Mishra, D r. Mohsin Aslam, Dr. NK Singh, Dr. Anil Virmani, Dr. Aravinda Jagadeesha, Dr. Shivashankar KN, Dr. Thomas Chacko, and Dr. D. K. Sreenivas—mere words cannot express what I owe to them.

My life has been made colorful and vibrant by the support of the strong women who I am fortunate to call my friends—Dr. Usha Sriram, Dr. Sudha Vidyasagar, Dr. Lily Rodrigues, Dr. Mary d Cruz, Dr. Kavita Gone, Dr. Sarala N, Dr. Vinutha Shankar, Dr. Savita Bhagavan, Dr. Shruthi Narayan, Dr. Vani, Dr. Vijayalakshmi, Dr Uma, Dr. Shailaja S., Dr. Sunitha Patil, Dr. Sudha Ramalingam, Dr. Archana Bhat, and my sister, Dr. Amritha Bhat.

The so-called gut feeling that many of us rely on while seeing patients is actually memory and intelligence and experience all working together. I hope the cases in this book stimulate both your intuition and your intelligence and make the process of diagnosis fun and fascinating.

Smitha Bhat

Competing Interests The author has no competing interests to declare that are relevant to the content of this manuscript.

Contents

Part I

Clinical Conundrums

1 Reversible Cause of Coma in a Previously Healthy Adult: The Miraculous Recovery

Grade Moderate

Abstract Young adult male with no prior comorbidities, not a consumer of ethanol or recreational drugs, with no history of trauma—brought to hospital in coma, with no apparent etiology detected.

The story You are about to finish your duty, so you are disappointed, but not surprised, when an unconscious patient is wheeled in just as you are about to leave. The patient is accompanied by a sobbing lady.

"I'm his sister." she informs you.

You attempt to console her and get a coherent history.

"He was ok last night, doctor. He returned from a party, went to bed and woke up vomiting since early morning, maybe 5 am. We thought it might be something he ate—maybe acidity, so I gave him some hot water and antacids, told him to take rest. He looked ok after that, so I went to work as usual. I went home to give him lunch, and I found him like this." She breaks down, sobbing.

"You said he went for a party. Is there any possibility that he might have taken too much alcohol or maybe recreational drugs?"

The sister refutes this—"He is a body builder, very careful about what he puts in his body. He permits himself no luxuries or comforts. He sleeps on the floor. He doesn't touch alcohol—he takes no stimulants—not even coffee. And he's a fitness fanatic—he exercises daily."

"I see. Please don't be upset—but I do have to ask this since he vomited so much. Is there a possibility that he consumed some poison or overdosed on something?"

"Absolutely not, doctor. There's no reason he would be sad or depressed. He is well known in the field of body building, he is making good money and is engaged to a wonderful girl."

S. Bhat, *Clinical Conundrums to Practice Diagnostic Reasoning*,
https://doi.org/10.1007/978-981-95-0636-1_1

You quickly examine the patient. The guy is impressively built—heavily tattooed, muscled, very striking in appearance.

The Glasgow coma scale is 3: E1V1M1.

Pulse: 100/min. BP 180/90 mmHg.

He looks mildly hypovolemic, which you ascribe to the vomiting.

Diaphoresis is present.

The pupils are dilated and fixed; you do not detect any other cranial nerve involvement.

You observe that there is generalized hypotonia; however, there are no lateralizing signs, and the neck is supple.

You are a little stumped.

"It might be a brainstem bleed. you tell the intern. "Get an urgent CT brain, and send a toxicology screen. Shift him to ICU."

You explain to the patient's sister that things don't look good, you will have to intubate to protect the airway, and the patient may need mechanical ventilation as well.

Your duty is over, and as you walk out of casualty, you hear the loud, harsh tones of the ancient general practitioner who has been employed to take care of the casualty at night. His fans claim he has outstanding clinical skills, but you beg to differ and find him more than a little irritating.

"I'll take care of everything!" he assures you heartily. "You go and enjoy the weekend."

You relax over the weekend and drive back to hospital 2 days later. As you sign in, you almost faint when you see the self-same GCS 3 guy leaning on a pillar, casually conversing with a friend.

Was this a ghost? Had the old GP accomplished a miraculous cure? Or have you lost your mind after years of hardwork and harder liquor?

Questions What might the diagnosis be?

Analysis

This is a case of coma with no lateralizing signs.

The following causes must be considered [1] (Fig. 1.1).

Analyzing this stepwise:

(a) The patient is a perfectly healthy young male—he has no risk factors for cerebrovascular accident like hypertension, previous ischemic or valvular heart disease, or transient ischemic accident. There is no past history of seizures.
(b) He goes to bed healthy and wakes up vomiting.
(c) He is deeply comatose with no lateralizing signs—thus, the possibility of structural lesions such as bleed, intracranial space occupying lesion decreases, and

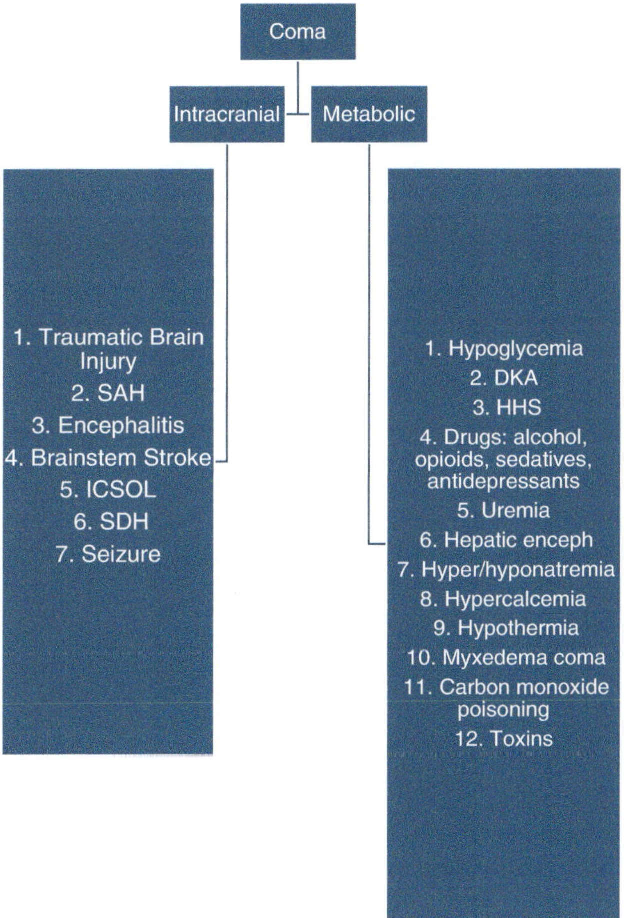

Fig. 1.1 Approach to coma.
SAH: subarachnoid hemorrhage. ICSOL: intracranial space occupying lesion. SDH: subdural hemorrhage. DKA: diabetic keto acidosis. HHS: hyperosmolar hyperglycemic state

that of metabolic/nutritional and toxic causes increases. The acute onset is a point against metabolic and nutritional; thus, the strongest possibility is a toxin. There are two points to be considered here. First, the possibility of overdose and consumption is low from the history given, and second, it is clearly mentioned that the man was sleeping on the floor.

Putting all these facts together: In a young healthy man who slept on the floor and woke up with vomiting, and then was discovered in coma with no structural lesions, an astute clinician would suspect a krait bite.

Differential Diagnosis

(a) Botulism.
(b) Acute abdomen.
(c) Guillain Barre syndrome: ascending rather than descending paralysis.
(d) Functional.
(e) Myasthenia gravis.
(f) Vasculotoxic snake bites may be complicated by intracerebral hemorrhage and present with neurological deficits—however, in these cases, clear lateralizing signs will be present.

Etiopathogenesis Beta-bungarotoxin [2] or beta-neurotoxin secreted by the krait is similar to botulinum toxin. It is a phospholipase A2 [3]. It differs from alpha-bungarotoxin secreted by the cobra in that its action is presynaptic rather than post-synaptic. Since it is a small molecule, it is rapidly transmitted from the tissues to the blood to the nerve terminals where it causes depletion of synaptic vesicles and decreases acetylcholine secretion [4] (Fig. 1.2).

What makes krait envenomation especially difficult to treat is that once the neuromuscular paralysis develops, it is prolonged in duration. Prolonged mechanical ventilation adds to the cost of therapy and the risk of infections, which led researchers to propose that all victims of krait bite must receive antivenom early, regardless of the presence or absence of signs of envenomation [5].

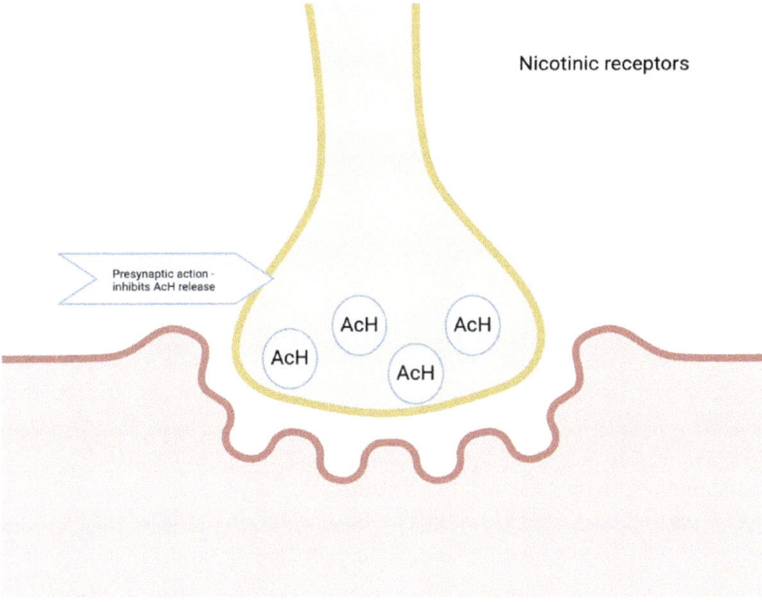

Fig. 1.2 Mechanism of action of toxin.
(Created in BioRender. Bhat (2025) https://BioRender.com/o5c1qug)

Clinical Features

History The diagnosis and treatment of krait bite is hampered by the fact that the bite is often occult and the history of bite is not forthcoming. Neuroparalytic symptoms, abdominal pain, and vomiting predominate as the presenting complaint—the typical history being a patient who goes to sleep healthy, wakes up with abdominal pain and vomiting, and develops descending paralysis within hours after waking up [6].

Examination A clear fang mark may not be seen in krait bite; careful examination with a magnifying glass may reveal a pinpoint bleed with perhaps a minimal surrounding rash. Ptosis, dysarthria, dysphonia, dysphagia, and diplopia may be present.

Single breath count and breath-holding time must be checked in cases of neuro toxic snake bites:

(i) Single breath count: The patient is made to sit upright and inhale deeply and then instructed to exhale while counting. A single breath count of more than 30 is normal and less than 25 is a cause for concern as it indicates possible respiratory muscle failure [7].

(ii) Breath-holding test: The patient must be able to hold their breath in inspiration for more than 45 s [8].

Investigations The whole blood clotting time (WBCT) is an easy bedside method of testing for hemotoxic envenomation. 2 mL of blood is kept in a clean dry glass tube and not shaken or disturbed. After 20 min, the tube is gently tilted, and if blood clots, there is no significant hemotoxic envenomation.

Treatment

(a) ASV 10 vials over 30 min, followed by reassessment at the end of 1 hour and repetition of 10 vials of ASV if signs of neurological envenomation persist [9].
(b) Atropine and neostigmine: 1.5 mg neostigmine preceded by 0.6 mg of atropine may be considered in the case of neurotoxic envenomation [10].
(c) Management of hypersensitivity reactions.
(d) Recent published literature suggests a role for melatonin receptor agonists (Ramelteon and Agomelatine) to hasten neuroregeneration [11].

To Note

(a) Exertion may worsen the severity of envenomation. Krait bite is especially tricky to diagnose as the signs of local envenomation viz. swelling, tenderness, and erythema are often absent or appear late.
(b) Bilateral dilated fixed pupil is NOT the sign of brain death in elapid bite.

Key Takeaway
In endemic areas, in patients with vomiting, followed by stupor with or without bilateral neurological deficits, neurotoxic envenomation must be ruled out.

References

1. Karpenko A, Keegan J. Diagnosis of coma. Emerg Med Clin North Am. 2021;39(1):155–72.
2. Rugolo M, Dolly JO, Nicholls DG. The mechanism of action of β-bungarotoxin at the presynaptic plasma membrane. Biochem J. 1986;233(2):519–23.
3. Prasarnpun S, Walsh J, Awad SS, Harris JB. Envenoming bites by kraits: the biological basis of treatment-resistant neuromuscular paralysis. Brain. 2005;128(12):2987–96.
4. Paniagua D, Vergara I, Boyer L, Alagón A. Role of lymphatic system on snake venom absorption. In: Inagaki H, Vogel CW, Mukherjee AK, Rahmy TR, Gopalakrishnakone P, editors. Snake venoms [Internet]. Dordrecht: Springer; 2017 [cited 2025 Jan 6]. p. 453–74. https://doi.org/10.1007/978-94-007-6410-1_10
5. French MA, Lenzo N, John M, Mallal SA, McKinnon EJ, James IR, Price P, Flexman JP, Tay-Kearney ML. Immune restoration disease after the treatment of immunodeficient HIV-infected patients with highly active antiretroviral therapy. HIV Med. 2000;1(2):107–15.

6. Jha S, Rr S, Ss T, Sk T, Pk Y. Clinical evaluation of patients with krait bites in the emergency department: a series of three cases. J Clin Diagn Res. 2023;17(11)
7. Bhandari SK, Bist A, Ghimire A. Single breath count test and its applications in clinical practice: a systematic review. Ann Med Surg. 2024;86(4):2130–6.
8. Parkes MJ. Breath-holding and its breakpoint. Exp Physiol. 2006;91(1):1–5.9. Snakebite_Full.pdf [Internet]. [cited 2025 Mar 19]. Available from: https://nhm.gov.in/images/pdf/guidelines/nrhm-guidelines/stg/Snakebite_Full.pdf
9. Anil A, Singh S, Bhalla A, Sharma N, Agarwal R, Simpson ID. Role of neostigmine and polyvalent antivenom in Indian common krait. Bungarus caeruleus:83–7.
10. D'Este G, Fabris F, Stazi M, Baggio C, Simonato M, Megighian A, Rigoni M, Negro S, Montecucco C. Agonists of melatonin receptors strongly promote the functional recovery from the neuroparalysis induced by neurotoxic snakes. PLoS Negl Trop Dis. 2024;18(1):e0011825.
11. Gutiérrez JM, R Casewell N, Laustsen AH. Progress and Challenges in the Field of Snakebite Envenoming Therapeutics. Annu Rev Pharmacol Toxicol. 2025 Jan;65(1):465–485. https://doi.org/10.1146/annurev-pharmtox-022024-033544. Epub 2024 Dec 17. PMID: 39088847.

2 A Group of People Presenting with Gastrointestinal Symptoms and Blurring of Vision: Mass Casualty

Grade Moderate.

Abstract A large number of people are admitted with vomiting, headache, and blurring of vision after attending a party.

Story It is Saturday night, you're manning the emergency department, and the room is surprisingly quiet. You decide to work on an article that has been pending for a while. As you sit down, a junior resident tells the nurse in charge "Oh, we're lucky—it's a calm night!"

You stand up furiously. "You should never say something like that! You are tempting fate!" Sure enough, in 5 min, the triage nurse runs up to you and says "It looks like something big, Doctor. There are 6 ambulances from Kalluruchi (a village 20 kilometres away)."

"See?! It's all your fault!" You snarl at the hapless junior resident and mentally prepare to deal with whatever is in store.

You obtain the history from a paramedical worker.

"There was a celebration in the village last night because a certain political party won in the panchayat elections. I don't know whether there was something wrong with the food, but almost everyone who went to the party started having severe abdominal pain and vomiting this morning. The staff at the primary health centre was overwhelmed and they referred the patients here."

You note that almost every bed in the emergency department is occupied. Troubled, you look around wondering with which bed to start. You ask the nurse to call in more staff, tell the junior residents to start triaging the patients, and begin to examine the patient who looks sickest to you.

Mr. Shankar is a man in his early thirties, writhing on the bed in pain.

"My stomach pains, Doctor!" he moans. You are just about to palpate his abdomen, when he has a violent bout of vomiting. You try to ignore the vomitus on your

S. Bhat, *Clinical Conundrums to Practice Diagnostic Reasoning*,
https://doi.org/10.1007/978-981-95-0636-1_2

pants and shoes as you endeavor to obtain intravenous access, and all around you can hear voices crying in pain.

"My head hurts, doctor... it feels like it is going to explode!"

"My tummy hurts!"

"I can't see anything! Please help me!"

The patient in the next bed appears extremely agitated—he leaps out of the bed and grabs the nurse by the shoulders and shakes her.

"Do something for my pain! I can't bear it!" he yells.

For a minute, you cannot move. You stand in the emergency department, looking around—patients are screaming, doctors and nurses are yelling instructions at each other, people are begging for some relief from their pain—you wonder what version of hell you are working in.

By dint of a half-an-hour of extremely concerted effort from every single doctor and nurse present, things calm down somewhat, patients are restrained, sedated, on intravenous fluids and antiemetics. You take a breath and try to figure out what is happening.

Mr. Shankar is no longer vomiting, but he appears very apprehensive.

"Please help me Doctor." he weeps.

You note that his heart rate is 110/min, blood pressure is 150/100 mm Hg, and the respiratory rate is 30 cycles per min. Auscultation of the chest reveals scattered crackles and tachycardia. You cannot perform a detailed nervous system examination since the patient is still restless, but you do note that the pupils are only sluggishly reactive.

You order lab investigations and proceed to the next patient. By the time you assess and stabilize patient number 4, the junior resident approaches you and says "Doctor, I think you should have a look at these reports."

Lab investigations are as follows:

Blood glucose: 104 mg%
pH: 7.3
Na: 143 mEq/L, K+: 4 mEq/L, Cl-: 105 mEq/L, HCO3-: 19 mEq/L
BUN: 36 mg/dL, s creat: 1.8 mg/dL
Urine ketones: negative
s. osmolality: 356 mOsm/kg

Questions What explains these symptoms and findings in multiple patients? Is it a simple case of food poisoning? Or is there something else going on? What do the lab investigations indicate?

Analysis

The tetrad of visual, gastrointestinal, nervous system, and respiratory system findings in a large group of people who attended a celebration together is suggestive of methanol poisoning [1].

This is further corroborated by the labs obtained.

Anion gap [2] = $Na^+ - (Cl^- + HCO3\text{-})$ = 143–105—19 = 19 mmol/L (High)

Calculated osmolality = (2× sodium) + (Blood glucose/18) + BUN/2.8

= (2 × 143) + (104/18) + (36/2.8)

= 286 + 5.7 + 12.85 = 304.5 mOsm/kg

However, measured osmolality = 356 mOsm/kg.

Hence, osmolar gap = measured osmolality—calculated osmolality = 356–304 = 52 mOsm/kg.

The normal osmolar gap is up till 10 [3].

Thus, this is a case of high anion gap metabolic acidosis with a significant osmolar gap.

Methanol is an organic solvent that when ingested accidentally or deliberately results in metabolic acidosis and visual and neurological sequalae.

Etiopathogenesis

Methanol is an organic solvent which, when ingested accidentally or deliberately results in metabolic acidosis and visual and neurological sequelae. Methanol poisoning can occur due to accidental or suicidal consumption. It is present in anti-freeze, paint stripper, perfumes, and windshield washer fluid. It is sometimes an adulterant in alcohol, especially affecting those of low socioeconomic status [4].

Methanol is oxidized by alcohol dehydrogenase to formaldehyde and then to formic acid (Fig. 2.1).

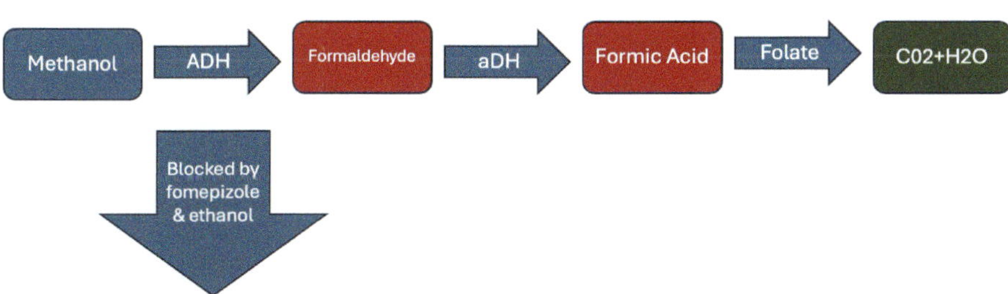

Fig. 2.1 Metabolism of methanol.
ADH: Alcohol dehydrogenase.
aDH: Aldehyde dehydrogenase

Formic acid affects the optic nerve by interfering with mitochondrial oxidative phosphorylation and by damaging myelin. It also injures the basal ganglia, especially the putamen [5].

Clinical Features [6]

(a) Drowsiness, disinhibition, ataxia
(b) Pain in abdomen, vomiting
(c) Blurring of vision
(d) Seizures, coma
(e) Tachycardia, tachypnea, hypertension, pulmonary edema
(f) Optic disk blurring and hyperemia

If the patient survives the initial phase, extrapyramidal features may be seen after 10–14 days [7].

The term "circulus hypoxicus" [8] has been used to refer to the toxicity of methanol. The initial metabolic acidosis due to methanol results in tissue hypoperfusion and lactic acidosis which further perpetuate the toxicity of methanol.

Diagnosis

High anion gap metabolic acidosis with elevated osmolar gap is a clue to methanol poisoning.

The osmolar gap may be used as a screening test for toxic alcohol consumption, for example, methanol and ethylene glycol [9, 10]. Osmolar gap >25 necessitates emergent therapy.

Treatment [11]

(a) Stomach wash with activated charcoal
(b) Fomepizole—inhibits alcohol dehydrogenase [12]
(c) Ethanol—if fomepizole is not available—orally or through nasogastric tube [13]
(d) Leucovorin/folic acid [14]
(e) Sodium bicarbonate if metabolic acidosis is present
(f) Hemodialysis may be required
(g) Supportive care: Intubation and mechanical ventilation, IV crystalloids
(h) Erythropoietin with methylprednisolone to protect against optic neuropathy [1].

To note: The anion gap may be falsely underestimated in patients with hypoalbuminemia

References

1. Nekoukar Z, Zakariaei Z, Taghizadeh F, Musavi F, Banimostafavi ES, Sharifpour A, Ghuchi NE, Fakhar M, Tabaripour R, Safanavaei S. Methanol poisoning as a new world challenge: a review. Ann Med Surg. 2021;66:102445.
2. Hovda KE, Hunderi OH, Rudberg N, Froyshov S, Jacobsen D. Anion and osmolal gaps in the diagnosis of methanol poisoning: clinical study in 28 patients. Intensive Care Med. 2004;30(9):1842–6.
3. Arora A. The 'gap'in the 'plasma osmolar gap'. Case Rep. 2013;2013:bcr2013200250.
4. Manning L, Kowalska A. Illicit alcohol: public health risk of methanol poisoning and policy mitigation strategies. Foods. 2021;10(7):1625.
5. Arora V, Nijjar IB, Multani AS, Singh JP, Abrol R, Chopra R, Attri R. MRI findings in methanol intoxication: a report of two cases. Br J Radiol. 2007;80(958):e243–6.
6. Ran M, Li Y, Zhang L, Wu W, Lin J, Liu Q, et al. Clinical features, treatment, and prognosis of acute methanol poisoning: experiences in an outbreak. Int J Clin Exp Med. 2019;12(5):5938–50.
7. Faizan R, Kumar A, Panhwar IA, Shamim B, Safeer T. MRI brain, featuring methanol intoxication: a rare case report. Pak J Radiology. 2021;31(4)
8. Drangsholt E, Vangstad M, Zakharov S, Hovda KE, Jacobsen D. The hypothesis of circulus hypoxicus and its clinical relevance in patients with methanol poisoning–an observational study of 35 patients. Basic Clin Pharmacol Toxicol. 2018;123(6):749–55.
9. Lynd LD, Richardson KJ, Purssell RA, Abu-Laban RB, Brubacher JR, Lepik KJ, Sivilotti ML. An evaluation of the osmole gap as a screening test for toxic alcohol poisoning. BMC Emerg Med. 2008;8:1.
10. Gallagher N, Edwards FJ. The diagnosis and management of toxic alcohol poisoning in the emergency department: a review article. Adv J Emerg Med. 2019;3(3):e28.
11. American Academy of Clinical Toxicology Ad Hoc Committee on the Treatment Guidelines for Methanol Poisoning, Barceloux DG, Randall Bond G, Krenzelok EP, Cooper H, Allister Vale J. American Academy of Clinical Toxicology practice guidelines on the treatment of methanol poisoning. J Toxicol Clin Toxicol. 2002;40(4):415–46.
12. Brent J, McMartin K, Phillips S, Aaron C, Kulig K. Fomepizole for the treatment of methanol poisoning. N Engl J Med. 2001;344(6):424–9.
13. Zakharov S, Pelclova D, Navratil T, Belacek J, Komarc M, Eddleston M, et al. Fomepizole versus ethanol in the treatment of acute methanol poisoning: comparison of clinical effectiveness in a mass poisoning outbreak. Clin Toxicol. 2015;53(8):797–806.
14. Pohanka M. Antidotes against methanol poisoning: a review. Mini Rev Med Chem. 2019;19(14):1126–33.

3 Patient Presenting with Vomiting, Hypovolemia, Kussmaul's Breathing, and Normal Blood Sugars: Pratik Decides to Party!

Grade Moderate

Abstract An adult male with Type 2 Diabetes Mellitus presents with symptoms and signs of diabetic ketoacidosis, but the blood sugars are normal.

Story Mr. Pratik is not usually a party-goer. After work, he likes to return home for a sedate cup of tea with his wife. However, missing the retirement party of his boss is not really an option. He absolutely does not want to get the dangerous reputation of not being a team player. Accordingly, barbered, suited, and bearing an expensive gift, he reaches the event venue. There, like many introverts forced out of their comfort zone, he proceeds to go a little crazy. He drinks a couple of glasses of wine, partakes liberally of the delicious snacks, and dances a clumsy and cringeworthy jig.

He pays for these excesses the next day, waking up with a pounding headache and a dry mouth. He vomits repeatedly. He treats himself with water and antacids, but that does not improve things noticeably. He feels weak and extremely fatigued and has a tummy ache too. His wife insists that he meet a doctor; he shows up at your clinic.

You note that other people who attended the party have not fallen ill, that Pratik has vomiting but no loose stools, and though there is a little abdominal discomfort, it is not severe and does not radiate to the back. He volunteers the history that he used to smoke and consume alcohol occasionally when he was a college student, but has been abstinent for the last 18 years. He also informs you that he has been on treatment for diabetes for the last 10 years and that his sugars are well controlled with tablets. He does not know the name of the tablet, but he remembers that his doctor said that it works by increasing the urinary excretion of glucose.

You examine Pratik and note that he looks ill and toxic. The pulse rate is 110 per minute, and the blood pressure is 100/70 mm Hg. His tongue is dry. Pratik is taking deep, sighing breaths, and the respiratory rate is 30 cycles per minute.

S. Bhat, *Clinical Conundrums to Practice Diagnostic Reasoning*, https://doi.org/10.1007/978-981-95-0636-1_3

The lungs are clear, SPO2 is 94% on room air, the abdomen is soft, and glucometer random blood sugar is 110 mg %.

Questions What do you think we are dealing with here? How would you proceed with investigations and treatment?

Analysis

The salient points here are as follows:

(a) Adult patient with T2DM being treated with oral antidiabetic drugs—perhaps an SGLT2 inhibitor (increased urinary excretion of glucose)
(b) Unaccustomed alcohol intake, followed by vomiting and volume depletion
(c) Abdominal pain, dehydration, and perhaps Kussmaul's breathing
(d) Blood sugar: 110 mg%

In other words, it is a clinical picture of diabetic ketoacidosis, but the sugars are not very elevated—hence, it is Euglycemic Diabetic Ketoacidosis (EDKA).

EDKA is an acute complication of diabetes, usually seen in patients treated with SGLT2 inhibitors, wherein there is a high-anion gap metabolic acidosis and ketonemia, but blood sugars do not generally exceed 200 mg% [1].

Etiopathogenesis The most common setting of EDKA is in a patient treated with SGLT2 inhibitors. In fact, SGLT2 inhibitors increase the risk of EDKA up to sevenfold [2]. Both SGLT2I and DKA cause volume loss, resulting in counter-regulatory hormone secretion, lipolysis, and ketosis [3] (Fig. 3.1).

Specifically, SGLT2 inhibitors increase glucagon levels and alter the glucagon: insulin ratio. This increases the level of circulating ketones even in the steady non-EDKA state [4]. The effect of SGLT2 inhibitors in promoting glucosuria limits hyperglycemia and exacerbates dehydration [5].

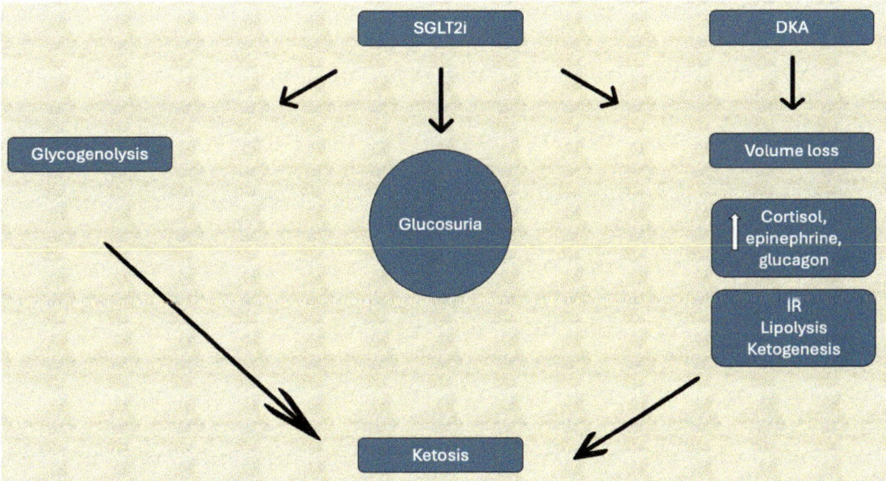

Fig. 3.1 Pathogenesis of EDKA.
SGLT2i—SGLT2 inhibitors. DKA—Diabetic ketoacidosis

In addition to SGTL2 inhibitor use, the following may be associated with EDKA [6]:

1. Pregnancy
2. Decreased caloric Intake
3. Heavy alcohol use
4. Insulin use prior to hospital admission
5. Cocaine abuse
6. Pancreatitis
7. Sepsis

Clinical Features

Risk Factors

1. Prolonged fasting
2. Low carbohydrate diet
3. Dehydration
4. Low BMI
5. Pregnancy
6. Over-exertion
7. Alcohol dependence syndrome

Symptoms and Signs [7]

(a) Anorexia, nausea, vomiting
(b) Fatigue
(c) Pain in abdomen
(d) Dyspnea
(e) Tachycardia

Polydipsia and polyuria that are characteristic of DKA are often absent here.

In fact, the patient may present only with nonspecific symptoms and signs like malaise, tachycardia, tachypnea, and fever [8].

Investigations [9]

Blood glucose—normally less than 200 mg%

Metabolic acidosis—one of the following—pH < 7.3, serum bicarb <18, anion gap >10

Blood glucose <200 mg%

Beta-hydroxybutyrate >3

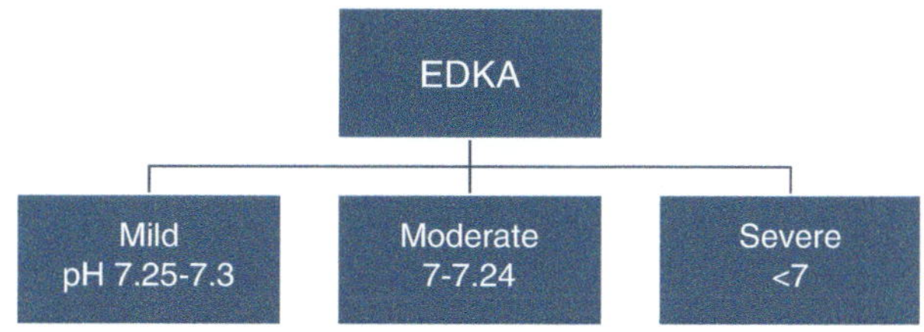

Fig. 3.2 Classification of EDKA

Classification EDKA is classified as per degree of acidosis (Fig. 3.2).

Treatment Insulin infusion at 1–2 units per hour until the anion gap and bicarbonate levels normalize. Dextrose must be infused concurrently.

Key Takeaway
When a sick-looking patient with T2DM who is on SGLT2 inhibitors presents with nausea, vomiting and abdominal pain, ketoacidosis must be excluded even if the blood sugars are not elevated more than 200 mg%.

References

1. Long B, Lentz S, Koyfman A, Gottlieb M. Euglycemic diabetic ketoacidosis: Etiologies, evaluation, and management. Am J Emerg Med. 2021;44:157–60.
2. Sodium-glucose co-transporter-2 inhibitors and the risk of diabetic ketoacidosis in patients with type 2 diabetes: A systematic review and meta-analysis of randomized controlled trials - Liu - 2020 - Diabetes, Obesity and Metabolism - Wiley Online Library [Internet]. [cited 2025 Jan 9]. Available from: https://dom-pubs.periclesprod.literatumonline.com/doi/10.1111/dom.14075.
3. Differences in metabolic and hormonal milieu in diabetic- and alcohol-induced ketoacidosis - PubMed [Internet]. [cited 2025 Jan 9]. Available from: https://pubmed.ncbi.nlm.nih.gov/10877365/.
4. Shift to Fatty Substrate Utilization in Response to Sodium-Glucose Cotransporter 2 Inhibition in Subjects Without Diabetes and Patients With Type 2 Diabetes - PubMed [Internet]. [cited 2025 Jan 9]. Available from: https://pubmed.ncbi.nlm.nih.gov/26861783/.
5. SGLT2 Inhibitors May Predispose to Ketoacidosis - PubMed [Internet]. [cited 2025 Jan 9]. Available from: https://pubmed.ncbi.nlm.nih.gov/26086329/.
6. Hyperglycemic Crises in Adult Patients With Diabetes - PMC [Internet]. [cited 2025 Jan 9]. Available from: https://pmc.ncbi.nlm.nih.gov/articles/PMC2699725/.
7. Euglycemic diabetic ketoacidosis: Etiologies, evaluation, and management - Science Direct [Internet]. [cited 2025 Jan 9]. Available from: https://www.sciencedirect.com/science/article/abs/pii/S0735675721001212.
8. Euglycemic Diabetic Ketoacidosis: A Potential Complication of Treatment With Sodium–Glucose Cotransporter 2 Inhibition | Diabetes Care | American Diabetes Association [Internet]. [cited 2025 Jan 9]. Available from: https://diabetesjournals.org/care/article/38/9/1687/37246/Euglycemic-Diabetic-Ketoacidosis-A-Potential.
9. Classic diabetic ketoacidosis and the euglycemic variant: Something old, something new | Cleveland Clinic Journal of Medicine [Internet]. [cited 2025 Jan 9]. Available from: https://www.ccjm.org/content/92/1/33.long.

Sudden Death in Polar Climes: The Arctic Trek

4

Grade Moderate.

Abstract A young fit man, with no prior comorbidities, well protected against the cold, is found dead in the Arctic region. He has no external injuries. The cause of death must be ascertained.

Story The ZZZ country football team is very excited that their captain is getting married. The 11 players, superbly trained and extremely fit, decide to have a stag party a little out of the ordinary. They do not want to go the usual degenerate route of drinking and clubbing. Instead, they charter a flight to go on a trek to explore Svalbard.

They start out one fine morning in a Gulfstream 450. The pilot, the co-pilot, 11 players, and the team captain's best friend are all in high spirits. Unfortunately, the jet hits bad weather a little after it crosses the Arctic circle, and radio contact is lost. When there is no news from the team for another day, the Sports and Aviation ministries spring in to action. They set up a group of four to travel to Svalbard and investigate. The pilot, the co-pilot, the sports secretary, and you—the medical expert.

You all board the helicopter to make the trip, hoping against hope that your worst fears do not come true. Unfortunately, 3 hours into the flight, the co-pilot spies wreckage at 10 o' clock. With great caution, the pilots land as close as they can to the crashed plane.

You make your way to the plane, wincing at the battered aircraft and wondering how anyone could possibly survive a crash of this magnitude.

You gingerly make your way into the aircraft and note sadly that both the pilots have not made it. In fact, no one seems to have survived the crash, you realize, looking at the bodies in each seat.

"Wait a minute! How many people were on this flight?" asks the sports secretary.

"Fourteen."

S. Bhat, *Clinical Conundrums to Practice Diagnostic Reasoning*,
https://doi.org/10.1007/978-981-95-0636-1_4

"Well, there are only 13 bodies! Maybe one of the team made it out alive!" exclaims the sports secretary.

You all jump off the plane shining your torchlights, looking desperately for the survivor. After a trek of about 10 km in the driving snow, you come across a tiny tent, designed to withstand the Arctic nights. You rush to it, hoping against hope, but when you reach it, you see a dead body—clad in survival gear designed for subzero temperatures. There is a blood-stained knife close by; however, there are no external injuries on the body.

You are unable to figure out what could have caused death in someone who was at the pinnacle of fitness, who could trek 10 km in tough terrain, and who was dressed in the best weatherproof apparel. There seem to be no external injuries. A quick survey of the body reveals no abnormalities apart from some peeling of skin on the palms. The surroundings do not yield much information apart from a pile of large animal bones and fur a short distance away. You are stymied.

Question What caused the death? It was not the cold; it was not injury.

Analysis

The first step is to list the possible causes of death in a situation like this:

(a) Injury due to the crash—this is an unlikely cause of death, considering that the player trekked 10 km after the plane went down.
(b) The cold—again, less likely. He was equipped with the best of survival gear; he was in a weatherproof tent.
(c) Could it have been a sudden myocardial infarction? Not impossible, but again, unlikely in a young fit male with no comorbidities.

Let us see if it is possible to reach a conclusion from the other clues provided:

(a) A blood-stained knife, a pile of bones, and fur near the body. That the player killed some animal is a fair supposition. Again, a not unreasonable conclusion is that he consumed the meat of the animal he killed, since it is unlikely that, after the plane crash, he would be in the mood to hunt for sport.
(b) It has been specified that the incident occurred in the Arctic circle. The clue here is in the location. Above the Arctic circle, in an around Svalbard, is where you would find polar bears. How do we connect the polar bears to the death of this fit young man with no external injuries at all? From the tale so far, it would appear that the man hunted and killed the polar bear for food. Regrettably, his survival training does not seem to have included information on the toxicity of polar bear liver, which contains enough Vitamin A to kill 50 adults [1]. An additional clue is the peeling of the palms—a not so common physical examination sign, which is seen in Vitamin A toxicity [2].

Pathogenesis (Fig. 4.1)

The fundamental mechanism of vitamin A toxicity stems from the saturation of cellular retinol-binding proteins (RBPs) and subsequent accumulation of unbound retinol in tissues. When intake exceeds the body's storage and metabolic capacity, free retinol and its metabolites can disrupt cell membrane stability through their detergent-like properties [3]. This leads to cellular dysfunction across multiple organ systems.

The liver, being the primary storage site for Vitamin A, experiences the initial impact. Hepatic stellate cells are damaged, leading to perisinusoidal fibrosis and portal hypertension [4]. Excess retinoids also interfere with bone remodeling by enhancing osteoclast activity while suppressing osteoblast function, potentially resulting in bone demineralization and increased fracture risk [5].

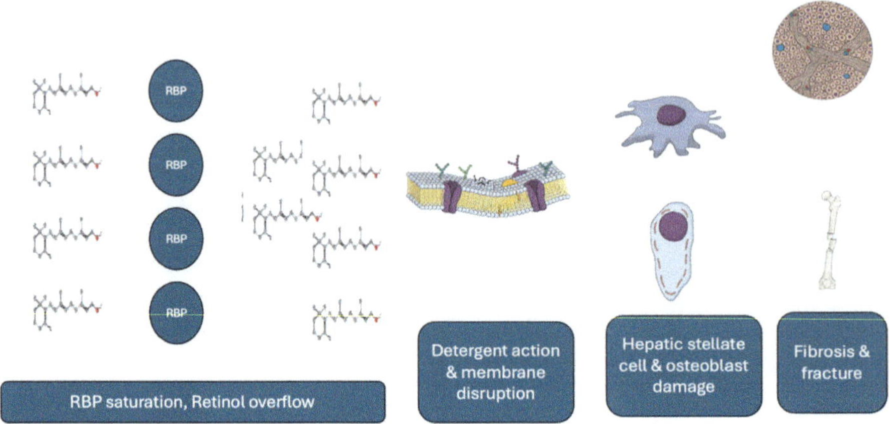

Fig. 4.1 Vitamin A toxicity.
RBP: Retinol-binding protein.
(Created by author on Microsoft Powerpoint using images from "Mindthegraph")

Clinical Features [10]

Acute hypervitaminosis A manifests within hours to days of ingesting large amounts of vitamin A (more than 660,000 IU).

Signs and Symptoms [6]

1. Neurological manifestations: Severe headache, blurred vision, papilledema, and increased intracranial pressure. Seizures may occur.
2. Gastrointestinal symptoms: Nausea, vomiting, and abdominal pain. The detergent-like effect of excess retinol on cell membranes can cause significant mucosal irritation.
3. Skin changes: Desquamation, particularly of palms and soles, and hair loss.

Chronic toxicity develops over months to years of excess intake (>10 times RDA). Additional features are as follows [7]:

1. Musculoskeletal complications: Bone pain, hyperostosis, and increased risk of fractures.
2. Pseudotumor cerebri.
3. Hepatomegaly, fibrosis, cirrhosis.
4. Growth retardation in children.
5. Vitamin A may be teratogenic in high doses [8].

Investigations [9] Diagnosis: Vitamin A levels >80 mcg/mL (25,000 IU/kg or more), hypercalcemia, and impaired renal function:

- Serum retinol levels (though these may not correlate well with toxicity)
- Liver function tests: may show transaminitis, hypertriglyceridemia
- Calcium and alkaline phosphatase levels
- Complete blood count

Imaging Studies

- Radiographic evaluation for bone changes
- Computed Tomography or Magnetic Resonance Imaging for suspected intracranial hypertension
- Liver imaging to assess hepatic involvement

Treatment [10]

1. Cessation of vitamin A intake.
2. Hypercalcemia may be managed by intravenous hydration, corticosteroids, and calcitonin.
3. Emollients for those with skin peeling.
4. Methylcellulose drops for those with dry eyes.
5. Treatment of increased intracranial pressure with mannitol or acetazolamide when indicated.

Long-Term Monitoring

- Regular assessment of liver function
- Bone density monitoring
- Ophthalmological follow-up

The prognosis generally improves with early recognition and intervention, though some changes, particularly hepatic fibrosis, may be irreversible.

Fascinating factoid In 1974, a scientist Basil Brown, from the UK consumed 70 million units of vitamin A over a 10-day span, washing down this magnificent amount with gallons of carrot juice. Unfortunately, he achieved the distinction of being one of the first cases of mortality secondary to vitamin supplementation [11].

Key Takeaway

Supposedly safe nutraceuticals and supplements which our patients obtain over the counter may be harmful—in themselves, in higher than advised doses, or by interacting with prescription drugs. Many patients do not volunteer a history of nutraceutical/supplement use, believing it is not relevant.

Advising women who are planning to conceive about the teratogenic potential of vitamin A is crucial.

References

1. Ball MD, Furr HC, Olson JA. Acyl coenzyme A: retinol acyltransferase activity and the vitamin A content of polar bear (Ursus maritimus) liver. Comp Biochem Physiol B. 1986;84(4):513–7.
2. Carazo A, Macáková K, Matoušová K, Krčmová LK, Protti M, Mladěnka P. Vitamin A update: forms, sources, kinetics, detection, function, deficiency, therapeutic use and toxicity. Nutrients. 2021;13(5):1703.
3. Howard WB, Willhite CC. Toxicity of retinoids in humans and animals. J Toxicol Toxin Rev. 1986;5(1):55–94.
4. Kowalski TE, Falestiny M, Furth E, Malet PF. Vitamin A hepatotoxicity: a cautionary note regarding 25,000 IU supplements. Am J Med. 1994;97(6):523–8.
5. Baineni R, Gulati R, Delhi CK. Vitamin A toxicity presenting as bone pain. Arch Dis Child. 2017;102(6):556–8.
6. Penniston KL, Tanumihardjo SA. The acute and chronic toxic effects of vitamin A. Am J Clin Nutr. 2006;83(2):191–201.
7. Chisholm JT, Abou-Jaoude MM, Hessler AB, Sudhakar P. Pseudotumor cerebri syndrome with resolution after discontinuing high vitamin A containing dietary supplement: case report and review. Neuro-Ophthalmology. 2018;42(3):169–75.
8. Bastos Maia S, Rolland Souza AS, Costa Caminha MD, Lins da Silva S, Callou Cruz RD, Carvalho dos Santos C, Batista FM. Vitamin A and pregnancy: a narrative review. Nutrients. 2019;11(3):681.
9. Shasho R, Shasho M. Diagnostic approach common cases of vitamins toxicity in children. Sch J Appl Med Sci. 2022;10(1):1–8.
10. Olson JM, Ameer MA, Goyal A. Vitamin A toxicity. In: StatPearls [Internet]; 2023.
11. Basil Brown | Fact | FactRepublic.com [Internet]. [cited 2025 Mar 23]. Available from: https://factrepublic.com/facts/15949/#google_vignette

5 Rash and Neuropathy in an Adult Male: The Retreat by the Ganges

Grade Moderate.

Abstract A stressed individual on a wellness vacation develops rash and unsteadiness of gait.

Story Mr. K was a hot shot marketing consultant in New York City—his days were busy making money, and his dreams at night were of how to make more. He lived on a steady diet of caffeine, nicotine, and stress. Was it any wonder that his health took a hit?

When he met his physician for an annual checkup, the good doctor told him to either make a change or reserve a hospital bed for himself.

"You don't understand, doc." K said. "I can't slow down now—there is too much at stake."

"That's all very well," the doctor said, "but if you want to be present at the autumn stockholders' convention, you will have to stay away from work for a while."

K reluctantly came to terms with the idea of taking his first break in 25 years.

Never one to do something by half measures, he did extensive research and found a wellness resort on the banks of the Ganges in the Indian state of Bihar which seemed to be just what the doctor prescribed.

Strangely, K fell in love with the resort, slowly but steadily. He spent mornings on the stone steps by the river, watching the mist dissolve into the sunshine and listening to the boatmen sing. His days were a blur of healthy meals and long walks and periods of quiet reflection.

By the end of his first month at the retreat, he could not believe how young and healthy and light he felt. He was not sure if it was the rest, the healthy diet, or the natural remedies doled out every day, but he was feeling like a new man, so he extended his stay by another 6 months.

S. Bhat, *Clinical Conundrums to Practice Diagnostic Reasoning*,
https://doi.org/10.1007/978-981-95-0636-1_5

Unfortunately, by the end of the fourth month, Mr. K felt his health take a downward trend, and he could not figure out why. He had a continuous tummy upset—sometimes loose stools, sometimes vomiting. His feet started feeling numb sometimes and painful at others. One evening, on his way back in the dark from the dining room to his cottage, he felt so unsteady he had to sit down and call for help.

Another strange thing he noticed was that his skin was darkening, but he ascribed this to the effect of the blazing Indian sun.

Things came to a head when he noticed his palms and his soles peeling—he decided that at this point, a nature cure could not be of much help, and decided to meet a doctor soon.

Mr. K meets you in your clinic at the end of a busy day. You listen to his story and proceed with the examination. You note that his palms and soles have a papular rash.

His liver is palpable three fingerprints below the right costal margin, and ankle jerks are absent bilaterally. There is a glove and stocking sensory loss and some weakness in the hands and feet.

Question What do you think is happening with Mr. K? Is it just an inability to adjust to the heat and humidity of India or is it something more specific?

Analysis

The key points here are:

(a) Indian state of Bihar
(b) Consumption of natural remedies
(c) Loose stools and vomiting
(d) Hyperpigmentation, rash, peeling of skin on palms and feet
(e) Clinical examination suggestive of a peripheral neuropathy

The intake of natural remedies for a prolonged period preceding the symptoms are a clue to chronic poisoning. The *triad of gastrointestinal, dermatological, and neurological symptoms* and signs point toward arsenic as the cause [1].

Chronic arsenic poisoning, also known as arsenicosis, arises from prolonged exposure to elevated levels of arsenic. Arsenic is a widely distributed element found in the earth's crust, air, and water [2]. Chronic arsenic poisoning is a global public health concern, with significant occurrences in areas where drinking water is contaminated with arsenic. Prevalence varies depending on regional arsenic levels, with some areas showing higher incidence due to natural deposits or industrial contamination.

Etiology

Arsenic exists in various forms, with inorganic arsenic compounds generally being more toxic than organic forms. Arsenic can be classified based on its

(a) Chemical form: Inorganic (e.g., arsenic trioxide and arsenic disulphide) or organic (e.g., arsenobetaine) [3]
(b) Valence state: Trivalent (As[III]) or pentavalent (As[V]), with trivalent arsenicals being more toxic [4]
(c) Source of exposure: Environmental, occupational, medicinal

The primary causes of chronic arsenic poisoning are:

(a) Contaminated drinking water: When the groundwater contains high levels of naturally occurring arsenic [5].
(b) Traditional medicines: Certain Ayurvedic and traditional medicines may contain arsenic. For example, "Talkeshwar Ras" contains "Manashila" (arsenic disulphide) and "Haritala" (arsenic trioxide) [6]. Chinese patent medicines may also contain realgar, a highly arsenical compound.
(c) Occupational exposure: In workers in industries such as smelting, mining, and pesticide production [7].
(d) Dietary exposure: Rice and rice-based products can accumulate arsenic from contaminated soil and water [8].

Pathogenesis [9]

Arsenic toxicity occurs through the following:

(a) Enzyme inhibition: Arsenic inhibits sulfhydryl group-containing cellular enzymes, disrupting cellular functions [10].
(b) Arsenolysis: Arsenic replaces phosphate in high-energy compounds, interfering with energy production [11].
(c) Oxidative stress: Arsenic induces oxidative stress, leading to cellular damage [12].
(d) DNA damage: Arsenic and its metabolites can cause DNA damage, gene mutation, and chromosomal aberrations, contributing to carcinogenesis [13].
(e) Disruption of cellular signaling: It can disrupt the cellular levels of tumor protein p5326 [14].

Trivalent arsenic compounds are more potent in inhibiting enzymes, while pentavalent compounds are more involved in arsenolysis.

Clinical Features

Chronic arsenic poisoning presents with a range of clinical manifestations:

Skin Melanosis, leukoderma, raindrop-like hypopigmentation, hyperkeratosis, especially on palms and soles [15]

Neurological Symmetrical sensorimotor polyneuropathy, toxic delirium and encephalopathy; verbal IQ and long-term memory affected [16]

Gastrointestinal Nausea, vomiting, diarrhea and metallic taste [16]

Cardiovascular Hypotension, arrhythmias, including prolonged QT interval, peripheral vascular disease

Hematological Anemia, pancytopenia, bone marrow depression

Renal Proteinuria, acute kidney injury

Hepatic Hepatitis, noncirrhotic portal hypertension

Arsenic is a carcinogen.

Investigations [17]

Urine: Elevated total arsenic levels, typically greater than 1000 mg/L in acute toxicity. It is the most commonly tested sample.
Blood: High serum or tissue total arsenic.
Hair and nails: Can confirm exposure over months.
Complete blood count: To assess anemia and pancytopenia.
Liver function tests: To evaluate liver damage.
Renal function tests: To assess kidney function.
Nerve conduction studies: Motor and sensory axonopathy.

Diagnosis

Two major criteria used for diagnosis are: (1) the presence of pigmentary and/or keratotic skin lesions and (2) evidence of exposure to elevated levels of arsenic established by the history of intake of arsenic-contaminated water or by significant arsenic concentrations in urine, hair, or nails.

Laboratory confirmation Measurement of arsenic levels in urine, blood, hair, and nails.

Treatment

The primary goals of treatment are to remove the source of exposure and manage symptoms.

(a) Exposure cessation: Eliminating ongoing and future exposure
(b) Chelation therapy [18]: Chelating agents like penicillamine, dimercaptosuccinic acid (DMSA), or British Anti-Lewisite (BAL) may be considered [19]. However, chelation is more useful in acute arsenic toxicity, and its effectiveness in chronic poisoning is debatable.

Symptomatic Management

(a) Neuropathy: Vitamin A analogues (retinoids) may be beneficial.
(b) Skin lesions: Keratolytic ointments for symptomatic relief.
(c) Supportive care: Intravenous fluids, cardiac monitoring, and management of organ dysfunction.
(d) Nutritional support: A high-protein diet with vitamins A, E, and C may aid recovery.

Key Takeaway

Nutraceuticals, native medications, and over-the-counter drugs may contain ingredients detrimental to health. Hence, the patient must always be asked about the use of these.

References

1. Ratnaike RN. Acute and chronic arsenic toxicity. Postgrad Med J. 2003;79(933):391–6.
2. Oremland RS, Stolz JF. The ecology of arsenic. Science. 2003;300(5621):939–44.
3. O'Day PA. Chemistry and mineralogy of arsenic. Elements. 2006;2(2):77–83.
4. Jain CK, Ali I. Arsenic: occurrence, toxicity and speciation techniques. Water Res. 2000;34(17):4304–12.
5. Prakash S, Verma AK. Arsenic: it's toxicity and impact on human health. Int J Biol Innov IJBI. 2021;3(1):38–47.
6. Yadav S, Kapoor R. A review on chronic toxicity of arsenic. 12(16).
7. Vimercati L, Gatti MF, Gagliardi T, Cuccaro F, De Maria L, Caputi A, et al. Environmental exposure to arsenic and chromium in an industrial area. Environ Sci Pollut Res. 2017;24(12):11528–35.
8. Davis MA, Signes-Pastor AJ, Argos M, Slaughter F, Pendergrast C, Punshon T, et al. Assessment of human dietary exposure to arsenic through rice. Sci Total Environ. 2017;586:1237–44.
9. Singh AP, Goel RK, Kaur T. Mechanisms pertaining to arsenic toxicity. Toxicol Int. 2011;18(2):87.
10. Nriagu LB. Molecular aspects of arsenic stress. J Toxicol Environ Health B Crit Rev. 2000;3(4):293–322.
11. Saha JC, Dikshit AK, Bandyopadhyay M, Saha KC. A review of arsenic poisoning and its effects on human health. Crit Rev Environ Sci Technol. 1999;29(3):281–313.
12. Lantz RC, Hays AM. Role of oxidative stress in arsenic-induced toxicity. Drug Metab Rev. 2006;38(4):791–804.
13. Bhadauria S, Flora SJ. Response of arsenic-induced oxidative stress, DNA damage, and metal imbalance to combined administration of DMSA and monoisoamyl-DMSA during chronic arsenic poisoning in rats. Cell Biol Toxicol. 2007;23:91–104.
14. Yan W, Zhang Y, Zhang J, Liu S, Cho SJ, Chen X. Mutant p53 protein is targeted by arsenic for degradation and plays a role in arsenic-mediated growth suppression. J Biol Chem. 2011;286(20):17478–86.
15. Shannon RL, Strayer DS. Arsenic-induced skin toxicity. Hum Toxicol. 1989;8(2):99–104.
16. Rodŕiguez VM, Jiménez-Capdeville ME, Giordano M. The effects of arsenic exposure on the nervous system. Toxicol Lett. 2003;145(1):1–18.
17. Saha KC. Diagnosis of arsenicosis. J Environ Sci Health A. 2003;38(1):255–72.
18. Bjørklund G, Oliinyk P, Lysiuk R, Rahaman MS, Antonyak H, Lozynska I, Lenchyk L, Peana M. Arsenic intoxication: general aspects and chelating agents. Arch Toxicol. 2020;94:1879–97.
19. Kosnett MJ. The role of chelation in the treatment of arsenic and mercury poisoning. J Med Toxicol. 2013;9:347–54.

6 Fatigue and Gait Disturbance: The Failed Assassination

Grade Difficult.

Abstract An elderly gangster is suffering from weakness, forgetfulness, palpitations, and unsteadiness. His body responds to toxins in an unexpected way.

Story Mr. PG is an aging gangster. Though he is 65 years old, he maintains his reputation of being unreasonable, unpredictable, and uncontrollably violent. His enemies can be counted in thousands. They have a lot to lose if PG continues his reign of terror.

In smoke filled clubs on dark rainy nights, you would find gentlemen with dead eyes planning, whispering, and wondering how and when to make PG meet his maker.

Though PG strikes fear into the hearts of all and sundry, the truth is, he is very afraid himself. For the last 4 months, his mind and body seem to be failing. He finds it difficult to concentrate and tends to get confused when he has to process information. He finds food tasteless and difficult to eat. Fatigue overwhelms him by the time he finishes his customary rounds of his factories, his bars, and his brothels, and he gets breathless when he walks too fast. PG finds it inconceivable that he should fall ill. Has not he lived a life of discipline for as long as he can remember? Exercises at the break of day, absolutely no alcohol or smoking—and as for recreational drugs—they are for PG's customers—he personally eschews anything that would impair his functioning.

S. Bhat, *Clinical Conundrums to Practice Diagnostic Reasoning*,
https://doi.org/10.1007/978-981-95-0636-1_6

He does not want to visit a doctor. Nothing brings down power like the rumor of infirmity or weakness. Thus, PG soldiers on, and no one can guess that he is not at the height of physical and mental well-being.

This morning, PG notes that the stormy sky is a particularly virulent shade of purple and worries that it is an omen of bad things coming. It is still not light as he walks to the kitchen for his customary pre-exercise glass of carrot juice. Tired and irritable, with his heart pounding, he stomps and staggers down the dark corridor.

His glass of juice awaits him; this time, however, his enemies had poisoned it. He drank it all, with no ill effects.

Questions

A. What is going on with Mr. PG?
B. What was the poison?

Analysis

If one takes away the details of PG's unlawful but exciting life, what remains is the following:

(a) Loss of appetite
(b) Fatigue and exertional palpitations (heart pounding)—suggestive of anemia
(c) Imbalance while walking in the dark (stomping and staggering down the dark corridor)—suggestive of posterior column involvement (this is the history counterpart of a positive Romberg's sign)

A diagnosis which integrates both anemia and posterior column involvement would be Vitamin B12 deficiency.

Considering this, how do we explain PG's resistance to poison? Is there any illness which would cause Vitamin B12 deficiency as well as resistance to a certain poison? Let us answer this question by asking this question: For Vitamin B12 deficiency to occur, where would the pathology be? Logically, it should be in the place where Vitamin B12 is absorbed. Though Vitamin B12 is absorbed in the ileum, this process requires the secretion of intrinsic factor (IF) by the gastric parietal cells, release of B12 from the bound protein by the action of gastric acid secreted by oxyntic cells, binding of B12 to IF, and thereafter absorption of Vitamin B12 in the ileum [1]. Can a disease in either the duodenum, ileum, or gastric mucosa protect against a certain poison? One possibility is achlorhydria, due to atrophic gastritis (AG).

Hydrochloric acid in the stomach converts cyanide into its active form, HCN. Patients who have achlorhydria do not often suffer the effects of cyanide poisoning [2].

The famous example here is Grigori Rasputin, from Russia:

"*Ra ra Rasputin, lover of the Russian queen*
They put some poison in to his wine
Ra ra Rasputin, Russia's greatest love machine
He drank it all and said 'I feel fine'"

One of the many theories of how Rasputin escaped from cyanide poisoning is that he suffered from achlorhydria, and thus cyanide did not convert into HCN.

Cyanide Poisoning

Cyanide binds and inhibits cytochrome oxidase, which is needed for oxidative phosphorylation [3]. Thus, tissue utilization of oxygen is inhibited, resulting in cellular dysfunction. Cyanide smells like bitter almonds. Interestingly, the ability to detect this smell is genetically determined and is not universal [4].

Cyanide poisoning presents as headache, nausea, metallic taste, drowsiness, dizziness, anxiety, mucous membrane irritation, and hyperpnoea [5]. Later, frank dyspnoea, bradycardia, hypotension, arrythmias, and periods of cyanosis and unconsciousness develop.

The following are antidotes to cyanide [6], though hopefully, we will not have the need to use them:

(a) Sodium thiosulphate
(b) Sodium nitrite
(c) 4-DMAP
(d) Dicobalt edetate
(e) Hydroxocobalamin

Vitamin B12

Among other functions, it is also required for RBC production and myelination of nerves. Hence, Vitamin B12 deficiency results in dyserythropoiesis and impaired myelination, causing anemia and posterior column dysfunction.

Pathophysiology of Vitamin B12 Deficiency in AG [7]

- Reduced Intrinsic Factor Production: In AG, the immune system targets and destroys parietal cells, leading to a decrease or absence of IF production. Without adequate IF, Vitamin B12 cannot be properly absorbed in the ileum.
- Impaired Release of Vitamin B12 from Food Proteins: Gastric acid and pepsin are necessary to release Vitamin B12 from food proteins. The reduction in gastric acid secretion in AG impairs this process, further reducing B12 absorption. Thus, individuals with atrophic gastritis may have difficulty absorbing B12 from food but may be able to absorb crystalline B12 from supplements.

Clinical Features of Vitamin B12 Deficiency in AG [8]

(a) Anemia: Vitamin B12 deficiency causes megaloblastic anemia, characterized by macrocytic red blood cells, hypersegmented neutrophils, and, in severe cases, pancytopenia. Symptoms include fatigue, weakness, light-headedness, and palpitations.
(b) Markers of autoimmunity like vitiligo.
(c) Beefy red tongue and hyperpigmented knuckles.
(d) Neurological manifestations: B12 deficiency can lead to various neurological symptoms, including:
    I. Peripheral neuropathy: This presents as paresthesias and sensory loss, often starting in the extremities.
    II. Optic neuropathy.
    III. Characteristic combination of absent ankle jerk and upgoing plantar.

IV. Loss of proprioception.
V. Positive Romberg's sign.
VI. Cognitive decline—memory loss and confusion.
VII. Neuropsychiatric manifestations: depression, psychosis, and dementia.
VIII. Gastrointestinal manifestation: Atrophic glossitis.

Treatment [9]

Vitamin B12 supplementation: Inj. B12 1000 ug IM daily for a week; then, weekly for a month and then monthly for 3 months, followed by high-dose oral supplementation lifelong.

Subacute Combined Degeneration of the Cord (SCD)

- SCD is a specific neurological syndrome that can occur as a result of chronic and severe Vitamin B12 deficiency [10].
- Pathophysiology: The deficiency of B12 causes abnormal lipid and protein methylation reactions, which are needed for myelination. Lack of B12 can lead to demyelination of the posterior and lateral columns of the spinal cord.
- Clinical presentation [11]: SCD presents with a combination of
  I. Sensory ataxia: Loss of proprioception, leading to gait disturbances
  II. Paresthesias: Numbness, tingling, and burning sensations in the extremities
  III. Spastic paraparesis
- The neurological manifestations of Vitamin B12 become irreversible if treatment is delayed.

Autoimmune Gastritis (AIG) and Achlorhydria [12]

Atrophic gastritis (AG) is characterized by the replacement of normal gastric with atrophic and metaplastic tissue. AG is a premalignant condition that increases the risk of gastric cancer [13].

Epidemiology

Autoimmune atrophic gastritis (AAG) has an estimated prevalence between 0.3% and 2.7% in the general population. The prevalence is higher in areas with a high incidence of *Helicobacter pylori* infection and gastric cancer.

Etiology: AG is classified into [14]:

- Autoimmune metaplastic atrophic gastritis (AMAG): This results from the production of autoantibodies against parietal cells and the intrinsic factor. AMAG spares the antral mucosa. It may be associated with other autoimmune conditions such as thyroid disease and type 1 diabetes. Parietal cell loss leads to reduced production of gastric acid and intrinsic factor, resulting in hypergastrinemia and potential B12 deficiency.
- Environmental metaplastic atrophic gastritis (EMAG): This form is caused by chronic *H. pylori* infection, leading to gastric mucosal atrophy and metaplasia.

Diagnosis [15]

- Endoscopy reveals a pale mucosa, loss of gastric folds, and prominence of submucosal blood vessels. The rugal folds are flattened, and submucosal vessels are visible.
- Biopsies: Two biopsies from the antrum and two from the corpus are recommended. Histology reveals atrophy of the oxyntic mucosa, intestinal metaplasia, enterochromaffin-like (ECL) cell, hyperplasia, and gastrin cell hyperplasia in the antrum [16].
- Vitamin B12 levels: Serum vitamin B12 levels are measured; however, these can fluctuate and may be normal in cases of cobalamin-responsive disorders.
- Homocysteine and methylmalonic acid (MMA): These are typically elevated in B12 deficiency.
- Serology [17]:
  - Antiparietal cell antibodies (APCA).
  - Anti-intrinsic factor antibodies (AIFA).
  - Pepsinogen I and II and Gastrin-17: A low pepsinogen I/II ratio and high gastrin-17 levels are suggestive of autoimmune gastritis.
  - *H. pylori* serology: Detection of antibodies to *H. pylori* can help determine if EMAG is the cause.

Treatment

- Iron supplementation.
- H. pylori eradication for EMAG.
- Proton pump inhibitors (PPIs) may worsen malabsorption. H2 receptor antagonists are used for symptom relief.
- Endoscopic surveillance is recommended for patients with AG, particularly those with AMAG, due to the increased risk of gastric cancer and NETs. Surveillance intervals should be based on risk stratification.
- Emerging therapies: Locally acting anti-inflammatory agents are under development to reduce gastric inflammation and prevent the progression of atrophy and metaplasia.

References

1. Guéant JL, Guéant-Rodriguez RM, Alpers DH. Vitamin B12 absorption and malabsorption. Vitam Horm. 2022;119:241–74.
2. JaypeeDigital | Hydrocyanic Acid [Internet]. [cited 2025 Feb 2]. Available from: https://www.jaypeedigital.com/book/9789351528647/chapter/ch55
3. Nelson L. Acute cyanide toxicity: mechanisms and manifestations. J Emerg Nurs. 2006;32(4):S8–11.
4. Kirk RL, Stenhouse NS. Ability to smell solutions of potassium cyanide. Nature. 1953;171(4355):698–9.
5. Yen D, Tsai J, Wang LM, Kao WF, Hu SC, Lee CH, Deng JF. The clinical experience of acute cyanide poisoning. Am J Emerg Med. 1995;13(5):524–8.
6. Reade MC, Davies SR, Morley PT, Dennett J, Jacobs IC, Australian Resuscitation Council. Management of cyanide poisoning. Emerg Med Australas. 2012;24(3):225–38.
7. Kryssia IR, Marilisa F, Antonino N, Chiara M, Antonio N, Gioacchino L, Tiziana M, Gian LD, Francesco DM. Clinical manifestations of chronic atrophic gastritis. Acta Bio Medica: Atenei Parmensis. 2018;89(Suppl 8):88.
8. Hunt A, Harrington D, Robinson S. Vitamin B12 deficiency. BMJ. 2014;349:349.
9. Nogueira-de-Almeida CA, Fernandes SL, de Almeida SE, Lourenço DM, Zotarelli Filho IJ, Junior NI, Ribas FD. Consensus of the Brazilian Association of Nutrology on diagnosis, prophylaxis, and treatment of vitamin B12 deficiency. Int J Nutrol. 2023;16(1)
10. Scalabrino G. Cobalamin (vitamin B12) in subacute combined degeneration and beyond: traditional interpretations and novel theories. Exp Neurol. 2005;192(2):463–79.
11. Linazi G, Abudureyimu S, Zhang J, Wulamu A, Maimaitiaili M, Wang B, Bakeer B, Xi Y. Clinical features of different stage subacute combined degeneration of the spinal cord. Medicine. 2022;101(37):e30420.
12. Neumann W, Coss E, Rugge M, et al. Autoimmune atrophic gastritis—pathogenesis, pathology and management. Nat Rev Gastroenterol Hepatol. 2013;10:529–41.
13. Vavallo M, Cingolani S, Cozza G, Schiavone FP, Dottori L, Palumbo C, Lahner E. Autoimmune gastritis and hypochlorhydria: known concepts from a new perspective. Int J Mol Sci. 2024;25(13):6818.
14. Lenti MV, Rugge M, Lahner E, Miceli E, Toh BH, Genta RM, De Block C, Hershko C, Di Sabatino A. Autoimmune gastritis. Nat Rev Dis Primers. 2020;6(1):56.
15. Minalyan A, Benhammou JN, Artashesyan A, Lewis MS, Pisegna JR. Autoimmune atrophic gastritis: current perspectives. Clin Exp Gastroenterol. 2017;10:19–27. https://doi.org/10.2147/CEG.S109123.
16. Shah SC, Piazuelo MB, Kuipers EJ, Li D. AGA clinical practice update on the diagnosis and management of atrophic gastritis: expert review. Gastroenterology. 2021;161(4):1325–32.
17. Botezatu A, Bodrug N. Chronic atrophic gastritis: an update on diagnosis. Med Pharm Rep. 2021;94(1):7.

Cluster of Unexplainable Symptoms: The Hysterical Wife

7

Grade Difficult.

Abstract An adult female presents with insidious onset, gradually progressive symptoms in the form of weakness, weight loss, breathlessness, swelling of feet, and bruising.

Story Mrs. Sampriti totters into your clinic in her silks and high heels. Accompanying her is her husband, Mr. Sahu, a bewhiskered gentleman who looks harassed and ill-tempered in equal measure.

You greet them both and walk forward to shake hands. Sampriti withdraws—"Sorry, my fingers hurt all the time—I've stopped shaking hands".

You ask them both to be seated and proceed to obtain a history where Sampriti complains, and her husband chimes in like a grumpy echo.

"What seems to be the problem?" you enquire politely.

"I'm feeling so tired all the time and I've lost so much weight, doctor" Sampriti says throatily.

"She's on a crazy diet half the time." says the husband.

"My feet are swollen." mutters the wife.

"It's those high heels she wears," counters the husband.

"I feel so short of breath while walking, maybe my tongue is blocking my throat." moans Sampriti.

"Yes, it has become huge with all the exercise you are giving it." Sahu sniggers.

"Have you had any other health issues like diabetes, high blood pressure, thyroid problems?"

S. Bhat, *Clinical Conundrums to Practice Diagnostic Reasoning*,
https://doi.org/10.1007/978-981-95-0636-1_7

"No, doctor. Everything has been tested and found normal."

"Any problem with passing urine? Or stool?"

"No, but my urine looks very bubbly when I pass it."

"You must be very concerned about these problems." you tell Sampriti sympathetically.

"Yes, I am. My mother had problems with her nerves in her early sixties and passed away well before her time."

You proceed to examine her.

Your findings are as follows:

BP: 120/80 mm Hg supine, 100/68 mm Hg standing.

You request Sampriti to lie down on the examination couch. As you begin to examine her, you notice a fair amount of bruising on her arms and thighs and a raccoon eye appearance too. This worries you—you ask Sahu to leave the room and discreetly ask Sampriti about domestic violence which she denies emphatically. You proceed with the examination and find increased Jugular venous pressure (JVP), a right ventricular third heart sound (RVS3) and hepatosplenomegaly.

Question

1. Were Mrs. Sampriti's problems real or imagined? What do you think is going on with her?
2. How would you like to proceed with the investigation and treatment?

Analysis

The problems were very real indeed. Reflect on the history and findings again:

(a) Throaty voice: hoarse voice
(b) Fatigue and loss of weight
(c) Pedal edema, perhaps proteinuria (frothing of urine present), Either Congestive cardiac failure or Right ventricular failure?
(d) Breathlessness on exertion? Because of heart failure? Because of lung disease?
(e) Sensation of tongue blocking the throat: macroglossia
(f) Family history suggestive of neuropathy
(g) Orthostatic hypotension
(h) Bruising and raccoon eyes—coagulopathy

Putting these features together—a multisystem disease causing neuropathy, coagulopathy, and macroglossia, with perhaps a hereditary component, one comes up with the possibility of amyloidosis.

Amyloidosis is a condition with protean manifestations involving multiple systems due to the deposition of insoluble beta-sheet fibrillar protein in various tissues [1].

Classification

The current classification of amyloid is based upon the protein deposited. Some of the major subtypes are as follows:

A. AL—immunoglobulin light chain [2]—characterized by nephrotic range proteinuria, carpal tunnel syndrome, and edema
B. AA—due to chronic inflammation (rheumatoid arthritis and inflammatory bowel disease)—this affects the kidney [3]
C. ATTR—hereditary or age-related—cardiomyopathy common [4]
D. Beta-2 microglobulin [5]

Misfolding of proteins, resulting in extracellular deposition of insoluble fibrils can occur due to various reasons [6]:

(a) Accumulation of excess protein: HD patients and beta-2 microglobulin.
(b) Tendency to acquire abnormal configuration with aging: ATTR.
(c) Alteration of amino acid composition in the protein leads to a. loss of function of b. pathological aggregation (hereditary amyloid).
(d) Acute-phase reactants associated with inflammation.

Clinical Features

a) Symptoms: fatigue, loss of appetite, loss of weight
b) General examination: macroglossia
c) Fat pad at shoulder
d) GIT: hepatosplenomegaly, malabsorption, constipation, bacterial overgrowth
e) Neurological—length-dependent peripheral neuropathy, particularly carpal tunnel syndrome, autonomic neuropathy leading to orthostatic hypotension
f) CVS: diastolic, followed by systolic dysfunction
g) Hematological: coagulopathy, ecchymoses, periorbital purpura

Labs would reveal proteinuria, sometimes in the nephrotic range.

Tissue biopsy shows the characteristic apple green birefringence on Congo red staining.

Treatment

1. AL amyloidosis—treatment of underlying plasma cell disease—stem cell transplant, bortezomib [2]
2. AA amyloidosis—management of the underlying infectious or immune disease [7]
3. Dialysis-related amyloidosis—to consider renal transplant [8]
4. Transthyretin amyloidosis—liver transplant
5. RNA-targeted therapies—patisiran, vutrisiran, inotersen, and eplontersen
6. Stabilization of transthyretin tetramers—Tafamidis and diflunisal [9]

Investigational Therapies

- RNA silencing
- Gene editing
- Inhibition of proteolysis
- Immunotherapy
- Targeting of serum amyloid P
- Fibril disruptor

Key Takeaway

Diseases with multisystem manifestations can masquerade as functional. They may have a disparate number of complaints, and an astute clinician's insights may be required to suspect and diagnose.

References

1. Kyle RA. Amyloidosis: a convoluted story. Br J Haematol. 2001;114(3):529.
2. Milani P, Merlini G, Palladini G. Light chain amyloidosis. Mediterr J Hematol Infect Dis. 2018;10(1):e2018022.
3. Papa R, Lachmann HJ. Secondary, AA, amyloidosis. Rheum Dis Clin. 2018;44(4):585–603.
4. Westermark P, Bergström J, Solomon A, Murphy C, Sletten K. Transthyretin-derived senile systemic amyloidosis: clinicopathologic and structural considerations. Amyloid. 2003;10(sup1):48–54.
5. Stoppini M, Bellotti V. Systemic amyloidosis: lessons from β2-microglobulin. J Biol Chem. 2015;290(16):9951–8.
6. Bellotti V, Nuvolone M, Giorgetti S, Obici L, Palladini G, Russo P, Lavatelli F, Perfetti V, Merlini G. The workings of the amyloid diseases. Ann Med. 2007;39(3):200–7.
7. Lachmann HJ, Goodman HJ, Gilbertson JA, Gallimore JR, Sabin CA, Gillmore JD, Hawkins PN. Natural history and outcome in systemic AA amyloidosis. N Engl J Med. 2007;356(23):2361–71.
8. Scarpioni R, Ricardi M, Albertazzi V, De Amicis S, Rastelli F, Zerbini L. Dialysis-related amyloidosis: challenges and solutions. Int J Nephrol Renov Dis. 2016:319–28.
9. Dorbala S, Ando Y, Bokhari S, Dispenzieri A, Falk RH, Ferrari VA, Fontana M, Gheysens O, Gillmore JD, Glaudemans AW, Hanna MA. ASNC/AHA/ASE/EANM/HFSA/ISA/SCMR/SNMMI expert consensus recommendations for multimodality imaging in cardiac amyloidosis: part 1 of 2—evidence base and standardized methods of imaging. Circulation. Cardiovasc Imaging. 2021;14(7):e000029.

Adult Male with Muscle Ache and Difficulty in Moving—Heavy Fuel

8

Grade Easy.

Abstract An adult male, regular consumer of ethanol and nicotine, who presents with difficulty in movement and muscle ache.

The Story Richard sits in your clinic with his wife, Sue. There are some bad vibes in the air, perhaps a disagreement between husband and wife.

"Good afternoon," you greet them. Richard has been your patient for a couple of years now, and you have a fair measure of the man. He is one of the jolly, gregarious types, but he does not look so happy today. You wonder if it is because of the strict warning you gave him when you met him last—no booze, no smoking, and no junk food.

"How are you, Richard?" you ask pleasantly.

"Not bad, not bad."

"I hope you've cut down on the nicotine and ethanol."

"Of course!" he says with a hearty laugh. "What's the point of having an excellent doctor, if I don't obey his instructions."

Sue snorts bitterly.

"This is apparently some new meaning of the word obey that I was not aware of. He continues to smoke, doctor, continues to imbibe."

"What's life without a little fun, eh doc?" Richard guffaws, nudging you with his bony elbow.

You wince and ask, "Have you come for a routine check-up or is there something else troubling you?"

S. Bhat, *Clinical Conundrums to Practice Diagnostic Reasoning*,
https://doi.org/10.1007/978-981-95-0636-1_8

"You know how Sue is—she fusses a lot."

"He has become old before his time, doctor. He groans and moans when he moves. In fact, my 90-year-old mother gets out of a chair faster than him."

"It's just that my muscles get cramped and achy quite often. It gets better once I walk for a while, doctor. It's just the initial few moments where I feel weak and find it difficult to move. I'm no longer the young man you married, my dear," Richard tells his wife roguishly.

"That's a fact. And see, doctor, we are discussing his health—such an important issue—he's sitting there with his eyes half closed as if he couldn't be less interested in what we are saying."

You glance at Richard and note that he is not uninterested—he appears to have ptosis of both eyes which makes him look sleepy and dull.

You proceed with the physical examination, and your findings are as follows:

- Ptosis bilaterally.
- No muscle wasting.
- Power 3/5 proximal lower limbs. Normal distally. Upper limbs are normal.
- Lower limb deep tendon reflexes are absent.

Questions What might Richard's diagnosis be? Are there any maneuvers you would like to do to narrow down the diagnosis further?

Analysis

When you remove all the frills and drama, what is left is essentially the following:
A chronic smoker who presents with

(a) Proximal muscle weakness (difficulty in rising from a chair).
(b) Weakness which improves with movement "It's just the initial few moments when I feel weak, and it is difficult to move. It gets better after I move a bit."
(c) Ptosis, absent tendon reflexes in lower limbs.

Diagnosis This is a case of Lambert-Eaton myasthenic syndrome (LEMS) , perhaps secondary to bronchogenic cancer in a chronic smoker. Checking the power again after voluntary muscle contraction might reveal post-exercise or post-activation facilitation.

Lambert-Eaton myasthenic syndrome (LEMS) is a disorder of neuromuscular junction transmission characterized by muscle weakness due to reduction in the release of acetylcholine (ACh) from presynaptic nerve terminals, despite normal ACh vesicle number and concentration and normal postsynaptic ACh receptors [1]. This reduction in ACh release is a consequence of impaired calcium influx into the presynaptic terminal, a process mediated by voltage-gated calcium channels (VGCCs).

Etiopathogenesis [2]: LEMS may be paraneoplastic, non-neoplastic, or toxic (Fig. 8.1). VGCCs are essential for the release of ACh. Upon arrival of a nerve impulse, depolarization opens VGCCs, allowing calcium ions to flow into the nerve terminal. This calcium influx triggers the fusion of ACh-containing vesicles with the presynaptic membrane, releasing ACh into the synaptic cleft (Fig. 8.2a). Antibodies directed against VGCCs located on the presynaptic nerve terminal disrupt the normal functioning of these channels, which is crucial for calcium influx. This reduces the calcium influx through the VGCCs, leading to diminished ACh release (Fig. 8.2b).

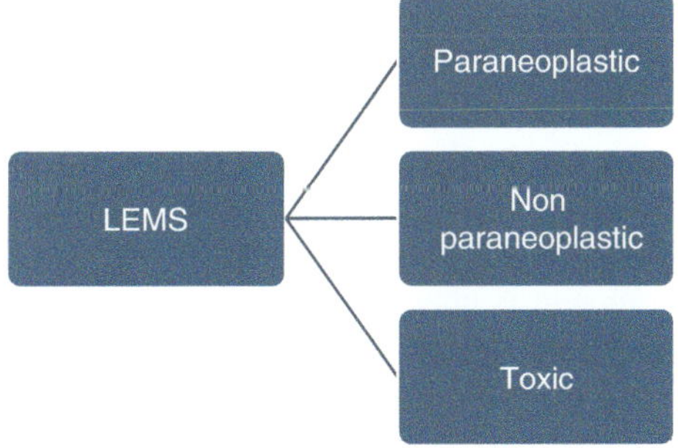

Fig. 8.1 Causes of LEMS

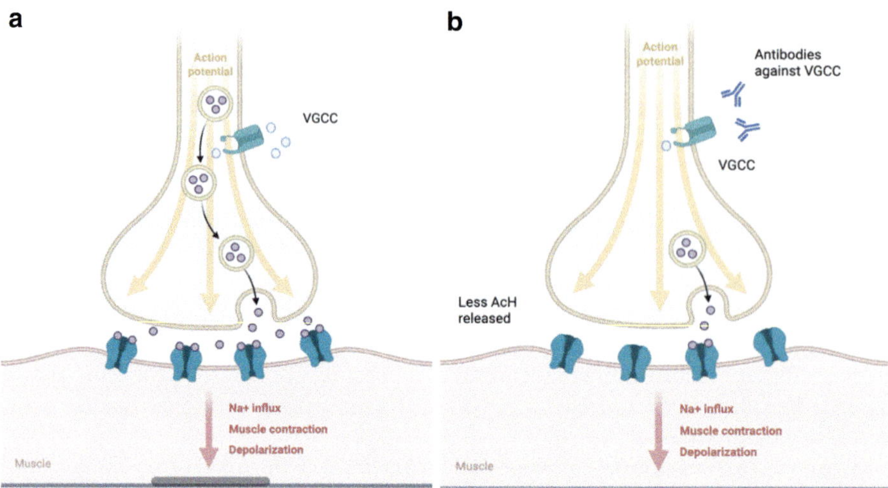

Fig. 8.2 (**a**) Transmission across the neuromuscular junction; (**b**) Antibodies against VGCC and the decreased release of AcH.
VGCC: Voltage-gated calcium channels.
(Created in BioRender. Bhat, S. (2025) https://BioRender.com/7axwu1x)

Clinical Features [3]: The classic presentation of LEMS involves a triad of symptoms: proximal muscle weakness, autonomic dysfunction, and diminished or absent deep tendon reflexes.

Muscle weakness typically manifests as an insidious onset, gradually progressive proximal muscle weakness, particularly affecting the lower limbs. Patients often report difficulty rising from a seated position, climbing stairs, or walking. The weakness tends to be symmetrical, progressing from proximal to distal and from caudal to cranial regions, eventually reaching the oculobulbar area. Upper extremity weakness is less prominent. Many patients describe a sensation of aching or stiffness in the muscles. It is also important to note that the degree of weakness is often less than the functional difficulty would lead one to expect, and patients might be suspected to be malingering. Deep tendon jerks are diminished or absent.

Ptosis and diplopia occur early in the disease, followed by dysphagia and dysarthria.

The prevalence of autonomic symptoms in LEMS varies from 80% to 96%. The most frequently reported symptoms are dry mouth, constipation, erectile dysfunction, orthostatic hypotension, and altered sweating.

The hallmark of LEMS is *post-exercise or post-activation facilitation* [4]. This phenomenon is characterized by enhanced muscle strength and deep tendon reflexes after a brief, vigorous muscle activity. It is caused by the increased calcium influx that occurs with repeated stimulation, thus increasing the amount of Ach that is released into the synapse.

It is important to note that the effect of post-exercise facilitation is temporary. More sustained physical activity can often induce muscle weakness.

Investigations

(a) Nerve conduction studies
(b) Repetitive nerve stimulation [5]
(c) Needle electromyography and single fiber electromyography if diagnosis is uncertain
(d) VGCC antibody testing [6]
(e) Meticulous search for malignancy to rule out paraneoplastic LEMS [7] (Fig. 8.3a–c)

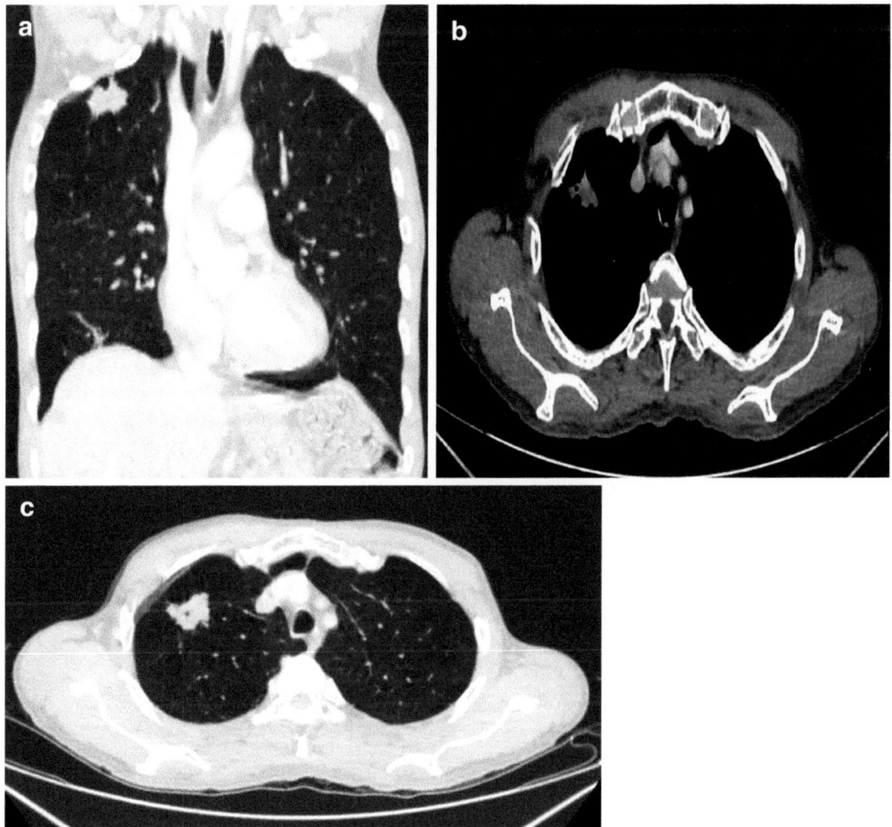

Fig. 8.3 (**a–c**) Small-cell carcinoma lung. (Image contributed by Dr. Ram Shenoy Basti, FMMC)

Diagnosis [8]

The following are the diagnostic criteria for LEMS:

1. *Clinical features*
   (a) Proximal muscle weakness
   (b) Reduced deep tendon reflexes
   (c) Autonomic symptoms
2. *VGCC antibodies*
3. *Repetitive nerve stimulation abnormalities*
   (a) Low compound muscle action potential
   (b) Decrement > 10%
   (c) Increment > 100% after maximum voluntary contraction

Differential Diagnosis

(a) Myasthenia gravis
(b) Inflammatory myositis

Treatment

Definitive management of paraneoplastic-associated LEMS is the treatment of the malignancy. Amifampridine (3,4-aminopyridine) [9] is the initial treatment for the patients of LEMS with significant weakness [10]. If improvement is not satisfactory, the algorithm in Fig. 8.4 can be followed for escalating treatment [11].

If the patient does not respond to cyclophosphamide and MMF, rescue therapy with rituximab [12] and plasmapheresis [13] may be considered.

Key Takeaway

(a) Always check for improvement/deterioration with physical activity in individuals who present with proximal muscle weakness.
(b) Consider and rule out paraneoplastic syndrome in patients with risk factors for malignancy and unexplained neurological symptoms.

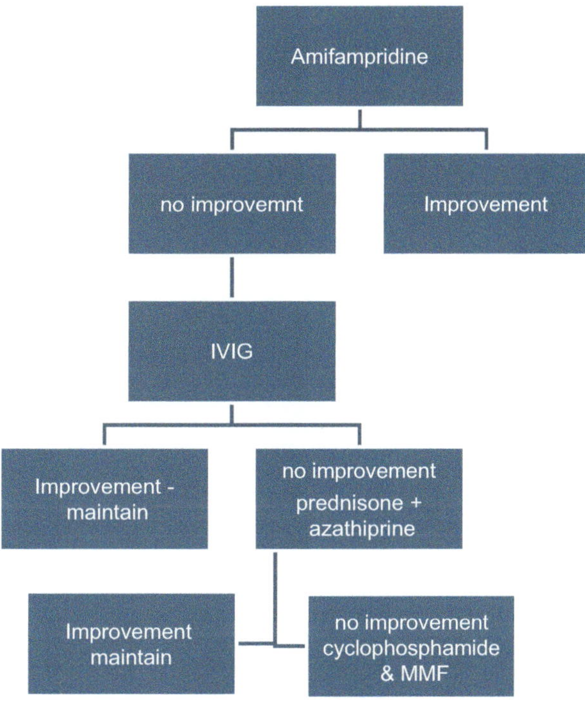

Fig. 8.4 Approach to the treatment of LEMS

References

1. Lambert EH, Elmqvist D. Quantal components of end-plate potentials in the myasthenic syndrome. Ann N Y Acad Sci. 1971;183(1):183–99.
2. Hülsbrink R, Hashemolhosseini S. Lambert–Eaton myasthenic syndrome – Diagnosis, pathogenesis and therapy. Clin Neurophysiol. 2014;125(12):2328–36.
3. Motomura M, Nakata R, Shiraishi H. Lambert–Eaton myasthenic syndrome: clinical review. Clin Exp Neuroimmunol. 2016;7(3):238–45.
4. Henriksson KG, Nilsson O, Rosén I, Schiller HH. Clinical, neurophysiological and morphological findings in eaton lambert syndrome. Acta Neurol Scand. 1977;56(2):117–40.
5. Oh SJ. Distinguishing features of the repetitive nerve stimulation test between lambert–Eaton myasthenic syndrome and myasthenia gravis, 50-year reappraisal. J Clin Neuromuscul Dis. 2017;19(2):66.
6. Majed M, Zekeridou A, Lennon V, Pittock S, McKeon A, Klein C, et al. Testing for N-type Voltage gated calcium channel antibody has limited utility in evaluating patients with suspected lambert-Eaton myasthenic syndrome. Neurology. 2022;99(23_Supplement_2):S31–2.
7. Titulaer MJ, Wirtz PW, Willems LN, van Kralingen KW, Smitt PA, Verschuuren JJ. Screening for small-cell lung cancer: a follow-up study of patients with Lambert-Eaton myasthenic syndrome. J Clin Oncol. 2008;26(26):4276–81.
8. Titulaer MJ, Lang B, Verschuuren JJ. Lambert–Eaton myasthenic syndrome: from clinical characteristics to therapeutic strategies. Lancet Neurol. 2011;10(12):1098–107.
9. Keogh M, Sedehizadeh S, Maddison P. Treatment for Lambert-Eaton myasthenic syndrome. Cochrane Database Syst Rev. 2011;2011(2):CD003279.

10. Yoon CH, Owusu-Guha J, Smith A, Buschur P. Amifampridine for the management of Lambert-Eaton myasthenic syndrome: a new take on an old drug. Ann Pharmacother. 2020;54(1):56–63.
11. Newsom-Davis J. Therapy in myasthenia gravis and Lambert-Eaton myasthenic syndrome. In: Seminars in neurology 2003, vol. 23, No. 02; 2003. p. 191–8. Copyright© 2002 by Thieme Medical Publishers, Inc., 333 Seventh Avenue, New York, NY 10001, USA. Tel.:+ 1 (212) 584-4662.
12. Boutin E, Rey C, Romeu M, Pouget J, Franques J. Favourable outcome after treatment with rituximab in a case of seronegative non-paraneoplastic Lambert-Eaton myasthenic syndrome. Rev Med Interne. 2013;34(8):493–6.
13. Motomura M, Hamasaki S, Nakane S, Fukuda T, Nakao YK. Apheresis treatment in Lambert-Eaton myasthenic syndrome. Ther Apher. 2000;4(4):287–90.

9 Young Woman with Agoraphobia, Anxiety, and Difficulty in Ambulation: Frankenstein's Sister

Grade Difficult.

Abstract A young woman is brought to you with an insidious onset, gradually progressive neuropsychiatric disorder in the form of reluctance to go outside her home, fearfulness, and difficulty in walking.

Story Your school classmate Sangeetha calls to ask for an appointment to see you.

"I really do need to meet you, Shruthi. I hope I'm not messing up your schedule."

"Of course not, Sangeetha. But you sound stressed. I hope all is well? Your health is ok?"

"Actually, it's about my sister, not me. She's not ok at all and I...." her voice breaks.

You wait quietly while Sangeetha collects herself.

"Sorry about that, Shruthi. It's just that Ritu is the only family I have left and she's not doing well at all. I'll bring her to see you tomorrow."

However, the next day, Sangeetha arrives alone at your clinic.

"I'm sorry, Ritu refused to budge. She's very anxious these days, Shruthi. She just doesn't want to leave home. I thought I'd come and discuss her problems with you."

"Of course. And then maybe, if you'd like, I can come to your place and examine her."

"You would do that? Thanks so much. It means a lot!"

"No problem at all! We've known each other for more than 2 decades now."

You order some coffee to the room and give Sangeetha the time and space to vent her woes.

"You may remember that Ritu had some health problems since the age of 17."

"Yes, I remember. She was diagnosed to have diabetes and you also learnt how to give her the insulin injections."

S. Bhat, *Clinical Conundrums to Practice Diagnostic Reasoning*,
https://doi.org/10.1007/978-981-95-0636-1_9

"Yes. Well, she was quite ok for a long time after that actually. She managed to get her bachelor's degree in dietetics and was working part time in a hospital close to our house. I don't know what went wrong. Maybe it was losing both our parents in that car crash."

"I heard about that. I'm so very sorry."

"She gradually started showing a disinclination to leave the house. And maybe the diabetes affected her nerves, but she started walking funny. So much so that the neighbourhood kids called her Frankenstein."

"Children can be cruel."

"So cruel."

"Sangeetha, I'm sorry—I forget how old Ritu is now?"

" She's 30 now. All the problems started maybe 5 years ago."

Sangeetha takes you to her small neat flat. You walk into the room where Ritu sits with the curtains drawn and the lights off. Sangeetha turns on the lights and says, "See Ritu, Doctor is here to see you."

Ritu stands up with difficulty and you observe an exaggerated lumbar lordosis. The book she is reading falls to the ground, and Sangeetha picks it up for her saying "She finds it difficult to bend."

"May I examine you?" you ask Ritu gently.

She looks at you fearfully and nods in the affirmative.

You note that there is rigidity in both upper limbs and lower limbs, especially proximally. While you are palpating the abdomen, there is a loud noise from outside the window, possibly a car engine backfiring. This surprises and terrifies poor Ritu. All her muscles spasm so much that the abdomen feels stiff and board-like.

Question What might be going on with Ritu? Is it the pain of losing her parents at a young age? Or is there another diagnosis? Is there something you may be able to do to make her feel better?

Analysis

This is a little bit of a tricky puzzle.

The clues are:

(a) The presence of what is most probably T1DM (diagnosed at a young age, on insulin since then).
(b) Rigidity, especially of proximal muscles.
(c) The "startle reflex" (muscle spasm when she was surprised by a sudden loud sound).

These features together suggest "Stiff man or stiff person syndrome" (SPS).

Stiff person syndrome (Moersch–Woltman syndrome) is an autoimmune neurological hyperexcitability disease causing muscle rigidity and axial muscle spasm [1].

Classification: (Fig. 9.1)

Etiopathogenesis [2, 9]: Stiff Person Syndrome falls under the glutamic acid decarboxylase (GAD) antibody disorders; other examples of GAD spectrum diseases include autoimmune epilepsy, cerebellar ataxia, and encephalitis. To a certain extent, SPS may be genetically determined, with the DQB1*0201 allele being more common in patients of SPS. There is a strong association with Type 1 Diabetes and anti-GAD antibodies.

GAD converts glutamate to GABA (Fig. 9.2). GABA is released through vesicles into the synaptic cleft and attaches to the GABA A2 receptor. These open the ion pores, allowing chloride to enter, increasing the negativity of the cell, and resulting in an inhibitory effect.

Antibodies in SPS inhibit the expression of GABA receptors on the surface and impair the functioning of GABA pathways [3]. Lower levels of brain GABA cause decreased GABAergic inhibition and cortical excitability which result in stiffness and phobias.

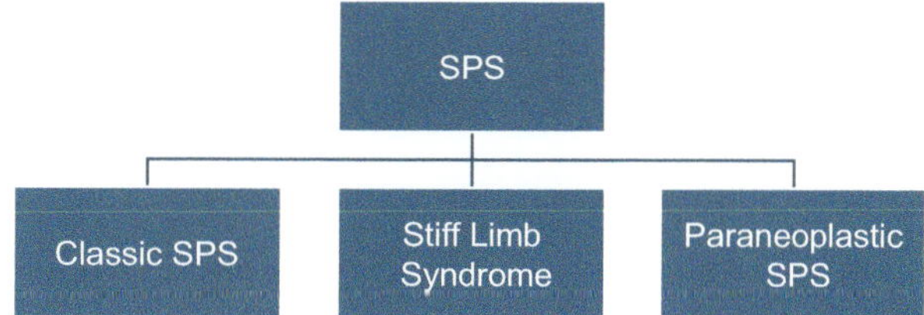

Fig. 9.1 Classification of SPS

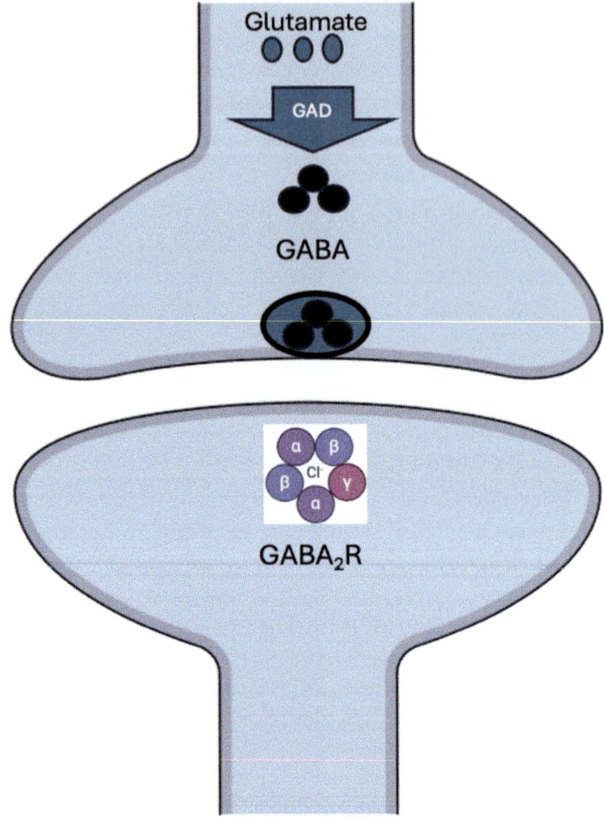

Fig. 9.2 Normal GABA inhibitory synapse

Clinical Features [4]

1. Excessive axial and proximal limb muscle rigidity [5]
2. Stiff gait
3. Frequent falls leading to fractures
4. Painful muscle spasms triggered by anxiety and surprise
5. "Startle" response [6]
6. Task-specific phobias [7]

Autoimmune disorders other than T1DM that are often seen in patients with SPS are vitiligo, thyroid disease, and celiac disease.

Complications

(a) Paroxysmal autonomic dysfunction causing tachycardia, tachypnea, hypertension, and pupil dilatation.
(b) Difficulty in swallowing leading to aspiration.

(c) Occasionally, the muscle spasm is generalized and lasts for hours. This is referred to as status spasticus. Status spasticus is treated with intravenous muscle relaxants.

Investigations

1. GAD antibody titers
2. CSF GAD antibody titers
3. Nerve conduction studies
4. Needle electromyography

Diagnostic Criteria [7]

1. Stiffness in the limb and axial muscles, prominent in the abdomen and thoracolumbar region
2. Painful spasms precipitated by unexpected tactile and auditory stimuli
3. Evidence of continuous motor unit activity in agonist and antagonist muscles demonstrated by EMG
4. Absence of other neurological impairments that could support an alternative diagnosis
5. Positive serology for anti-GAD65 or anti-amphiphysin autoantibodies
6. Clinical response to therapy with benzodiazepines

Treatment [8]

A. *To reduce muscle spasm*
   (a) Benzodiazepines
   (b) Baclofen
   (c) Gabapentin

B. *To reduce autoantibodies*
   (a) IV Ig
   (b) Rituximab
   (c) Plasmapheresis
   (d) Efgartigimod

Key Takeaway
Unfortunately, the symptoms may be misdiagnosed as a functional or psychiatric illness. Hence, a high index of suspicion is required for the diagnosis of this condition.

References

1. Baizabal-Carvallo JF, Jankovic J. Stiff-person syndrome: insights into a complex autoimmune disorder. J Neurol Neurosurg Psychiatry. 2015;86(8):840–8.
2. Burton AR, Baquet Z, Eisenbarth GS, Tisch R, Smeyne R, Workman CJ, Vignali DA. Central nervous system destruction mediated by glutamic acid decarboxylase-specific CD4+ T cells. J Immunol. 2010;184(9):4863–70.
3. Manto MU, Laute MA, Aguera M, Rogemond V, Pandolfo M, Honnorat J. Effects of anti–glutamic acid decarboxylase antibodies associated with neurological diseases. Ann Neurol. 2007;61(6):544–51.
4. Tsiortou P, Alexopoulos H, Dalakas MC. GAD antibody-spectrum disorders: progress in clinical phenotypes, immunopathogenesis and therapeutic interventions. Ther Adv Neurol Disord. 2021;14:17562864211003486.
5. Sarva H, Deik A, Ullah A, Severt WL. Clinical spectrum of stiff person syndrome: a review of recent reports. Tremor Hyperkinetic Mov. 2016;6:340.
6. Termsarasab P, Thammongkolchai T, Katirji B. Startle syndromes. In: Termsarasab P, Thammongkolchai T, Katirji B, editors. Stiff-person syndrome and related disorders: a comprehensive, practical guide. Cham: Springer International Publishing; 2020. p. 159–77. [cited 2025 Mar 25] Available from: https://doi.org/10.1007/978-3-030-43059-7_15.
7. Henningsen P, Meinck HM. Specific phobia is a frequent non-motor feature in stiff man syndrome. J Neurol Neurosurg Psychiatry. 2003;74(4):462–5.
8. Dalakas MC. Stiff person syndrome: advances in pathogenesis and therapeutic interventions. Curr Treat Options Neurol. 2009;11(2):102–10.
9. Alexopoulos H, Dalakas MC. A critical update on the immunopathogenesis of Stiff Person syndrome. Eur J Clin Investig. 2010;40(11):1018–25.

10 Dysphagia in a Young Male with No Pallor or Lymphadenopathy—Hard to Swallow

Grade Moderate.

Abstract A young man with no other markers of malignancy presenting with dysphagia to solids.

Story K has an appointment at 3 pm, but he turns up a little early. You are working on an article, but you say, "Watch out!" as he walks in, almost hitting his head on the door frame. He ducks and smiles—"I'm used to this, doc. The world wasn't designed for very tall people."

He sits down, folding his long lean body into the chair like a spider curling up and sits down with his knees crossed.

"Please sit down. Tell me why you are here today."

"Frankly, doctor you are my last resort."

"Really? Well, I certainly will try my very best to help. What's the problem?"

"For the last say 5–6 months, I have been having a little difficulty in swallowing."

"That's worrying . For liquids or solids?"

"For solids, and it seems to have become just a little worse lately."

"Have you lost weight?"

"A little, I think."

"Are there any other problems? Vomiting—or lumps and bumps anywhere in the body?"

"None at all. In fact, my appetite is good—it's just that eating is difficult because it is tough to swallow. Also, I'm feeling very low and blue that no one can help me. The only thing that is keeping me sane is my job."

S. Bhat, *Clinical Conundrums to Practice Diagnostic Reasoning*,
https://doi.org/10.1007/978-981-95-0636-1_10

"May I ask what you do?"
" I'm a musician."
" A pianist?" you ask, observing his long, beautiful fingers.
"No," he smiles "I play the sax."

You are trying to concentrate on what he says but you are distracted by the fact that he keeps shaking his leg really fast, more than once a second, in fact. It is a throwback to your childhood when your mother used to go on and on about how disgusting it was to shake your legs and how that was not something that a gentleman would ever do. You ask him to lie down and proceed to examine him.

His blood pressure is 150/70 mm Hg. There is no pallor/lymphadenopathy. A forceful apex is palpable at the left 6th intercostal pace, half an inch lateral to the midclavicular line. The abdomen is soft. There is no palpable organomegaly.

A point-of-care ultrasound is noncontributory except for simple renal cysts.

Questions What should you do next? Ask for an endoscopy? Or something else?

Analysis

These are the clues:

(a) A very tall man, long thin fingers: both together suggest Marfan's syndrome.
(b) Leg shaking at a rate more than once per second is suggestive of synchrony with heartbeat; taken together with the wide pulse pressure (150 − 70 = 80 mm Hg), it is suggestive of Lincoln sign in aortic regurgitation (AR). How do we correlate dysphagia with aortic regurgitation? The answer lies in the fact that AR is associated with thoracic aortic aneurysm [1] which can cause extrinsic compression of the oesophagus resulting in dysphagia.

Dysphagia aortica is dysphagia due to compression of the oesophagus by aortic aneurysm. Dysphagia is difficulty in swallowing caused by impaired progression of matter from the oropharynx to the stomach. Aneurysm is defined as an increase in the size of the aorta more than 1.5 times its usual size.

Marfan's syndrome (MFS) is a connective tissue disorder transmitted by autosomal dominant inheritance, with the prevalence ranging from 1.5 to 17.2 per 100,000 individuals [2].

Etiopathogenesis

The fibrillin gene encodes a glycoprotein, FBN1, which is the major component of microfibrils in the extracellular matrix. A mutation in this gene located on chromosome 15q21 results in the defective formation of microfibrils leading to defective connective tissue synthesis and affecting the heart, eyes, and musculoskeletal system [3].

Clinical Features [4]

Persons with MFS are tall, have kyphosis, and bilateral ectopia lentis. They tend to have disproportionate growth of the limbs, with an armspan more than 1.05 times their height, and elongated fingers (arachnodactyly) as well . Thoracolumbar scoliosis is present in over 60% of patients. Cardiovascular manifestations are a leading cause of mortality, with aortic root and proximal ascending aorta dilation being characteristic, potentially leading to aortic aneurysm and dissection, often before the age of 40.

Investigations

The 2010 modified Ghent criteria are used to diagnose MFS based on parameters such as cardiovascular, eye, and musculoskeletal disorders [5].

Molecular testing for FBN1 gene mutations [6] is also available and can aid in diagnosis, although a definitive diagnosis often requires more than just the presence of a mutation, considering clinical features and family history. Echocardiography, computed tomography (CT), and magnetic resonance imaging (MRI) are used to assess aortic dimensions.

Treatment

Beta-blockers and angiotensin receptor blockers to reduce the risk of aortic aneurysm [6].

Thoracic Aortic Aneurysm

Thoracic aortic aneurysm (TAA) is a permanent localized dilation of the thoracic aorta having at least a 50% increase in diameter compared with the expected normal diameter for that aortic segment [7].

Classification

TAAs are classified either based on the segment of the aorta that is involved: the ascending aorta, the aortic arch, the descending thoracic aorta, or a combination of these, or morphologically as fusiform or saccular [8].

Etiopathogenesis [9]

The etiology of TAA is multifactorial. Most TAAs are degenerative and associated with risk factors for atherosclerosis, such as hypertension, smoking, and hyperlipidemia. In the young, Marfan's syndrome and bicuspid aortic valve are more frequent causes.

Weakening of the aortic valve may be due to elastin degradation and alterations in the extracellular matrix. Endothelial dysfunction and imbalances in the angiotensin II and TGF-beta pathways play a role in the progression of TAA, especially in patients with Marfan's syndrome. The aneurysm typically grows slowly, at an average rate of about 0.1 cm per year.

Clinical Features: Most patients with TAA are asymptomatic until the aneurysm expands rapidly, dissects, or ruptures. Symptomatic TAAs can present with chest pain, which may indicate rapid expansion, dissection, infection, or impending rupture. Other symptoms may arise due to compression of adjacent structures, including dysphagia (oesophageal compression), dyspnea (tracheal or pulmonary compression), cough, hoarseness (recurrent laryngeal nerve compression), and superior vena cava syndrome [10].

Investigations

Computed tomography angiography (CTA) and magnetic resonance angiography (MRA) are the gold standards for assessing aortic diameter, extent, and morphology [11]. Transthoracic echocardiography (TTE) can be useful for evaluating the ascending aorta and aortic root. Chest radiography may reveal a widened mediastinum.

Treatment

The management of TAA depends on the size, location, etiology, and the patient's overall clinical condition. Surgical repair [12] (open or endovascular [13]) is the definitive treatment for significant TAAs to prevent rupture or dissection. Decision to intervene is based on aortic diameter thresholds, and these thresholds vary depending on the aortic segment and the presence of risk factors or genetic conditions.

Symptomatic aneurysms should be repaired regardless of size. Endovascular thoracic aortic repair (TEVAR) [14] has become an increasingly accepted alternative to open surgery for many indications due to its lower perioperative morbidity. Beta-blockers and angiotensin receptor blockers may reduce the rate of aneurysm growth by controlling blood pressure [15], although evidence for their benefit in non-Marfan aneurysms is less robust. Regular imaging surveillance is essential for monitoring the aneurysm size and growth rate.

Dysphagia Aortica

Dysphagia aortica is due to external compression of the oesophagus by an aortic aneurysm—most commonly a thoracic aortic aneurysm (TAA) or tortuous or ectatic aorta, even without a discrete aneurysm [16].

Pathogenesis

Dysphagia aortica develops when the enlarged aorta (aneurysm or tortuosity) compresses the oesophagus, leading to mechanical obstruction of the food bolus. The compression typically occurs anterolaterally, often pushing the oesophagus against the crural diaphragm or the left atrium.

Investigations [17]

Chest X-ray

Chest CT scan with oral and intravenous contrast

Upper GI endoscopy—shows pulsatile external compression of the oesophagus

Barium swallow

Differential Diagnosis

(a) Dysphagia due to intrinsic oesophageal disease: Strictures, webs, rings, motility disorders (e.g., achalasia, oesophageal spasm), esophagitis, and malignancy
(b) Other mediastinal masses: Tumors, cysts, lymphadenopathy
(c) Cardiovascular causes of dysphagia: Dilated left atrium (dysphagia megalatriensis), aberrant subclavian artery (dysphagia lusoria) causing vascular ring compression

Treatment [18]

(a) Conservative management: For mild symptoms, dietary modifications (e.g., softer foods and smaller bites) may be sufficient .
(b) Ryles tube feeding may be necessary to ensure adequate nutrition.
(c) Surgical repair of the aortic aneurysm.

Past US president Abraham Lincoln once had asked a journalist why his foot appeared blurry in photographs; the journalist Noah Brooks suggested it might be due to the throbbing of his artery causing a vibration of the crossed leg. Lincoln tested this out and found it to be true [19]. Fittingly, therefore, this sign of aortic regurgitation where the tremor of the foot when one leg is crossed above the other, caused by excessive pulsation of the popliteal artery, is called Lincoln's sign.

References

1. Aortic Regurgitation | Current Cardiology Reports [Internet]. [cited 2025 Apr 1]. Available from: https://link.springer.com/article/10.1007/s11886-019-1144-6.
2. Chiu HH, Wu MH, Chen HC, Kao FY, Huang SK. Epidemiological profile of Marfan syndrome in a general population: a national database study. Mayo Clin Proc. 2014;89(1):34–42.
3. Zeigler SM, Sloan B, Jones JA. Pathophysiology and pathogenesis of Marfan syndrome. In: Halper J, editor. Progress in heritable soft connective tissue diseases [Internet]. Cham: Springer International Publishing; 2021. [cited 2025 Apr 1]. p. 185–206. Available from: https://doi.org/10.1007/978-3-030-80614-9_8.
4. Marfan syndrome: clinical diagnosis and management | European Journal of Human Genetics [Internet]. [cited 2025 Apr 1]. Available from: https://www.nature.com/articles/5201851.
5. Faivre L, Collod-Beroud G, Adès L, Arbustini E, Child A, Callewaert B, et al. The new Ghent criteria for Marfan syndrome: what do they change? Clin Genet. 2012;81(5):433–42.
6. Loeys B, De Backer J, Van Acker P, Wettinck K, Pals G, Nuytinck L, et al. Comprehensive molecular screening of the FBN1 gene favors locus homogeneity of classical Marfan syndrome. Hum Mutat. 2004;24(2):140–6.
7. Senser EM, Misra S, Henkin S. Thoracic aortic aneurysm: a clinical review. Cardiol Clin. 2021;39(4):505–15.
8. Pressler V, Judson MNJ. Thoracic aortic aneurysm Natural history and treatment. J Thorac Cardiovasc Surg. 1980;79(4):489–98.
9. Etiology, pathogenesis and management of thoracic aortic aneurysm | Nature Reviews Cardiology [Internet]. [cited 2025 Apr 1]. Available from: https://www.nature.com/articles/ncpcardio0937.

10. Klein DG. Thoracic aortic aneurysms. J Cardiovasc Nurs. 2005;20(4):245.
11. Elefteriades JA. Thoracic aortic aneurysm: reading the enemy's playbook. Curr Probl Cardiol. 2008;33(5):203–77.
12. Elefteriades JA, Botta DM. Indications for the treatment of thoracic aortic aneurysms. Surg Clin. 2009;89(4):845–67.
13. Thurnher SA, Grabenwöger M. Endovascular treatment of thoracic aortic aneurysms: a review. Eur Radiol. 2002;12(6):1370–87.
14. Desai ND, Burtch K, Moser W, Moeller P, Szeto WY, Pochettino A, et al. Long-term comparison of thoracic endovascular aortic repair (TEVAR) to open surgery for the treatment of thoracic aortic aneurysms. J Thorac Cardiovasc Surg. 2012;144(3):604–11.
15. Chun AS, Elefteriades JA, Mukherjee SK. Medical treatment for thoracic aortic aneurysm – much more work to be done. Prog Cardiovasc Dis. 2013;56(1):103–8.
16. Wilkinson JM, Euinton HA, Smith LF, Bull MJ, Thorpe JA. Diagnostic dilemmas in dysphagia aortica. Eur J Cardiothorac Surg. 1997;11(2):222–7.
17. Dysphagia Aortica | Annals of Internal Medicine [Internet]. [cited 2025 Apr 1]. Available from: https://www.acpjournals.org/doi/abs/10.7326/0003-4819-142-3-200502010-00031?journalCode=aim.
18. Choi SHJ, Yang GK, Gagnon J. Dysphagia aortica secondary to thoracoabdominal aortic aneurysm resolved after endograft placement. J Vasc Surg Cases Innov Tech. 2019;5(4):501–5.
19. Did Abraham Lincoln Have Marfan Syndrome? – Clinical Correlations [Internet]. [cited 2025 Apr 1]. Available from: https://www.clinicalcorrelations.org/2013/04/19/did-abraham-lincoln-have-marfan-syndrome/.

Adult Male Presenting with Anxiety, Palpitations, and Diaphoresis—Anxious Allen

11

Grade Moderate.

Abstract A young adult male presents to the emergency ward with anxiety, palpitations, and sweating. Worrying findings are picked up on physical examination.

Story Allen is a software engineer in a busy multinational company. Every single day, roles are delegated to AI, and jobs are lost—maybe that is what is worrying Allen so much. Sometimes, he cannot tolerate the stress of it all—he breaks out in a sweat, his heart races, and he feels terrified. One of these attacks hits him when he is having dinner with his brother Aaron. Aaron says, "Nothing doing , we're not ignoring this anymore" and brings him to the hospital where you are in charge of the Emergency Department.

"Good evening, Doctor," Aaron says. " I've just witnessed my brother have a terrifying attack of sweating and breathlessness—he says his heart was racing too. I hope you can do something to help."

"Certainly." You request Allen to lie down and connect him to a monitor. You note that he is hemodynamically stable, and the acute attack has settled. This gives you some time to take a detailed history.

"Can you tell me a little more about these attacks?"

Allen clears his throat. "Sorry, my voice has been hoarse for a while now. I've been having the attacks for the last 4–5 months. I thought they were because of work stress initially."

"What exactly happens?"

"Suddenly, without any kind of warning at all, my heart starts beating very fast, I sweat like a horse, and my head starts hurting. This happened at work last Friday, and my colleagues took me to the company health centre. The doctor there measured my blood pressure and said it was very high—200/120 mm Hg. He said that

S. Bhat, *Clinical Conundrums to Practice Diagnostic Reasoning*,
https://doi.org/10.1007/978-981-95-0636-1_11

since I am only 30 years old, I need some tests to find out why I have high blood pressure at a young age."

"Ok, may I examine you?"

You note that the pulse and blood pressure are well within the normal range at 80/min and 130/80 mm Hg, respectively.

There appears to be a swelling on the right side of the neck which moves with deglutition. You palpate three firm to hard lymph nodes in the right deep cervical chain.

Questions Is it work stress which is causing the palpitations and anxiety or is it something else? How do you fit in the neck swelling and cervical nodes into the diagnosis?

Analysis

In itself, the palpitations and diaphoresis might be ascribed to stress. However, stress alone would not explain a blood pressure of 200/110 mm Hg. The headache, tachycardia , paroxysmal hypertension (paroxysmal, rather than sustained, since the documented high BP initially is completely normal when you examine the patient), and anxiety are clues to the presence of pheochromocytoma. Pheochromocytoma along with a neck mass (perhaps malignant—a medullary carcinoma thyroid) would make the diagnosis of MEN 2A a possibility. The hoarseness of voice that Allen mentions is worrying, as it might indicate recurrent laryngeal nerve involvement.

Multiple Endocrine Neoplasia type 2 (MEN2) is an autosomal dominant disorder characterized by a predisposition to tumors in organs which express the RET proto-oncogene [1]. The main features include medullary thyroid carcinoma (MTC), pheochromocytoma, and primary parathyroid hyperplasia [2].

MEN2 has an estimated prevalence of 1 per 30,000 in the general population [3]. MTC itself accounts for 1 to 5% of all thyroid cancers but contributes to a disproportionately high 13% of thyroid cancer-related deaths. About 25% of all MTC cases are familial, often linked to MEN2A.

Classification [3]

MEN2 is subclassified into two main syndromes: MEN2A and MEN2B. Within MEN2A, there are four variants:

(a) Classical MEN2A
(b) MEN2A with cutaneous lichen amyloidosis (CLA)
(c) MEN2A with Hirschsprung disease (HD)
(d) Familial MTC (FMTC)

Etiopathogenesis

MEN2A arises from germline mutations in the RET proto-oncogene. These mutations lead to constitutive activation of the RET tyrosine kinase receptor [4]. These mutations are present in all hereditary cases of MTC and in some sporadic cases as well. The penetrance of MTC in MEN2A is nearly 100%, though there is variability in the onset and other manifestations within and between families.

The RET proto-oncogene encodes a tyrosine kinase receptor involved in cell growth and differentiation. Mutations in RET lead to uncontrolled activation of

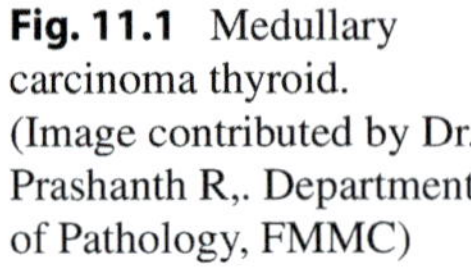
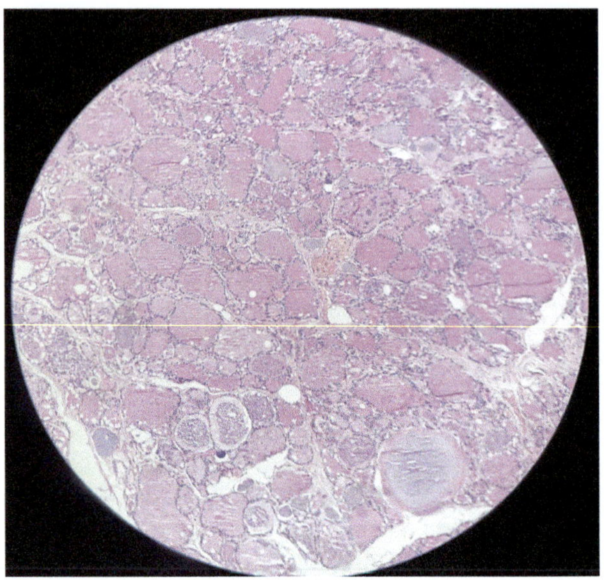

Fig. 11.1 Medullary carcinoma thyroid. (Image contributed by Dr. Prashanth R,. Department of Pathology, FMMC)

signaling pathways, which in turn causes parafollicular C-cell hyperplasia, a precursor to MTC.

Medullary Thyroid Carcinoma (MTC)

MTC is a neuroendocrine tumor originating from the parafollicular or C cells of the thyroid gland and accounts for 1–2% of all thyroid cancers (Fig. 11.1). MTC can be sporadic or familial.

Clinical Presentation

Sporadic MTC accounts for approximately 75% of MTC cases, typically presenting between the fourth and sixth decades of life. The most common presentation is a solitary thyroid nodule, observed in 75–95% of patients. C cells are mainly in the upper thyroid lobes, which explains the location of most tumors. About 70% of patients have cervical lymph node involvement at diagnosis, and 5–10% have distant metastases. Distant metastatic sites include the liver, lungs, bones, and less often, the brain and skin.

Familial MTC is associated with MEN2A and MEN2B.

MEN2A includes medullary thyroid cancer (MTC), pheochromocytoma, and primary parathyroid hyperplasia.

MEN2B includes inherited predisposition to MTC and pheochromocytoma, mucosal neuromas, intestinal ganglioneuromas, and a Marfanoid habitus [5].

Diagnosis

Diagnosis of MTC is typically achieved via fine-needle aspiration (FNA) biopsy of a solitary thyroid nodule. The sensitivity of FNA ranges from 50% to 80% but can be increased with immunocytochemical staining for calcitonin. Molecular testing of indeterminate nodules may also identify MTC markers.

Serum calcitonin and carcinoembryonic antigen (CEA) levels are measured to confirm hormone hypersecretion by the tumor. Preoperative calcitonin levels correlate with the tumor size.

Preoperative Evaluation

Preoperative evaluation includes testing for coexisting tumors by measuring serum calcium to rule out hyperparathyroidism and plasma-fractionated metanephrines to screen for pheochromocytoma [6]. If pheochromocytoma is identified, it should be removed before thyroidectomy, following appropriate alpha-adrenergic blockade.

Patients newly diagnosed with MTC should undergo biochemical and radiological staging. For patients with local lymph node metastases on ultrasound or with preoperative serum basal calcitonin >500 pg/mL, further imaging is needed to assess for metastatic disease.

Treatment

Total thyroidectomy is advised for hereditary MTC as it addresses the multicentric and bilateral nature of MTC and C-cell hyperplasia [7]. In MTC patients, death occurred in 50% of those with MEN2B and 9.7% of those with MEN2A.

Cervical nodal metastases are common in patients with palpable MTC or high calcitonin levels. Prophylactic dissection of nodal tissue in the central compartment is performed routinely, except in patients with very low calcitonin levels [5]. Lateral jugular and mediastinal nodes are carefully evaluated, followed by modified neck and/or mediastinal dissections if positive nodes are identified.

RET kinase inhibitors have been approved for use in MTC [8–10].

Postoperative monitoring for hypoparathyroidism or injury to the recurrent or superior laryngeal nerves is essential. Postoperative management and long-term monitoring are similar to those for sporadic MTC.

Staging and Management [11]

Initial staging is based on the tumor size, extrathyroidal invasion, nodal metastases, and distant metastases. Dynamic risk stratification helps modify initial risk estimates based on the tumor behavior and therapy response.

After surgery, thyroxine therapy should be initiated to maintain a euthyroid state. TSH suppression is not indicated in MTC.

Pheochromocytoma

Pheochromocytomas are catecholamine-secreting tumors derived from the chromaffin cells of the adrenal medulla. Tumors arising from sympathetic ganglia are referred to as catecholamine-secreting paragangliomas [12].

Clinical Presentation

The clinical presentation of pheochromocytoma results from the excessive and episodic secretion of catecholamines [13]. Symptoms include headache, palpitations, sweating, pallor, anxiety, tachycardia, and hypertension. Hypertension may be paroxysmal or sustained.

Metabolic complications such as hyperglycemia, lactic acidosis, and weight loss may also occur. Stress, medication, pain, or tumor manipulation can trigger symptoms.

Severe hypercatecholaminemia and longstanding hypertension can lead to congestive heart failure, myocardial infarction, shock, cerebrovascular accidents, hemorrhage, or dissecting aneurysms.

Diagnosis [14]

Biochemical testing is required to detect elevated catecholamine metabolite production in blood and/or urine.

Computed tomography and magnetic resonance imaging are commonly used for preoperative localization. Functional imaging, including MIBG scintigraphy and positron emission tomography, can improve tumor characterization.

Preoperative Evaluation

Once diagnosed, all patients should undergo resection of the pheochromocytoma following appropriate medical preparation.

Preoperative medical preparation with an alpha-blockade is required [15]. Drugs known to provoke a pheochromocytoma crisis should be avoided (e.g., beta-adrenergic blocker in the absence of alpha-adrenergic blockade, glucagon, histamine, metoclopramide, and high-dose corticosteroids)

Treatment

Surgery is the definitive treatment for pheochromocytoma. The transition to laparoscopic techniques has reduced perioperative morbidity and mortality [16].

For MEN2 patients with bilateral disease >2 cm, complete bilateral adrenalectomy is suggested due to the risk of recurrent pheochromocytoma.

Postoperative Management

Annual postoperative follow-up should include blood pressure measurement and testing for urinary metanephrines.

References

1. Thakker RV, Newey PJ, Walls GV, Bilezikian J, Dralle H, Ebeling PR, Melmed S, Sakurai A, Tonelli F, Brandi ML. Clinical practice guidelines for multiple endocrine neoplasia type 1 (MEN1). J Clin Endocrinol Metab. 2012;97(9):2990–3011.
2. Brandi ML, Gagel RF, Angeli A, Bilezikian JP, Beck-Peccoz P, Bordi C, et al. CONSENSUS: guidelines for diagnosis and therapy of MEN Type 1 and Type 2. J Clin Endocrinol Metab. 2001;86(12):5658–71.
3. Mathiesen JS, Peter KJ, Vestergaard P, Stochholm K, Poulsen PL, Rasmussen ÅK, et al. Incidence and prevalence of multiple endocrine neoplasia 2A in Denmark 1901–2014: a nationwide study. Clin Epidemiol. 2018;10:1479–87.
4. Lips CJ, Ball DW. Classification and genetics of multiple endocrine neoplasia type 2. UpToDate. Waltham: UpToDate; 2008.
5. Frank-Raue K, Rondot S, Raue F. Molecular genetics and phenomics of RET mutations: Impact on prognosis of MTC. Mol Cell Endocrinol. 2010;322(1–2):2–7.
6. Tuttle RM, Ross DS. Medullary thyroid cancer: surgical treatment and prognosis. UpToDate [Internet]; 2019.
7. Yasir M, Mulji NJ, Kasi A. Multiple endocrine neoplasias type 2. [Updated 2023 Aug 14]. In: StatPearls [Internet]. Treasure Island (FL): StatPearls Publishing; 2025. Available from: https://www.ncbi.nlm.nih.gov/books/NBK519054/.

8. Kaliszewski K, Ludwig M, Ludwig B, Mikuła A, Greniuk M, Rudnicki J. Update on the diagnosis and management of medullary thyroid cancer: what has changed in recent years? Cancers. 2022;14(15):3643.
9. Bradford D, Larkins E, Mushti SL, Rodriguez L, Skinner AM, Helms WS, Price LS, Zirkelbach JF, Li Y, Liu J, Charlab R. FDA approval summary: selpercatinib for the treatment of lung and thyroid cancers with RET gene mutations or fusions. Clin Cancer Res. 2021;27(8):2130–5.
10. Wells SA Jr, Asa SL, Dralle H, et al. Revised American Thyroid Association guidelines for the management of medullary thyroid carcinoma. Thyroid. 2015;25:567.
11. Jayasinghe R, Basnayake O, Jayarajah U, Seneviratne S. Management of medullary carcinoma of the thyroid: a review. J Int Med Res. 2022;50(7):03000605221110698.
12. Lenders JW, Kerstens MN, Amar L, Prejbisz A, Robledo M, Taieb D, Pacak K, Crona J, Zelinka T, Mannelli M, Deutschbein T. Genetics, diagnosis, management and future directions of research of phaeochromocytoma and paraganglioma: a position statement and consensus of the Working Group on Endocrine Hypertension of the European Society of Hypertension. J Hypertens. 2020;38(8):1443–56.
13. Lo CY, Lam KY, Wat MS, Lam KS. Adrenal pheochromocytoma remains a frequently overlooked diagnosis. Am J Surg. 2000;179(3):212–5.
14. Sbardella E, Grossman AB. Pheochromocytoma: an approach to diagnosis. Best Pract Res Clin Endocrinol Metab. 2020;34(2):101346.
15. Patel D. Surgical approach to patients with pheochromocytoma. Gland Surg. 2020;9(1):32–42.
16. Pacak K, Linehan WM, Eisenhofer G, Walther MM, Goldstein DS. Recent advances in genetics, diagnosis, localization, and treatment of pheochromocytoma. Ann Intern Med. 2001;134(4):315–29.

12 Cluster of Patients with Unexplained Jaundice: The Great Indian Wedding

Grade Moderate.

Abstract At a lavish wedding banquet in India, a particular subset of guests is affected by nausea, backache, and headache, though the food they consumed was not dissimilar to the food consumed by other guests.

Story Madhumitha, daughter of an incredibly wealthy business magnate, was studying at Harvard Business School when she fell in love with a man who seemed to be the ideal mate. Yiannis, from Naxos, was as handsome as he was intelligent, was as rich as he was kind. On a visit home to Mumbai, Madhumitha sat with her parents in the balcony of their massive penthouse flat, and as they partook of evening tea, she hesitantly told them about Yiannis. Her parents were initially a little skeptical, especially her dad.

"We did not expect, when you crossed the oceans to study, that you would ignore the boundaries of country, language and religion," her Papa said sternly. When Madhumitha explained that he was an excellent scholar, an astute businessman, and was the scion of a famous industrialist family in Greece, her Papa was a little mollified. But was he, really?

Her parents planned a gala wedding ceremony—sangeet, mehndi, banquet, and dancing into the wee hours on a yacht moored on the Mumbai marina. The guests were the A-listers of Mumbai high society, as well as the extremely good-looking, very well-dressed, gregarious friends and family of Yiannis, who had arrived in Mumbai by a private jet. A famous band had been paid a staggering amount of money to play at the banquet. Alcohol was not served, and the sumptuous dinner—the breads, the side dishes, and the protein—was exclusively vegetarian, as befitted the family ethos. The well-heeled crowd danced and dined like there was no tomorrow.

S. Bhat, *Clinical Conundrums to Practice Diagnostic Reasoning*,
https://doi.org/10.1007/978-981-95-0636-1_12

Yiannis and his group loved the party too! Yiannis and his three brothers were good sports, gamely trying a few Bollywood dance steps, applying mehndi, and partaking heartily of the Indian food extravaganza.

Was it because of these excesses that 2 days later, Yiannis, his father, and one of his brothers fell sick? They were rushed to hospital, complaining of unbearable back ache, headache, and nausea. The groom's mother, sisters, and other invitees were quite well. The physician informed the concerned family that all the patients had "jaundice".

Questions What was the cause for this mysterious illness that selectively affected only a few of the attendees at the party? Was it black magic? Foul play on the part of possessive parents who were not happy with their daughter's choice of a life partner?

Analysis

There are specific clues that point toward the diagnosis:

1. The severe back ache, followed by jaundice
2. The Greek ethnicity of Yiannis
3. The symptoms which afflicted only Yiannis, one brother and the father of Yiannis and, importantly, not the mother or sisters
4. The fact that even the protein was vegetarian
5. The mehndi (henna)

Back ache, followed by jaundice is a clue to hemolysis (similar to what occurs during an acute hemolytic transfusion reaction).

Certain diseases are more likely to affect specific ethnic groups. For example, sickle cell anemia is more common in those of African descent, Tay Sach's disease is seen in Ashkenazi Jews, and G6PD deficiency is more common in the Mediterranean and Africa. Yiannis is from Greece in the Mediterranean.

The symptoms did not affect all the invitees, so it is unlikely to be food poisoning. Yiannis, his father, and one of his brothers fell sick, while the other brothers, the sisters, and mother remain unaffected, giving a clue to an X-linked recessive condition (the pattern of illness in this instance suggests that the father had the condition, and the mother was a carrier).

So, at this point of the analysis, we have a hemolytic disorder affecting those of Mediterranean descent and inherited in an X-linked recessive manner, pointing toward G6PD deficiency. The mehndi and vegetarian protein (fava beans) precipitating the hemolysis are indirect clues.

Definition, Classification, and Epidemiology

G6PD deficiency is the most common enzymatic RBC defect [1] and is an X-linked recessive disorder [2]. It is especially common in malaria-endemic areas and the Mediterranean [3].

X-linked inheritance: Figs. 12.1 and 12.2.

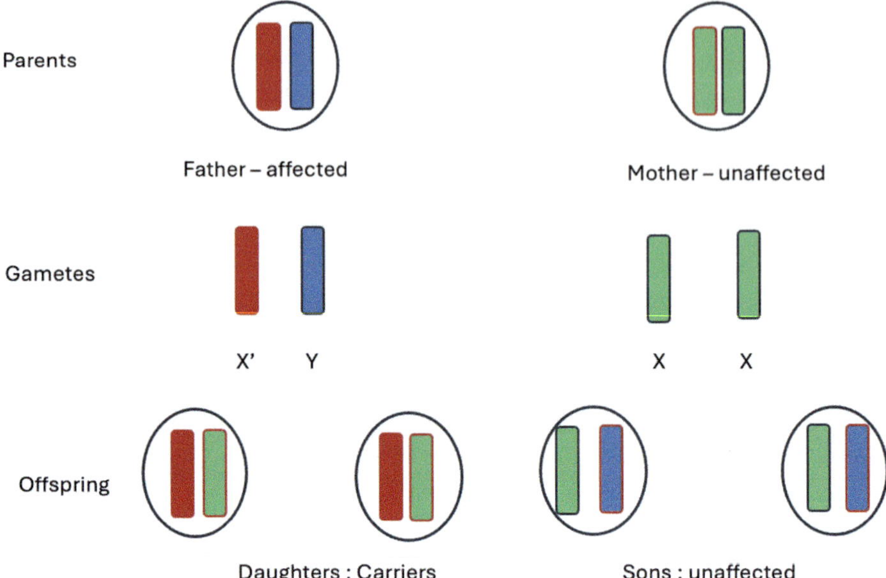

Fig. 12.1 Father—diseased. Mother: unaffected

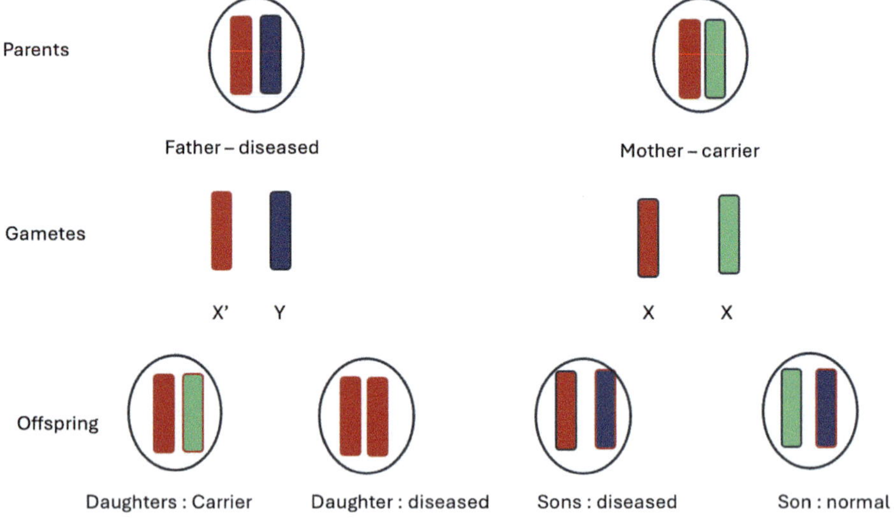

Fig. 12.2 Father: diseased; mother: carrier

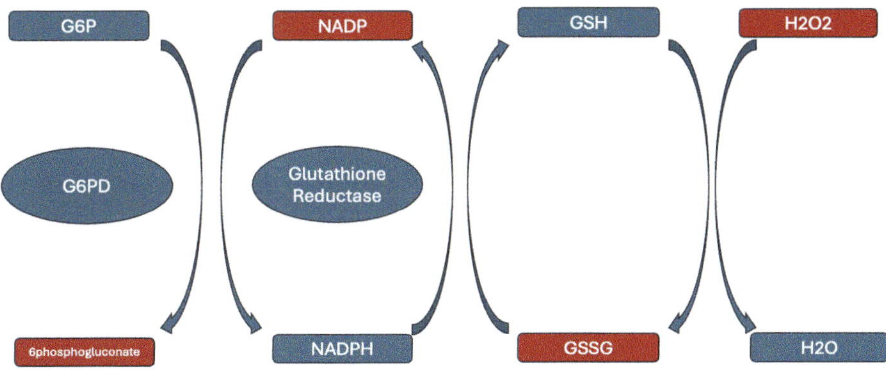

Fig. 12.3 Pentose phosphate pathway

Etiopathogenesis [4]

Oxidizing agents lead to oxidation of the sulfhydryl bridges in the Hb molecule, decreasing its solubility. A normal concentration of reduced glutathione (GSH) is the main mechanism to protect against oxidative damage (Fig. 12.3). Glutathione is reduced by glutathione reductase while converting NADPH to NADP. The rate-limiting step of this reaction is the oxidation of glucose-6-phosphate to 6-phosphogluconate by glucose-6-phosphate dehydrogenase. Hence, in G6PD deficiency, sufficient glutathione is unavailable to protect against the oxidative damage of hemoglobin [5].

Patients may be asymptomatic between the episodes of hemolysis though anemia may be detected. Signs and symptoms of hemolysis appear 2–4 days after the precipitating event. Patients may present with fever, chills, back ache, nausea, and high colored urine [6].

Investigations [7]

(a) Quantitative G6PD assay
(b) Qualitative G6PD assay

Treatment [8]

The key to management of individuals with G6PD deficiency is avoidance of exposure. Common precipitants of hemolysis include certain drugs like sulfonylureas, primaquine, fava beans, and henna compounds.

Acute episodes of hemolysis are managed by [9]:

(a) Removal of inciting agent.
(b) IV hydration.
(c) Transfusion may be required if hemolysis is severe.

References

1. Luzzatto L, Ally M, Notaro R. Glucose-6-phosphate dehydrogenase deficiency. Blood. 2020;136(11):1225–40.
2. Beutler E. The genetics of glucose-6-phosphate dehydrogenase deficiency. In: Seminars in hematology, vol. 27, No. 2; 1990. p. 137–64.
3. Howes RE, Piel FB, Patil AP, Nyangiri OA, Gething PW, Dewi M, Hogg MM, Battle KE, Padilla CD, Baird JK, Hay SI. G6PD deficiency prevalence and estimates of affected populations in malaria endemic countries: a geostatistical model-based map. PLoS Med. 2012;9(11):e1001339.
4. Hirono A, Kuhl W, Gelbart T, Forman L, Fairbanks VF, Beutler E. Identification of the binding domain for NADP+ of human glucose-6-phosphate dehydrogenase by sequence analysis of mutants. Proc Natl Acad Sci USA. 1989;86(24):10015–7.
5. Genetic variants of glucose-6-phosphate dehydrogenase and their associated enzyme activity: a systematic review and meta-analysis – PubMed [Internet]. [cited 2025 Jan 18]. Available from: https://pubmed.ncbi.nlm.nih.gov/36145477/.
6. Pfeffer DA, Satyagraha AW, Sadhewa A, Alam MS, Bancone G, Boum Y, Brito M, Cui L, Deng Z, Domingo GJ, He Y. Genetic variants of glucose-6-phosphate dehydrogenase and their associated enzyme activity: a systematic review and meta-analysis. Pathogens. 2022;11(9):1045.
7. Frank JE. Diagnosis and management of G6PD deficiency. Am Family Phys. 2005;72(7):1277–82.
8. Lee SW, Chaiyakunapruk N, Lai NM. What G6PD-deficient individuals should really avoid. Br J Clin Pharmacol. 2016;83(1):211.
9. Sonbol MB, Yadav H, Vaidya R, Rana V, Witzig TE. Methemoglobinemia and hemolysis in a patient with G6PD deficiency treated with rasburicase. Am J Hematol. 2013;88(2):152–4.

13 Adult Male Presenting with Left Foot Drop and Tingling Numbness in Both Feet: Nervous Norman

Grade Moderate.

Abstract An adult male who presents with tingling numbness and foot drop is found, on evaluation, to have various systemic manifestations.

Story Mr Norman, a skinny 40-year-old gentleman, makes his way hesitantly into your consultation chamber.

"Please sit down," you tell him and smile, trying to put him at ease.

"What seems to be the problem today?"

He coughs nervously and says "I'm sure I'm making a big fuss about nothing..."

"Maybe, maybe not. Please tell me what is troubling you. It's my job to help."

"Oh, nothing really. It's just that I'm feeling quite tired most of the time. My wife said my clothes are getting loose on me. She asked me to come and get a check-up."

"Is there anything else apart from the fatigue?"

"My muscles ache too. Also, my feet—especially my left foot—hurt."

"Could you lie down on the couch so I can examine you?" Mr Norman slowly rises and walks to the couch, his left foot slapping on the floor as he does so.

He lies down, and as you commence your examination, he whispers something to you.

"Sorry, what was that? I couldn't hear what you said."

"I have some pain in my balls too."

"Oh, I can see how that might be distressing. Do you have any problem with your waterworks or your bowels?"

"Not with my bowels, but my tummy hurts quite a bit, especially after a heavy meal. My pee looks really bubbly and pink, but I think that's because of the water supply here."

"Ok. Have you had any illness in the past that I should be aware of? High blood sugar or blood pressure or anything?"

S. Bhat, *Clinical Conundrums to Practice Diagnostic Reasoning*,
https://doi.org/10.1007/978-981-95-0636-1_13

"No diabetes or hypertension. I did have Hepatitis C two years ago and was treated for the same."

"Give me a moment to complete my examination."

Further examination reveals:

HR: 110/min
BP: 160/100 mm Hg
Respiratory rate: 30 cycles per min

You note that the JVP is elevated and there is bipedal edema. There are non-blanching purpura on both lower limbs.

Higher mental functions are normal, but you detect a left foot drop with absent ankle jerk and diminished sensation on the left foot.

Questions Do you think Mrs. Norman was justified in her concern for her husband's health? What might he be ailing from?

Analysis

The information we have obtained may be summarized as follows:

(a) Neuropathy—tingling numbness in both feet and left foot drop
(b) Renal involvement—proteinuria and hematuria (frothing of urine and pinkish discoloration of urine)
(c) Blood vessels—nonblanching purpura

These along with the constitutional symptoms point toward a vasculitis, most probably a medium vessel vasculitis. The history of hepatitis C in the past increases the likelihood of Polyarteritis nodosa (PAN). Though hepatitis B is more commonly associated with PAN, PAN can also follow hepatitis C infection, even in the absence of cryoglobulinemia [1].

PAN is a systemic necrotizing vasculitis that primarily affects medium-sized muscular arteries, with occasional involvement of small arteries [2, 3]. It is characterized by inflammation and loss of integrity of vessel walls. PAN is typically not associated with antineutrophil cytoplasmic antibodies (ANCA) and does not usually involve the lungs.

Classification [4]

PAN may be classified into the following:

(a) Idiopathic generalized PAN: The most common form, where the cause is unknown.
(b) Hepatitis B virus (HBV)-associated PAN: A form linked to HBV infection.
(c) Cutaneous PAN: A skin-limited form of the disease.
(d) Drug-induced PAN: A less common variant associated with certain medications.
(e) Adenosine deaminase 2 (ADA2) deficiency-associated PAN.

Epidemiology

PAN is a rare disease, most commonly seen in middle-aged or older adults, with a peak in the sixth decade of life.

Etiology

The exact cause of idiopathic PAN remains unclear. However, it is thought to involve complex interactions between genetic and environmental factors. HBV infection is a major environmental factor associated with PAN. Other viral infections such as hepatitis C virus (HCV) and human immunodeficiency virus (HIV) have also been implicated. Additionally, certain medications, such as minocycline, have been linked to drug-induced PAN.

Pathogenesis

The pathogenesis of PAN involves the necrotizing inflammation of medium and small arteries [5]. This inflammation leads to weakening of the arterial wall and the formation of microaneurysms, which can rupture or occlude the vessel. The inflammatory infiltrate typically consists of lymphocytes, macrophages, neutrophils, and eosinophils, without granulomas or giant cells. Active lesions display fibrinoid necrosis. Thrombosis and intimal hyperplasia worsen vessel occlusion.

Clinical Features [6]

A. Fever, weight loss, myalgias, and arthralgias.
B. Nodules, livedo reticularis, and ulcers [7].
C. Postprandial abdominal pain (intestinal angina), nausea, vomiting, diarrhea, hematochezia, and melena [8].
D. Renal involvement can lead to hypertension, hematuria, and proteinuria [9].
E. Stroke, seizures, or cognitive impairment.
F. Peripheral nerve involvement is due to the involvement of the vasa nervorum and may manifest as mononeuritis multiplex, peripheral neuropathy, asymmetric distal polyneuropathy, radiculopathy, plexopathy, and cranial neuropathy [10]. Mononeuritis multiplex involves damage to multiple individual peripheral nerves, causing asymmetric weakness, sensory loss, and pain. Foot drop, wrist drop, or numbness may be seen.
G. Myalgias and arthralgias.
H. Testicular pain due to testicular artery vasculitis [11].

Diagnosis

Electrophysiological studies, nerve biopsy.

Investigations

Increased ESR and CRP
Histopathology: skin or nerve biopsy
Visceral angiography if histology not confirmatory

Treatment [12]

1. Treat hepatitis B, C if present.
2. Oral glucocorticoids.
3. Azathioprine methotrexate or mycophenolate mofetil as steroid-sparing agents.
4. Cyclophosphamide may be added to glucocorticoids for severe disease.
5. Pulsed methylprednisolone may be required for acutely worsening mononeuritis multiplex.
6. Rituximab and tocilizumab [13, 14] may be required for resistant disease.

References

1. Saadoun D, et al. Hepatitis C virus-associated polyarteritis nodosa. Arthritis Care Res. 2011;63(3):427–35. https://doi.org/10.1002/acr.20381.
2. Springer JM, Byram K. Polyarteritis nodosa: an evolving primary systemic vasculitis. Postgrad Med. 2023;135(sup1):61–8.
3. Hughes LB, Bridges SL Jr. Polyarteritis nodosa and microscopic polyangiitis: etiologic and diagnostic considerations. Curr Rheumatol Rep. 2002;4(1):75–82.
4. Hernández-Rodríguez J, Alba MA, Prieto-González S, Cid MC. Diagnosis and classification of polyarteritis nodosa. J Autoimmun. 2014;48–49:84–9.
5. Ozen S. The changing face of polyarteritis nodosa and necrotizing vasculitis. Nat Rev Rheumatol. 2017;13(6):381–6.
6. Rohmer J, Nguyen Y, Trefond L, Agard C, Allain JS, Berezne A, Charles P, Cohen P, Gondran G, Groh M, Huscenot T. Clinical features and long-term outcomes of patients with systemic polyarteritis nodosa diagnosed since 2005: data from 196 patients. J Autoimmun. 2023;139:103093.
7. Pagnoux C, Seror R, Henegar C, Mahr A, Cohen P, Le Guern V, Bienvenu B, Mouthon L, Guillevin L. Clinical features and outcomes in 348 patients with polyarteritis nodosa: a systematic retrospective study of patients diagnosed between 1963 and 2005 and entered into the French Vasculitis Study Group Database. Arthritis Rheum. 2010;62(2):616–26.
8. Pagnoux C, Mahr A, Cohen P, Guillevin L. Presentation and outcome of gastrointestinal involvement in systemic necrotizing vasculitides: analysis of 62 patients with polyarteritis nodosa, microscopic polyangiitis, Wegener granulomatosis, Churg-Strauss syndrome, or rheumatoid arthritis-associated vasculitis. Medicine (Baltimore). 2005;84(2):115–28.
9. Maritati F, Iannuzzella F, Pavia MP, Pasquali S, Vaglio A. Kidney involvement in medium-and large-vessel vasculitis. J Nephrol. 2016;29:495–505.
10. Halabi C, Williams EK, Morshed RA, Caffarelli M, Anastasiou C, Tihan T, et al. Neurological manifestations of polyarteritis nodosa: a tour of the neuroaxis by case series. BMC Neurol. 2021;21(1):205.
11. Kolar P, Schneider U, Filimonow S, Burmester GR, Buttgereit F. Polyarteritis nodosa and testicular pain: ultrasonography reveals vasculitis of the testicular artery. Rheumatology (Oxford). 2007;46(8):1377–8.
12. Ribi C, Cohen P, Pagnoux C, Mahr A, Arène JP, Puéchal X, et al. Treatment of polyarteritis nodosa and microscopic polyangiitis without poor-prognosis factors: a prospective randomized study of one hundred twenty-four patients. Arthritis Rheum. 2010;62(4):1186–97.
13. Akiyama M, Kaneko Y, Takeuchi T. Tocilizumab for the treatment of polyarteritis nodosa: a systematic literature review. Correspondence on 'Tofacitinib for polyarteritis nodosa: a tailored therapy' by Rimar et al. Ann Rheum Dis. 2022;81(10):e204–4.
14. Conticini E, Sota J, Falsetti P, Lamberti A, Miracco C, Guarnieri A, et al. Biologic drugs in the treatment of polyarteritis nodosa and deficit of adenosine deaminase 2: a narrative review. Autoimmun Rev. 2021;20(4):102784.

Sudden Loss of Consciousness in a Fit, Young Patient: The Cricketer Who Collapsed

14

Abbreviations

DCM	Dilated cardiomyopathy
HOCM	Hypertrophic obstructive cardiomyopathy
MI	Myocardial infarction
VF	Ventricular fibrillation

Grade Easy.

Abstract A young fit cricket player faints after sudden exertion while at play. Medics are unable to resuscitate him.

Story It is the last ball of a nail-biting finish of a cricket match—you are at the edge of your seat! India requires 2 runs to win. The batsman KK takes a big risk and calls the second batsman for a second run—the stakes are so high! There is pin drop silence in the stadium as the batsman runs and the ball flies. The batsman falls on the ground, and the edge of the bat just touches the crease. Who will reach first? The third umpire is called.

The stadium explodes in cheers—India has won!

The air punches, the yelling, the celebrations dwindle into a puzzled silence—the batsman is not getting up (Fig. 14.1). Medicos run on to the field, and the young player—team treasure, health icon, the face of a hundred fitness products—is rapidly wheeled out to a waiting ambulance. The victory seems hollow, and a country sits waiting for news of the young champion batsman. Unfortunately, the news is not good—viewers sit in stunned silence as somber news anchors convey the sad news that KK is no more.

S. Bhat, *Clinical Conundrums to Practice Diagnostic Reasoning*,
https://doi.org/10.1007/978-981-95-0636-1_14

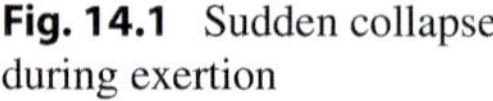

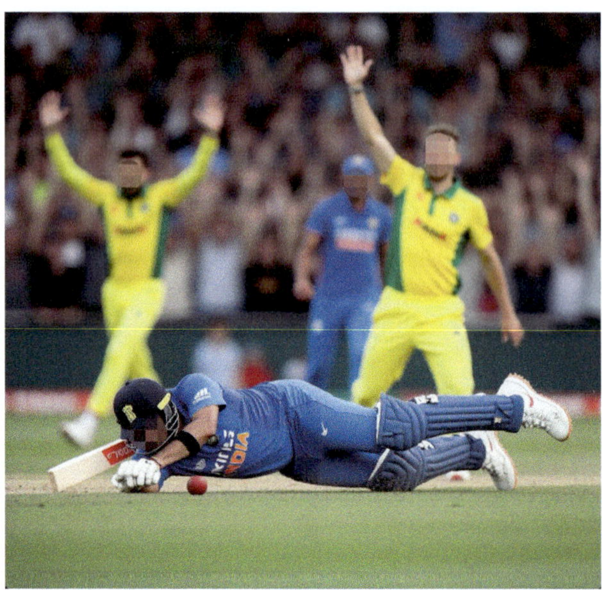

Fig. 14.1 Sudden collapse during exertion

Questions KK is a young healthy adult, not a diabetic, smoker, or hypertensive. What caused his sudden collapse?

Analysis

This is a fairly straightforward case of sudden cardiac death.

"Sudden cardiac arrest is the sudden cessation of cardiac activity—the victim becomes unresponsive, with no normal breathing and no signs of circulation. If corrective measures are not taken rapidly, this condition progresses to sudden death. Cardiac arrest should be used to signify an event as described above, that is reversed, usually by CPR and/or defibrillation or cardioversion, or cardiac pacing. Sudden cardiac death should not be used to describe events that are not fatal" [1].

Cardiac causes of sudden death may be ischemic, structural, or nonstructural (Fig. 14.2).

Noncardiac causes of sudden death include:

1. Massive intracranial hemorrhage
2. Pulmonary embolism

However, the most likely cause in the present situation is HOCM as HOCM is the most common cause of sudden death in athletes during exertion [2].

Hypertrophic obstructive cardiomyopathy (HOCM) is defined as left ventricular outflow tract obstruction secondary to asymmetrical septal hypertrophy [3] (Fig. 14.3).

Epidemiology and Etiopathogenesis

HOCM is the most common inherited monogenic cardiac condition [4]. In half the cases, HOCM is genetic in origin, with an autosomal dominant pattern of inheritance. 50% of the cases are sporadic. Left ventricular hypertrophy, hypercontractile myocardium, reduced compliance, and fibrosis are the pathological hallmarks [5]. An abnormal subvalvular mitral apparatus results in systolic anterior motion of mitral leaflets, which contributes to outflow obstruction.

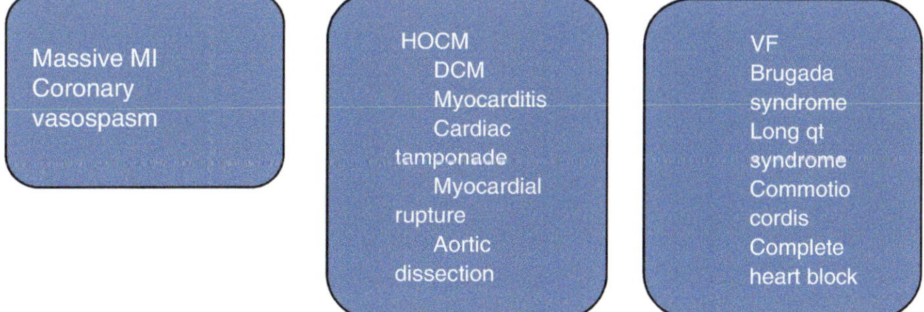

Fig. 14.2 Sudden cardiac death.
HOCM Hypertrophic obstructive cardiomyopathy,
DCM Dilated cardiomyopathy, VF Ventricular fibrillation

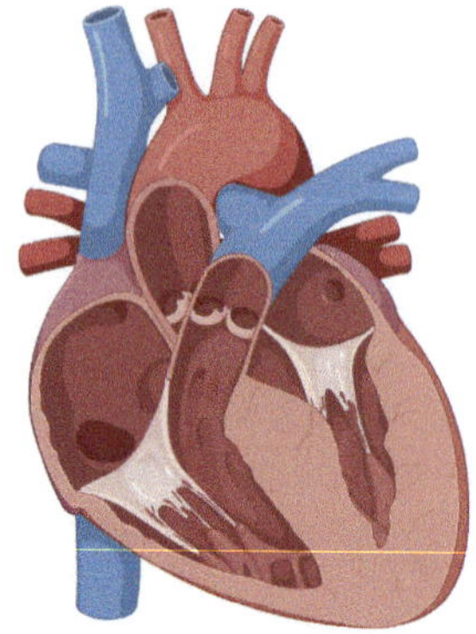

Fig. 14.3 Created in BioRender. (Bhat, S. (2025) https://BioRender.com/9lt3v00)

Asymmetrical septal hypertrophy causing LVOT obstruction

Clinical Features [6]

Unfortunately, the diagnosis of HOCM is very often made postmortem, with the patient being asymptomatic till sudden death. In those who present earlier, symptoms include palpitations, exertional chest pain, dyspnea, and sometimes presyncope and syncope, prompting the physician to consider ischemic heart disease or aortic stenosis.

O/E

(a) Jerky pulse
(b) Double carotid pulse
(c) Prominent “a” wave in jugular venous pulse (decreased right ventricular compliance because of the thickened interventricular septum)
(d) Double apical impulse
(e) S4
(f) Ejection systolic murmur at the left lower sternal border
(g) Pan-systolic murmur at the apex due to mitral regurgitation

Investigations

The diagnosis of HOCM may be made by ECG and echocardiogram; however, cardiac catheterization may be required to grade the severity [5].

Holter monitoring and exercise testing (for prognostication).

ECG: LVH with dagger Q waves [7].

Treatment

1. Beta-blockers to decrease cardiac contractility [8].
2. Verapamil—when beta-blockers are contraindicated. However, they must be administered cautiously as they are associated with sudden death in those with severe outflow obstruction [9].
3. Disopyramide [10].
4. Anticoagulation [11].
5. Implantable defibrillator [12].
6. "Mavacamten", an inhibitor of cardiac myosin ATPase, received FDA approval for use in HOCM [13].
7. For patients refractory to medical treatment, septal myomectomy and septal ablation [14].
8. To note: Patients with HOCM must be managed cautiously when admitted into the intensive care unit. Their condition worsens when there is volume depletion or inotropic agents are administered [15].

Prevention

First-degree relatives of affected patients must be screened by physical examination, ECG, and echocardiogram every 5 years [16].

Point of interest: Sudden cardiac death among athletes has been reported most often in football and basketball players. After a series of sudden deaths over 3 years, precompetition screening of players was made mandatory, and AEDs and trained medicos are present at all soccer matches.

Key Takeaway

If a young adult presents with syncope or ECG suggestive of LVH, do not dismiss as hypertension. Echo and cardiac catheterization must be done. If HOCM is confirmed, beta-blockers have mortality benefit.

References

1. Zipes DP, John Camm A, Borggrefe M, Buxton AE, Chaitman B, et al. Authors/Task Force Members, ESC Committee for Practice Guidelines, ACC/AHA (Practice Guidelines) Task Force Members, ACC/AHA/ESC 2006 guidelines for management of patients with ventricular arrhythmias and the prevention of sudden cardiac death—executive summary: a report of the American College of Cardiology/American Heart Association Task Force and the European Society of Cardiology Committee for Practice Guidelines (Writing Committee to develop guidelines for management of patients with ventricular arrhythmias and the prevention of sudden cardiac death) developed in collaboration with the European Heart Rhythm Association and the Heart Rhythm Society. Eur Heart J. 2006;27(17):2099–21402.

2. Maron BJ, Doerer JJ, Haas TS, Tierney DM, Mueller FO. Sudden deaths in young competitive athletes: analysis of 1866 deaths in the United States, 1980–2006. Circulation. 2009;119(8):1085–92.
3. Nishimura RA, Holmes DR. Hypertrophic obstructive cardiomyopathy. N Engl J Med. 2004;350(13):1320–7.
4. Semsarian C, Ingles J, Maron MS, Maron BJ. New perspectives on the prevalence of hypertrophic cardiomyopathy. J Am Coll Cardiol. 2015;65(12):1249–54.
5. Hughes SE. The pathology of hypertrophic cardiomyopathy. Histopathology. 2004;44(5):412–27. https://doi.org/10.1111/j.1365-2559.2004.01835.x.
6. Maron MS, Olivotto I, Zenovich AG, Link MS, Pandian NG, Kuvin JT, et al. Hypertrophic cardiomyopathy is predominantly a disease of left ventricular outflow tract obstruction. Circulation. 2006;114(21):2232–9.
7. Finocchiaro G, Sheikh N, Biagini E, Papadakis M, Maurizi N, Sinagra G, et al. The electrocardiogram in the diagnosis and management of patients with hypertrophic cardiomyopathy. Heart Rhythm. 2020;17(1):142–51.
8. Monda E, Lioncino M, Palmiero G, Franco F, Rubino M, Cirillo A, et al. Bisoprolol for treatment of symptomatic patients with obstructive hypertrophic cardiomyopathy. The BASIC (bisoprolol AS therapy in hypertrophic cardiomyopathy) study. Int J Cardiol. 2022;354:22–8.
9. Taha M, Dahat P, Toriola S, Satnarine T, Zohara Z, Adelekun A, et al. Metoprolol or verapamil in the management of patients with hypertrophic cardiomyopathy: a systematic review. Cureus [Internet]. 2023 Aug 9 [cited 2025 Mar 23].
10. Maurizi N, Chiriatti C, Fumagalli C, Targetti M, Passantino S, Antiochos P, et al. Real-world use and predictors of response to disopyramide in patients with obstructive hypertrophic cardiomyopathy. J Clin Med. 2023;12(7):2725.
11. Zhu X, Wang Z, Ferrari MW, Ferrari-Kuehne K, Bulter J, Xu X, Zhou Q, Zhang Y, Zhang J. Anticoagulation in cardiomyopathy: unravelling the hidden threat and challenging the threat individually. ESC Heart Fail. 2021;8(6):4737–50.
12. Francia P, Olivotto I, Lambiase PD, Autore C. Implantable cardioverter-defibrillators for hypertrophic cardiomyopathy: the Times They Are a-Changin. EP Europace. 2022;24(9):1384–94.
13. Bishev D, Fabara S, Loseke I, Alok A, Al-Ani H, Bazikian Y. Efficacy and safety of Mavacamten in the treatment of hypertrophic cardiomyopathy: a systematic review. Heart Lung Circ. 2023;32(9):1049–56.
14. Maron BJ. Role of alcohol septal ablation in treatment of obstructive hypertrophic cardiomyopathy. Lancet Lond Engl. 2000;355(9202):425–6.
15. Maron MS, Masri A, Nassif ME, Barriales-Villa R, Arad M, Cardim N, Choudhury L, Claggett B, Coats CJ, Düngen HD, Garcia-Pavia P. Aficamten for symptomatic obstructive hypertrophic cardiomyopathy. New England Journal of Medicine. 2024;390(20):1849–61.
16. Silajdzija E, Rasmus Vissing C, Basse Christensen E, Lamiokor Mills H, Olivia Kock T, Andersen LJ, Snoer M, Thune JJ, Daniel Bartels E, Axelsson Raja A, Hørby Christensen A. Family screening in hypertrophic cardiomyopathy: identification of relatives with low yield from systematic follow-up. J Am Coll Cardiol. 2024;84(19):1854–65.

Tachycardia, Hypotension, and Agitation in a Postpartum Mother: The Mother in Distress

15

Grade Difficult.

Abstract A young lady deteriorates after a normal vaginal delivery. She develops tachycardia, hypotension, and extreme agitation.

Story You are on the night shift in the emergency unit, and you get a call from an obstetrician at a small hospital in a village 50 km away.

"Doctor, this is Dr. Deepa. One of my patients has become extremely ill post-delivery and may require care in a higher centre. We are preparing to shift her to your hospital very soon."

"Please tell me a little bit about the patient."

"My patient, Mrs. Aparna, delivered a live female baby 3 hours ago by normal vaginal delivery. Placenta was delivered normally and there was no post-partum haemorrhage. We shifted her out of the labour room; vital signs were stable at shift. For the last half hour, however, she has become extremely agitated—almost violent, in fact. At present her heart rate is 150/minute. The pulse is irregularly irregular. Blood pressure is 90/60 mm Hg. Oral temperature is 104 degree F and bibasilar crackles are auscultable."

"Is there still a possibility that it could be a post-partum haemorrhage?"

"No, definitely not. The uterus is well contracted, she does not look pale and there is no bleeding per vaginally."

"I see. Are there any known comorbidities? And was the antenatal period uneventful?"

"There were no comorbidities." Dr. Deepa says, "She was a little on the lighter side, though, with BMI at first booking appointment being 18. At age 34, this is her first pregnancy—they were trying to conceive for 2–3 years at least. The antenatal period was fairly uneventful."

S. Bhat, *Clinical Conundrums to Practice Diagnostic Reasoning*,
https://doi.org/10.1007/978-981-95-0636-1_15

You ask the patient to be shifted to your hospital with utmost dispatch and prepare your team for her arrival.

She reaches your emergency department in an hour, and the paramedic who accompanies her mentions that she vomited repeatedly on the way to the hospital.

You examine Mrs. Aparna and note that she is still extremely agitated and tremulous. Her pulse rate is 160/minute, irregular in rhythm. The blood pressure is holding at 90/60 mm Hg, and her temperature is now 105°.

Bilateral basal crackles and scattered rhonchi are present.

Question What might the potential diagnosis be? With this diagnosis in mind, would there be anything you would have liked to change in the antenatal or preconception management?

Analysis

The key features in this story are as follows:

(a) Tachycardia
(b) Hypotension
(c) Agitation
(d) Hyperpyrexia
(e) GI symptoms—vomiting
(f) Features of cardiac failure—basal crackles

A postpartum hemorrhage might account for the hypotension and tachycardia, but it does not explain the extreme agitation and the high fever. It is too early for postpartum sepsis.

This clinical picture on a background of the lower BMI and the history of difficulty in conception make us consider thyroid storm on a background of unrecognized thyroid disease.

Ideally, this would have been recognized preconception. Not all countries recommend universal preconception screening; however, considering the high prevalence of thyroid disease in India, Indian Thyroid Society guidelines recommend universal screening for thyroid disease either prepregnancy or in the first antenatal visit [1]. Apart from the fact that unrecognized maternal thyroid disease can precipitate a thyroid storm during parturition, it can result in adverse consequences to the fetus as well [2].

Thyroid storm is a severe and life-threatening exacerbation of thyrotoxicosis on a background of either recognized or unrecognized hyperthyroidism. It is characterized by a constellation of multisystem manifestations resulting from an abrupt surge in thyroid hormones and a hyperadrenergic state [3].

Thyroid storm is a clinical diagnosis. Severity rating scales, such as the Burch–Wartofsky Point Scale (BWPS) [4] and the Japanese Thyroid Association (JTA) scale [5], help to categorize severity. A BWPS score of ≥45 or JTA categories of Thyroid Storm 1 (TS1) or Thyroid Storm 2 (TS2) with evidence of systemic decompensation requires aggressive therapy.

A thyroid storm is rare, accounting for about 1–2% of admissions for hyperthyroidism. The incidence of thyroid storm ranges from 0.57 to 0.76 cases per 100,000 per year in the general population and 4.8 to 5.6 cases per 100,000 per year in hospitalized patients [6]. Mortality rates may approach 10–20%.

Etiopathogenesis

Several factors can precipitate thyroid storm in individuals with pre-existing hyperthyroidism [7]:

(a) Abrupt discontinuation of antithyroid medications.

(b) Infections.
(c) Surgery: Thyroid or nonthyroid surgery.
(d) Trauma.
(e) Iodine load: Administration of large quantities of exogenous iodine or iodine-containing contrast agents.
(f) Childbirth: Pregnancy and parturition.
(g) Systemic illness like myocardial infarction and diabetic ketoacidosis (DKA) can induce thyroid storm.

Thyroid storm often occurs in a patient with pre-existing Graves' disease.

Pathogenesis [8]

The pathogenesis of thyroid storm involves a complex interplay of factors, ultimately leading to an excessive action of thyroid hormones on target tissues. Key elements in the pathogenesis include:

(a) Increased thyroid hormone levels: A sudden increase in free thyroxine (T4) and triiodothyronine (T3) levels
(b) Hyperadrenergic state: Increased sensitivity to catecholamines and elevated levels of circulating catecholamines
(c) Cytokine release: A possible role for inflammatory cytokines in exacerbating the hypermetabolic state

The increased sympathetic nervous system activity causes increased metabolic rate, metabolic fuel consumption, and oxygen consumption. Additionally, the cytokines secreted in systemic illness may displace thyroid hormones from their binding sites, causing an increase in free thyroid hormones [9].

Clinical Features [10]

The clinical presentation of thyroid storm is marked by a rapid onset of the following signs:

Fever: Often high-grade, exceeding 102 °F or 39 °C
Tachycardia: Usually out of proportion to the fever, with heart rates often above 130 bpm
Arrhythmias: Including atrial fibrillation
Congestive heart failure and pulmonary edema
Blood pressure: Systolic hypertension initially, followed by hypotension
Neurological manifestations: Altered mental status, including agitation, delirium, psychosis, seizures, and coma
Gastrointestinal symptoms: Nausea, vomiting, diarrhea, and abdominal pain

Investigations

Thyroid function tests: Measurement of TSH, free T4, and free T3 levels
Serum electrolytes and liver function tests
Blood glucose
Complete blood count
Electrocardiogram ECG
Urinalysis

Diagnosis

The diagnosis of thyroid storm is primarily clinical, relying on the recognition of characteristic signs and symptoms.

Principles of Treatment [11]

1. Reducing thyroid hormone synthesis and release
2. Blocking the effects of thyroid hormones
3. Identifying and addressing the precipitating cause

Treatment

1. General support: Prompt assessment and management of airway, breathing, and circulation.
2. Inhibit thyroid hormone synthesis:
   (a) Thionamides: Methimazole or propylthiouracil (PTU) is used to block the synthesis of new thyroid hormones.
   (b) PTU also has the added benefit of inhibiting the peripheral conversion of T4 to T3.
   (c) Glucocorticoids: Administration of a glucocorticoid.
   (d) Methimazole is recommended in pregnant patients with thyroid storm in the second and third trimesters, though PTU is recommended in the first trimester.
3. Block thyroid hormone release:
   Iodine: After thionamide therapy is initiated, iodine solutions (Lugol's solution) can be administered to block the release of preformed thyroid hormones.
4. Block the effects of thyroid hormones:
   Beta-blockers: Propranolol or esmolol are used to control adrenergic deatures such as tachycardia, hypertension, and tremor [12].
5. Supportive care:
   Fluid resuscitation
   Cooling

Electrolyte correction
Blood sugar management

6. Treat complications:
   Heart failure: Diuretics and other appropriate heart failure therapies.
   Arrhythmias: Treat with antiarrhythmic medications or cardioversion if necessary.
   Delirium/Agitation: Benzodiazepines or antipsychotics.
7. Treat the precipitating illness.
8. Cholestyramine: Cholestyramine can further reduce thyroid hormone levels [13].
9. Infection: Administer appropriate antibiotics.
10. Drug-induced: Discontinue the offending medication.
11. Plasma exchange has been used [14].

Thyroid Storm in Pregnancy

The symptoms of thyroid storm in pregnancy are similar to those in nonpregnant individuals but may be more difficult to recognize due to the overlapping symptoms of pregnancy. Key features include:

Severe tachycardia: Usually >140 bpm
High fever: >103 °F
Cardiac arrythmias
Congestive heart failure: Shortness of breath and edema
Nausea, vomiting, and diarrhea
Confusion/Restlessness

Management

The management of thyroid storm in pregnancy requires a multidisciplinary approach involving endocrinologists, obstetricians, and neonatologists.

References

1. Guidelines for Diagnosis and Management of Thyroid Disease During Pregnancy [Internet]. [cited 2024 Dec 30]. Available from: https://www.thyroid.org/association-guidelines-management/.
2. Dave A, Maru L, Tripathi M. Importance of universal screening for thyroid disorders in first trimester of pregnancy. Indian J Endocrinol Metab. 2014;18(5):735–8.
3. Sarlis NJ, Gourgiotis L. Thyroid emergencies. Rev Endocr Metab Disord. 2003;4(2):129–36. https://doi.org/10.1023/a:1022933918182.
4. Abdullah Fahmi NM. The predictive value of the Burch-Wartofsky Point Scale (BWPS) in clinically diagnosing thyroid storm. J ASEAN Fed Endocr Soc. 2019;34:27.

5. Satoh T, Isozaki O, Suzuki A, Wakino S, Iburi T, Tsuboi K, et al. 2016 guidelines for the management of thyroid storm from the Japan Thyroid Association and Japan Endocrine Society (first edition). Endocr J. 2016;63(12):1025–64.
6. De Groot LJ, Bartalena L, Feingold KR. Thyroid storm. Endotext [Internet]. 2022 June 1.
7. Farooqi S, Raj S, Koyfman A, Long B. High risk and low prevalence diseases: thyroid storm. Am J Emerg Med. 2023;69:127–35.
8. Elmenyar E, Aoun S, Al Saadi Z, Barkumi A, Cander B, Al-Thani H, El-Menyar A. Data analysis and systematic scoping review on the pathogenesis and modalities of treatment of thyroid storm complicated with myocardial involvement and shock. Diagnostics. 2023;13(19):3028.
9. Carroll R, Matfin G. Endocrine and metabolic emergencies: thyroid storm. Ther Adv Endocrinol Metab. 2010;1(3):139–45.
10. Akamizu T, Satoh T, Isozaki O, Suzuki A, Wakino S, Iburi T, Tsuboi K, Monden T, Kouki T, Otani H, Teramukai S. Diagnostic criteria, clinical features, and incidence of thyroid storm based on nationwide surveys. Thyroid. 2012;22(7):661–79.
11. Guerrero-Pita LM, González-Macía A, Lozano-Quintero C, López-Herrero E. Tormenta tiroidea precipitada por administración de contrastes yodados en paciente con tirotoxicosis tipo II por toma de amiodarona. Revista Española de Casos Clínicos en Medicina Interna. 2024;9(3):153–6.
12. Tetsuya T, Yuko Y, Tsuyoshi T, Takashi T, Atsushi O, Hideyuki Y, Kazuo K, Kiichiro H, Makito T, Satoko S, Takeshi U. Short-term effects of β-adrenergic antagonists and Methimazole in new-onset thyrotoxicosis caused by graves' disease. Intern Med. 2012;51(17):2285–90.
13. Kaykhaei MA, Shams M, Sadegholvad A, Dabbaghmanesh MH, Omrani GR. Low doses of cholestyramine in the treatment of hyperthyroidism. Endocrine. 2008;34:52–5.
14. Simsir IY, et al. Therapeutic plasmapheresis in thyrotoxic patients. Endocrine. 2018;62(1):144–8. https://doi.org/10.1007/s12020-018-1661-x.

16 Young Lady with Abdominal Cramps and Difficulty in Breathing: The Shy Bride

Grade Easy.

Abstract A previously healthy young woman presents with episodic abdominal pain and breathlessness. She is admitted to hospital with profuse loose stools and hypovolemic shock.

Story Vijeth has been your patient for a long time—he is meticulous about his health and meets you annually for routine checks. You are happy to see that he is your first patient on a Monday morning.

"Doctor Prabhu, I've come to invite you for my wedding," he says smiling shyly.

"That's wonderful news! Congratulations! Who's the lucky lady?"

"She's my childhood friend, Mira. She's very gentle and shy," he says, showing you a photo of a sweet-faced young lady.

"Congratulations once more."

"Please do come for the wedding, Doctor."

Three weeks later, you stand in line to wish the young couple as they embark on the adventure of life together. You are happy to see them—obviously very much in love. Mira seems a little shyer than the usual bride, blushing furiously when you wish her a happy married life. Vijeth is incandescent with joy and very glad that you have come.

"Please have lunch before you leave, doctor," he says.

A couple of months later, Vijeth is at your clinic again for his annual check. You are alarmed to see that he has lost weight, has lost his characteristic ebullience—he looks deflated and dull.

"I hope all is well, Vijeth," you say as you check his blood pressure. "You don't look your usual self, if I may say so."

"I'm ok, doctor. But I am worried about Mira."

"Why? What happened?"

S. Bhat, *Clinical Conundrums to Practice Diagnostic Reasoning*, https://doi.org/10.1007/978-981-95-0636-1_16

"She doesn't seem happy. She misses work very often—saying she is feeling ill, has a tummy upset, feels that her breathing isn't right sometimes. I just don't know what is wrong, doctor."

"Maybe you should bring her to me for a quick check up," you suggest.

"No doctor, I don't think there's anything wrong with her physically. Maybe she is disappointed in me. I should try to be a better husband", he says sadly.

You watch, perturbed, as your happy, confident patient shuffles out of the room dispiritedly.

It is a couple of months later that you get a call from the secondary care hospital in town. "Doctor, this is Dr Mukund from Chinmay hospital. We have a patient, Mrs Mira admitted with us. Frankly, we are a little puzzled about her. We would welcome a second opinion; besides which her husband Mr Vijeth is requesting your advice."

"Certainly," you say and start off to the hospital as soon as you finish your morning clinic.

On your way, you wonder what ails Mira. Were there some clues you should have picked up from what Vijeth said? You hope you can help, as you are very worried that Vijeth will not be able to cope, should something go wrong.

Vijeth is standing at the door of his wife's ward, and he greets you with a relief that you think is disproportionate. You begin to feel the pressure of what is perhaps an inflated opinion of your prowess.

Mrs Mira is in the high-dependency unit. The monitor shows that her heart rate is 110/min, and BP is 90/60 mm Hg.

You note that there is a generalized erythema, most prominent on the face, neck, and trunk. There is a rash on the upper chest.

The tongue is dry, and the jugular veins are collapsed. You mention this to the nurse at the bedside, and she says "We are trying to replace the volume, Doctor, but profuse watery loose stools continue."

You see that the oxygen saturation is 90% on room air and understand the cause of the hypoxia when you auscultate extensive bilateral polyphonic rhonchi.

Suddenly everything—the history, the examination findings, and the patient's appearance coalesce in your mind, and you blurt out a diagnosis.

"Of course! You must be right!" Dr. Mukund says, shaking his head at your brilliance. He orders some investigations to confirm the diagnosis.

Questions What's happening with Mira? Are there investigations available to confirm the diagnosis? What are the therapeutic options available?

Analysis

The history of episodic cramps, loose stools, and breathlessness is a fairly obvious pointer, but another clue is given by the fact that she blushes excessively. The blush is a clue to vasodilatation; the breathlessness and rhonchi signify bronchoconstriction. What condition causes bronchoconstriction, vasodilatation, abdominal cramps, and loose stools? It is carcinoid syndrome. At present, Mira appears to be in carcinoid crisis.

Carcinoid syndrome (CS) is a complex paraneoplastic disorder that arises from the excessive secretion of various hormones and bioactive substances by well-differentiated neuroendocrine tumors (NETs) [1] characterized by a constellation of clinical manifestations including flushing and diarrhea [2].

NETs, the underlying cause of CS, are relatively uncommon, with small intestinal NETs occurring in approximately 1 out of 100,000 individuals. Carcinoid syndrome develops in 10–40% of patients with well-differentiated NETs. The overall incidence of NETs is around 6 per 100,000 per year [3]. Carcinoid syndrome is frequently associated with midgut NETs that have metastasized to the liver. Notably, the number of patients with neuroendocrine neoplasms (NENs) and carcinoid syndrome has increased over time. Carcinoid heart disease (CHD), a serious complication, may occur in up to 20–70% of patients with CS. Mortality is higher in patients with NETs and CHD.

Etiopathogenesis (Fig. 16.1)

Carcinoid syndrome (CS) is caused by the secretion of various humoral factors by NETs. These tumors arise from neuroendocrine cells which are part of the diffuse neuroendocrine system [4]. The small intestine is the most common primary tumor

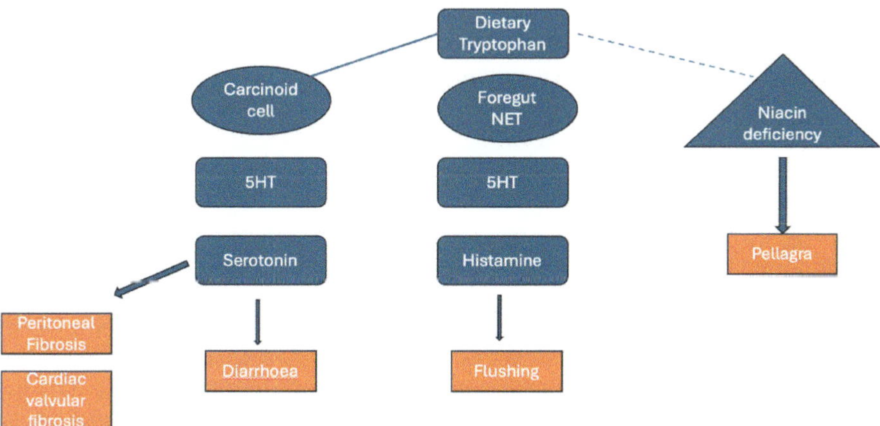

Fig. 16.1 Dietary tryptophan is diverted away from niacin production, causing niacin deficiency and pellagra. It is metabolized to serotonin, histamine, and various other kinins which result in the clinical features of carcinoid

site associated with carcinoid, with metastases to the liver being common. However, CS may also occur with bronchial and pancreatic NETs.

The pathogenesis of CS is multifactorial (Fig. 16.1) [5] with several key mediators.

Serotonin is considered the most significant mediator, as tumors synthesize, store, and release serotonin. Elevated levels of serotonin or its metabolite, 5-hydroxyindoleacetic acid (5-HIAA), cause the diarrhea observed in carcinoid and are implicated in the pathogenesis of other symptoms as well.

Other bioactive substances such as tachykinins, histamine, prostaglandins, and bradykinin are also implicated. However, their exact contribution to the clinical features remains less clear [6].

Carcinoid Heart Disease (CHD)

Long-term exposure to humoral factors, particularly serotonin, leads to the formation of plaque-like deposits of fibrous tissue in the heart. This most often affects the right heart valves and endocardium, causing tricuspid regurgitation and pulmonic stenosis. The 5-HT2 receptor, overexpressed in the heart, can lead to abnormal mitochondrial function and ventricular hypertrophy [7].

The clinical presentation of CS is variable—common manifestations include:

(a) Flushing: Episodic red or violaceous flushing of face, neck, and upper chest, accompanied by a burning sensation, hypotension, and tachycardia [8].
(b) Diarrhea: Chronic secretory diarrhea is common, with stools being typically watery and nonbloody [6]. Abdominal cramps may occur due to mesenteric fibrosis or intestinal obstruction.

Additional clinical features include hypotension, tachycardia, bronchoconstriction, venous telangiectasia, dyspnea, and fibrotic complications such as mesenteric and retroperitoneal fibrosis and carcinoid heart disease. Persistent brawny edema of the face and extremities may occur with severe flushing attacks [9].

Investigations

1. Serum serotonin, urinary 5-HIAA, fasting plasma 5-HIAA, NT-pro BNP
2. CT scan (Fig. 16.2) and MRI
3. Echocardiography: to screen for carcinoid heart disease

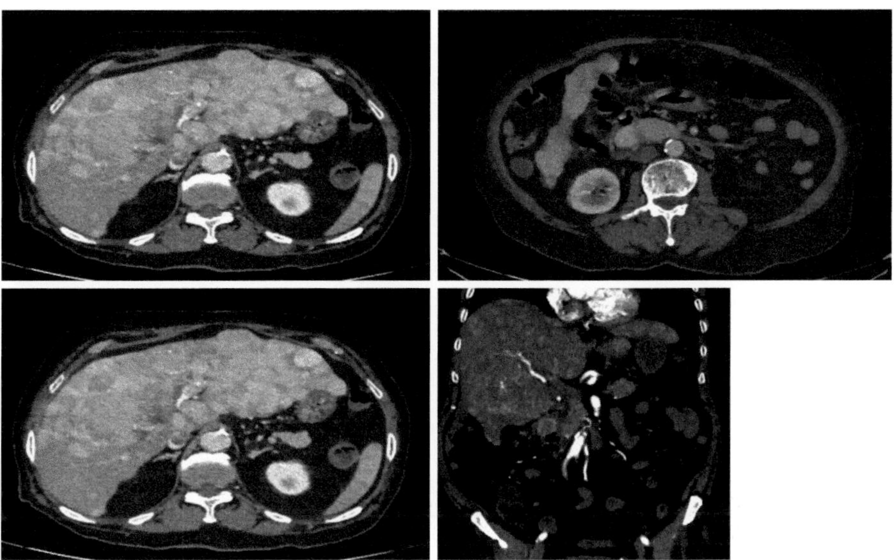

Fig. 16.2 CT abdomen showing carcinoid tumor. (Contributed by Dr. Ram Shenoy Basti, FMMC)

Treatment [2]

(a) *Somatostatin analogs (SSAs):* Including octreotide and lanreotide. Long-acting SSAs may be combined with short-acting SSAs, such as subcutaneous octreotide, for patients with moderate or severe symptoms.
(b) *Telotristat ethyl:* This tryptophan hydroxylase inhibitor is used for patients with diarrhea not adequately controlled by SSAs alone.
(c) *Surgical resection:* If feasible, surgical removal of the primary tumor.
(d) *Liver-directed therapies:* These include embolization, radiofrequency ablation, and resection of liver metastases.
(e) *Peptide receptor radionuclide therapy (PRRT):* This is a targeted therapy that uses radiolabeled somatostatin analogues to target tumor cells [10].
(f) *Carcinoid heart disease management:* Consideration for valve replacement.
(g) *Supportive care:* Nutritional support and antidiarrheal agents such as loperamide.

Treatment of Carcinoid Crisis

This acute release of vasoactive hormones, which can occur during surgery or biopsy, should be treated with intravenous fluids, corticosteroids, and intravenous octreotide. Vasopressors should be used cautiously due to their potential to paradoxically worsen a carcinoid crisis.

References

1. Vitale G, Carra S, Alessi Y, Campolo F, Pandozzi C, Zanata I, Colao A, Faggiano A, NIKE Group. Carcinoid syndrome: preclinical models and future therapeutic strategies. Int J Mol Sci. 2023;24(4):3610.
2. Grozinsky-Glasberg S, Davar J, Hofland J, Dobson R, Prasad V, Pascher A, Denecke T, Tesselaar ME, Panzuto F, Albåge A, Connolly HM. European Neuroendocrine Tumor Society (ENETS) 2022 guidance paper for carcinoid syndrome and carcinoid heart disease. J Neuroendocrinol. 2022;34(7):e13146.
3. Subash N, Papali MM, Bahadur KP, Avanthika C, Jhaveri S, Thannir S, Joshi M, Valisekka SS. Recent advances in the diagnosis and management of carcinoid syndrome. Dis Mon. 2022;68(7):101304.
4. Öberg K. Neuroendocrine gastrointestinal and lung tumors (carcinoid tumors), the carcinoid syndrome, and related disorders. In: Williams Textbook of Endocrinology. Elsevier; 2016. p. 1833–53.
5. de Celis R, Ferrari AC, Glasberg J, Riechelmann RP. Carcinoid syndrome: update on the pathophysiology and treatment. Clinics. 2018;73:e490s.
6. Mulders MC, de Herder WW, Hofland J. What is carcinoid syndrome? A critical appraisal of its proposed mediators. Endocr Rev. 2024;45(3):351–60.
7. Nebigil CG, Jaffré F, Messaddeq N, Hickel P, Monassier L, Launay JM, Maroteaux L. Overexpression of the serotonin 5-HT2B receptor in heart leads to abnormal mitochondrial function and cardiac hypertrophy. Circulation. 2003;107(25):3223–9.
8. Van Der Lely AJ, Herder WW. Carcinoid syndrome: diagnosis and medical management. Arq Bras Endocrinol Metabol. 2005;49:850–60.
9. Strosberg JR, Whitcomb DC. Diagnosis of carcinoid syndrome and tumor localization. Waltham, MA: UpToDate; 2017.
10. Cook R, Hendifar AE. Evidence-based policy in practice: management of carcinoid syndrome diarrhea. P T. 2019;44(7):424. https://pmc.ncbi.nlm.nih.gov/articles/PMC6590927/.

Adult Male Admitted to Intensive Care Unit with Tachycardia, Hypertension, and Agitation: It's Where My Demons Hide

17

Grade Difficult.

Abstract An anxious individual treated for infected wound, followed shortly thereafter by admission to hospital with tachycardia, hypertension, and agitation.

Story Shridar is a high-ranking official in a government office. That he has reached this position is a testament both to his will power and to the efficacy of psychotherapeutics. He used to suffer from debilitating anxiety for years in high school, as a college student, and at the Administrative Service Training Academy. He came under the care of a kind and efficient psychiatrist, Dr. Amritha, and was finally able to function effectively in the real world.

He was on an official tour of an industrial township, when he sustained an injury from a jagged piece of metal. Unfortunately, after this, he developed a skin and soft tissue infection, for which he required incision and drainage. He was sent home with strict instructions to complete his course of antibiotics.

The very next day, his wife noticed that his anxiety seemed to have increased again. She wondered if it was because of the pain of the injury. She tried to reassure him, but his unease only got worse.

Over the next day, he became extremely agitated—so much so that his colleagues called his wife to pick him up from work. She noticed that he was trembling, upset, and sweating profusely. She brought him to hospital where the ER doctor shifted him to the ICU in view of the extremely high blood pressure, high temperature, and tachycardia.

You are the doctor in charge of the ICU. You approach Mr. Shridar's bed and greet him gently. He looks at you fearfully. You observe that his heart rate is 150 beats/min. The temperature documented in the case file is 105 °F and blood pressure is 190/120 mm Hg. He appears extremely agitated, tremulous, and diaphoretic. His pupils are 4 mm dilated, reactive to light. Interestingly, his eyes have a strange

S. Bhat, *Clinical Conundrums to Practice Diagnostic Reasoning*,
https://doi.org/10.1007/978-981-95-0636-1_17

side-to-side movement which you have not seen before and cannot figure out. You do a detailed nervous system examination and find generalized hypertonia, brisk reflexes, and ankle clonus bilaterally. With this picture, you are wondering if it is alcohol withdrawal, cocaine intoxication, or—very low on the list of differentials—tetanus. You come outside to speak to Mrs. Shridhar. You take a detailed history and find that he has never consumed alcohol in his life and does not use recreational drugs either. You send blood biochemistry and toxicology panels and start immediate measures for sedation and cooling the patient.

Questions What do you think is wrong with Mr. Shridhar?

Analysis

The past history is provided for a reason

(a) He is on treatment for anxiety
(b) He is on antibiotics for a skin and soft tissue infection

When a patient already on treatment for a particular illness develops a new complaint, the dictum is to consider a side effect of the treatment as a cause for the new symptoms. Especially when the patient is on multiple medications, the possibility of drug interaction arises.

The drugs prescribed for generalized anxiety disorder (GAD) include duloxetine, escitalopram, pregabalin, quetiapine, and venlafaxine. Duloxetine and venlafaxine are Serotonin Noradrenalin Reuptake Inhibitors (SNRIs), escitalopram is a Selective Serotonin Reuptake Inhibitor (SSRI), and quetiapine is an atypical antipsychotic. One possible adverse effect of SNRIs and SSRIs is the serotonin syndrome, especially if there is an unintended, unrecognized drug interaction.

Serotonin syndrome is a triad of mental status abnormalities, autonomic instability, and neuromuscular manifestations. It may be classified into the following [1]:

(a) Mild serotonin syndrome: Autonomic hyperactivity
(b) Moderate serotonin syndrome: Autonomic hyperactivity with neuromuscular excitation
(c) Severe serotonin syndrome: Autonomic hyperactivity with neuromuscular excitation with agitated delirium, and the core temperature exceeding 41.1 °C

Epidemiology

Serotonin syndrome can occur in all age groups. Its increasing incidence is thought to be associated with the increased use of serotonergic agents. One study of hospitalized patients who were prescribed at least one serotonergic medication found that 7.8% met the diagnostic criteria for the serotonin syndrome [2].

Etiopathogenesis

Serotonin syndrome results from excessive serotonergic neurotransmission [3]. This can occur due to:

(a) Medication use: Therapeutic use of antidepressants and other serotonergic agents
(b) Drug interactions: Interactions between medications
(c) Overdose: Intentional or accidental overdose of serotonergic medications

A variety of medications are associated with serotonin syndrome [4], including SSRIs, SNRIs, serotonin modulators, tricyclic and tetracyclic antidepressants, MAOIs, antiemetics, some illicit drugs, opioids, and triptan migraine medications (Fig. 17.1).

Serotonin syndrome is caused by overstimulation of 5-HT receptors in the central gray nuclei and the medulla and perhaps by overstimulation of 5-HT receptors in other areas.

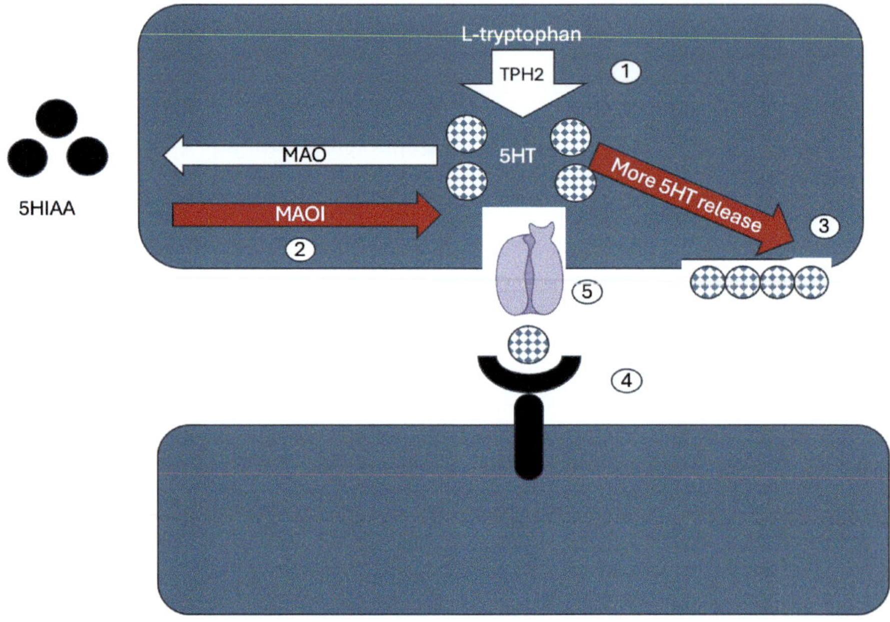

Fig. 17.1 Increased serotonergic neurotransmission can occur due to
(1) Increased levels of l-tryptophan—tryptophan, oxitriptan.
(2) MAO inhibitors decreasing conversion of serotonin to 5HIAA—linezolid, methylene blue, selegiline,
(3) Increased 5HT release—amphetamines, cocaine, mirtazapine.
(4) Increased stimulation of 5HT postsynaptic receptors—direct serotonin receptor agonist—triptans, fentanyl, ergot derivatives, LSD.
(5) SERT inhibition—increased synaptic 5HT because of decreased reuptake of 5HT into presynaptic cell—tramadol, SSRIs, SNRIs, TCAs, lamotrigine, bupropion.
TPH2 tryptophan hydroxylase,
MAO mono-amine oxidase, MAOI mono amine oxidase inhibitors, 5HT serotonin,
5HIAA 5- hydroxy indole acetic acid

Clinical Features [5]

The classic presentation involves a triad of clustered symptoms: Altered mental status, neuromuscular abnormalities, and autonomic hyperactivity

1. Altered mental status: Anxiety, agitation, restlessness, disorientation, delirium, and coma.
2. Neuromuscular abnormalities: Hyperreflexia, clonus, muscle rigidity, tremor, myoclonus, hypertonia, and incoordination.
3. Autonomic hyperactivity: Tachycardia, hyperthermia, diaphoresis, hypertension, vomiting, diarrhea, and mydriasis.

The diagnosis is confirmed by applying the Hunter Serotonin Toxicity Criteria [6]: Spontaneous clonus; inducible clonus with agitation or diaphoresis; ocular clonus with agitation or diaphoresis; tremor and hyper-reflexia; or hypertonia, with temperature above 100.4 °F (38 °C), and ocular or inducible clonus. Differential diagnoses include neuroleptic malignant syndrome, thyroid storm, malignant hyperthermia, and sympathomimetic intoxication (Table 17.1).

Table 17.1 Differential diagnosis of serotonin syndrome

	SS	NMS	Thyroid storm	Malignant hyperthermia	Sympathomimetic intoxication	Anticholinergic toxicity
Onset	Within 24 h	Days to weeks				
Vital signs	Hypertension, tachycardia Fever above 100.4 °F (38 °C)	Hypertension, tachycardia, tachypnea, hyperthermia	High fevers (40 °C [104 °F] or greater) tachycardia, agitation, confusion, obtundation and coma.	Hypertension, tachycardia, tachypnea, hyperthermia (up to 114.8 °F [46 °C])	Presents as CNS excitation (agitation, anxiety, tremors, delusions, and paranoia), along with tachycardia, hypertension, mydriasis, hyperpyrexia, diaphoresis, and *seizures*, in the presence of increased catecholamines[22]	Tachycardia, tachypnea, hyperthermia (usually *102.2 °F [39 °C] or below*
Signs	*Agitation* Restlessness Diaphoresis Diarrhea Hyperreflexia Ataxia Mental status change Myoclonus Ocular clonus Seizures Rhabdomyolysis	Sialorrhea diaphoresis, pallor, *stupor*, mutism, coma, normal or decreased bowel sounds, lead-pipe rigidity, bradyreflexia		Diaphoresis, mottled skin, agitation, decreased bowel sounds, muscular rigidity, *hyporeflexia*		Dry mouth, blurred vision, mydriasis, flushed skin, agitation/delirium, decreased bowel sounds

Treatment [7]

1. Discontinuation of all serotonergic agents.
2. Supportive care: Management of agitation with benzodiazepines, control of hyperthermia, and maintenance of hemodynamic stability.
3. Serotonin antagonists: Cyproheptadine (a serotonin antagonist) 12 mg orally or via nasogastric tube, followed by 2 mg every 2 h until clinical response is seen.
4. In severe cases, immediate sedation, paralysis, and endotracheal intubation.
5. Treat hyperthermia with standard cooling measures.

Key Takeaway
Consider the adverse effects of treatment and drug interaction as the cause for new complaints developing when the patient is already on therapy.

References

1. Birmes P, Coppin D, Schmitt L, Lauque D. Serotonin syndrome: a brief review. CMAJ. 2003;168(11):1439–42.
2. Nguyen CT, Xie L, Alley S, McCarron RM, Baser O, Wang Z. Epidemiology and economic burden of serotonin syndrome with concomitant use of serotonergic agents: a retrospective study utilizing two large US claims databases. Prim Care Companion CNS Disord. 2017;19(6):23092.
3. Buckley NA, Dawson AH, Isbister GK. Serotonin syndrome. Bmj. 2014:348.
4. Volpi-Abadie J, Kaye AM, Kaye AD. Serotonin Syndrome. Ochsner J. 2013;13(4):533–40.
5. Basu T, Gillman PK, Gnanadesigan N, Espinoza RT, Smith RL, Claassen JA, Gelissen HP, Boyer EW, Shannon M. The serotonin syndrome. N Engl J Med. 2005;352(23):2454–6.
6. Dunkley EJC, Isbister GK, Sibbritt D, Dawson AH, Whyte IM. The hunter serotonin toxicity criteria: simple and accurate diagnostic decision rules for serotonin toxicity. QJM. 2003;96(9):635–42.
7. Chiew AL, Isbister GK. Management of serotonin syndrome (toxicity). Br J Clin Pharmacol. 2025;91(3):654–61.

Fever, Rash, and Arthritis in a Young Female: Andrea Is Angry!

18

Grade Moderate.

Abstract An adult female with symptoms of fever and rash but almost no physical examination findings presents to you after being dismissed as functional by many physicians.

Story Ms Andrea is your last patient before a very late lunch break.

"I need a medical certificate," she says brusquely before she even sits down.

"Oh God it's one of those..." you tell yourself with a mental eye roll. "Good afternoon, Ms Andrea. Do sit down. Tell me exactly what the problem is."

"Like I said... I need a medical certificate!"

"I'll need to know a little bit about the specific health concerns before I issue a certificate."

"Fine," she barks out tersely. "No one believes me when I say I'm sick, but I'll tell you anyway. I have high fever, almost every day. Twice a day! And a rash too."

You look at Andrea's extremely clear skin and say skeptically, "I see."

"The rash comes only when I have the fever," Andrea says with hostility.

"All right...is there anything else troubling you?"

"So many things! But what's the point in my telling you, doctor. I can see in your face that you don't believe what I am saying."

"I assure you that I am taking everything you say very seriously indeed. Please tell me if there are any other health concerns."

"My knees hurt! My muscles pain! My tummy hurts and I have lost my appetite! I've lost weight!"

"When did all these problems start?"

"About 4 months ago when I had a really bad sore throat. I've been running from pillar to post over the last couple of months searching for some doctor to believe

S. Bhat, *Clinical Conundrums to Practice Diagnostic Reasoning*,
https://doi.org/10.1007/978-981-95-0636-1_18

what I'm saying. For someone to help me. But everyone thinks I'm making things up."

"I believe you." you tell Ms. Andrea, ignoring the smirk and raised eyebrows of the postgraduate resident sitting opposite you.

"Can you please lie down? May I examine you?"

The examination does not reveal much. There is mild hepatomegaly, and there are a couple of slightly tender enlarged cervical nodes. However, the patient is afebrile at the time of examination, and there is no rash. There is a slight painful restriction of movement on both knees, but you suspect osteoarthritis, since Andrea's BMI is 32 (even after the supposed weight loss), making her prone to the mechanical complications of obesity. You search carefully for a possible source of infection—however, the throat is normal, the neck is supple, the lungs are clear, and the abdomen is soft. You ask for a history of genitourinary symptoms or contact with tuberculosis, but she denies both.

Questions Are Andrea's symptoms functional? Is she malingering to get a medical certificate? Or is there actually a pathology that can be diagnosed and treated?

Analysis

The absence of fever and rash during examination might make you skeptical—but the hepatomegaly and lymphadenopathy indicate that there is an organic disease.

The following points may be noted:

1. Quotidian fever with two spikes a day
2. Evanescent rash simultaneous with the fever
3. Myalgia and arthritis
4. Hepatomegaly and lymphadenopathy

The fever indicates that an infectious/inflammatory process is at play—however, in the absence of a septic focus, the pendulum swings more toward an inflammatory disease. The rash and arthritis should prompt one to consider an autoimmune disease or vasculitis.

With this background and the history of rash which appears with fever and disappears with defervescence, Adult-Onset Still's Disease is a possibility.

Adult-Onset Still's Disease (AOSD) is characterized by a clinical triad of quotidian (daily) fevers, arthritis, and an evanescent rash [1]. The signs and symptoms of AOSD may be seen below the age of 16 when it is referred to as "systemic onset idiopathic juvenile arthritis." The prevalence ranges from 3.9 to 6.9 per 100,000 [2, 3]. AOSD is more common in females and has a bimodal age distribution, most commonly seen between the ages of 15–25 and 35–45 [4].

Etiopathogenesis [5]

AOSD may be triggered by an infection (generally pharyngitis) in a genetically predisposed individual. HLA-B17, HLA-B18, HLA-B35, and HLA-DR2 have been associated with Still's disease. Bacterial infections [6]—M. pneumoniae, C. pneumonia, Y. enterecolitica, Brucella abortus, Borrelia burgdoferi, and viral infections—rubella, measles, echovirus 7, coxsackiévirus B4, cytomegalovirus, and Epstein–Barr virus have been implicated [7].

Intense innate immune cell activation and the ensuing overproduction of various proinflammatory cytokines, such as interleukin-1 (IL-1), interleukin-6 (IL-6), and interleukin-18 (IL-18), precipitate AOSD [8].

Clinical Features

Fever: High-spiking quotidian fevers with temperature $\geq$ 39 °C with one or two peaks each day. The temperature typically returns to baseline or near baseline between spikes [9].

Arthritis: Can range from arthralgias to polyarthritis. The joints most frequently involved are knees, wrist, and ankle [10].

Rash: The rash is an evanescent, salmon-pink maculopapular rash which is located on the trunk and proximal extremities. It is typically nonpruritic. The rash characteristically appears and disappears with fever and defervescence [11].
Sore throat: Many patients with AOSD volunteer a history of preceding pharyngitis.
Myalgias.
Lymphadenopathy, hepatomegaly, and splenomegaly.
Serositis: Commonly pleuritis and pericarditis.

Investigations [12]

1. Increased ESR and CRP.
2. Neutrophilic leukocytosis.
3. Atypically for an immune disease, rheumatoid factor and antinuclear antibodies (ANAs) are generally negative.
4. Hyperferritinemia: Markedly elevated serum ferritin levels and a low fraction of glycosylated ferritin support the diagnosis of AOSD [13, 14].
5. Transaminitis.
6. ^{18}F-fluoro-deoxyglucose positron emission tomography/computed tomography (PET/CT) may have a role in evaluating patients with fever of unknown origin and suspected AOSD.

Diagnosis

Yamaguchi Criteria [15]

The presence of at least five criteria (including at least two major criteria) is suggestive of AOSD

Major Criteria

(a) Fever of 39 °C or higher lasting for at least 1 week
(b) Arthritis
(c) Evanescent rash
(d) Leukocytosis with $\geq$10,000/mm^3

Minor Criteria

A. Sore throat
B. Lymphadenopathy
C. Splenomegaly
D. Transaminitis
E. Negative tests for rheumatoid factor and ANA

Treatment [16]

(a) Nonsteroidal anti-inflammatory drugs (NSAIDs)
(b) Glucocorticoids
(c) Conventional disease-modifying antirheumatic drugs (DMARDs): methotrexate, sulfasalazine, leflunomide, and hydroxychloroquine.
(d) Biologicals [17]:

1. Interleukin-1 (IL-1) inhibitors: Anakinra (recombinant human IL-1 receptor antagonist), canakinumab (anti-IL-1β monoclonal antibody), and rilonacept (IL-1 trap).
2. Interleukin-6 (IL-6) inhibitors: Tocilizumab and sarilumab (anti-IL-6 receptor antibodies).
3. Tumor necrosis factor-alpha (TNF-α) inhibitors: While less consistently effective than IL-1 and IL-6 inhibitors, agents like infliximab and etanercept may be beneficial in some patients, especially for managing refractory AOSD.

Complications [18]

A. Macrophage activation syndrome (MAS) or secondary hemophagocytic lymphohistiocytosis (sHLH) [19]
B. Pulmonary involvement—interstitial lung disease and pulmonary arterial hypertension
C. Cardiac involvement (myocarditis and pericarditis)
D. Amyloidosis (renal AA amyloidosis)

References

1. Bywaters EG. Still's disease in the adult. Ann Rheum Dis. 1971;30(2):121.
2. Magadur-Joly G, Billaud E, Barrier JH, Pennec YL, Masson C, Renou P, et al. Epidemiology of adult Still's disease: estimate of the incidence by a retrospective study in West France. Ann Rheum Dis. 1995;54(7):587–90.
3. Wakai K, Ohta A, Tamakoshi A, Ohno Y, Kawamura T, Aoki R, et al. Estimated prevalence and incidence of adult still's disease: findings by a Nationwide Epidemiological Survey in Japan. J Epidemiol. 1997;7(4):221–5.
4. Chen PD, Yu SL, Chen S, Weng XH. Retrospective study of 61 patients with adult onset Still's disease admitted with fever of unknown origin in China. Clin Rheumatol. 2012;31(1):175–81.
5. Bindoli S, Baggio C, Doria A, Sfriso P. Adult-onset Still's disease (AOSD): advances in understanding pathophysiology, genetics and emerging treatment options. Drugs. 2024;84(3):257–74.x.
6. Perez: Adult Still's disease associated with Mycoplasma... – Google Scholar [Internet]. [cited 2025 Mar 24]. Available from: https://scholar.google.com/scholar_lookup?title=Adult%20Stills%20disease%20associated%20with%20Mycoplasma%20pneumoniae%20infection&publication_year=2011&author=C.%20Perez&author=V.%20Artola.
7. Wouters JM, Van Der Veen J, Van de Putte LB, de Rooij DJ. Adult onset Still's disease and viral infections. Ann Rheum Dis. 1988;47(9):764–7.

8. Choi JH, Suh CH, Lee YM, Suh YJ, Lee SK, Kim SS, et al. Serum cytokine profiles in patients with adult onset Still's disease. J Rheumatol. 2003;30(11):2422–7.
9. Ahn EY, Kwon HM, Hwang W, Lee EY, Lee EB, Song YW, et al. FRI0487 association between fever pattern and clinical manifestations in adult onset of still's disease: unbiased analysis of fever pattern using hierarchical clustering. Ann Rheum Dis. 2016;75:615.
10. Kontzias A, Efthimiou P. Adult-onset still's disease. Drugs. 2008;68(3):319–37.
11. Yamamoto T. Cutaneous manifestations associated with adult-onset Still's disease: important diagnostic values. Rheumatol Int. 2012;32(8):2233–7.
12. Efthimiou P, Paik PK, Bielory L. Diagnosis and management of adult onset Still's disease. Ann Rheum Dis. 2006;65(5):564–72.
13. Lian F, Wang Y, Yang X, Xu H, Liang L. Clinical features and hyperferritinemia diagnostic cutoff points for AOSD based on ROC curve: a Chinese experience. Rheumatol Int. 2012;32(1):189–92.
14. Kaur M, Lo SWS, Liu Y, Yip K. Hyperferritinemia: important differentials for the rheumatologists. Cureus [Internet]. 2024 Sep 3 [cited 2025 Mar 24]; Available from: https://www.cureus.com/articles/277121-hyperferritinemia-important-differentials-for-the-rheumatologists.
15. Yamaguchi M, Ohta A, Tsunematsu TO, Kasukawa RE, Mizushima YU, Kashiwagi HE, Kashiwazaki SA, Tanimoto KI, Matsumoto YO, Ota TO. Preliminary criteria for classification of adult Still's disease. J Rheumatol. 1992;19(3):424–30.
16. Fautrel B, Mitrovic S, De Matteis A, Bindoli S, Antón J, Belot A, Bracaglia C, Constantin T, Dagna L, Di Bartolo A, Feist E. EULAR/PReS recommendations for the diagnosis and management of Still's disease, comprising systemic juvenile idiopathic arthritis and adult-onset Still's disease. Ann Rheum Dis. 2024;83(12):1614–27.
17. Galozzi P, Bindoli S, Doria A, Sfriso P. Progress in biological therapies for adult-onset Still's disease. Biol Targets Ther. 2022;16:21–34.
18. Mitrovic S, Fautrel B. Complications of adult-onset Still's disease and their management. Expert Rev Clin Immunol. 2018;14(5):351–65.
19. Wang R, Li T, Ye S, Tan W, Zhao C, Li Y, et al. Macrophage activation syndrome associated with adult-onset Still's disease: a multicenter retrospective analysis. Clin Rheumatol. 2020;39(8):2379–86.

Young Female with Polyuria: The Painful Co-Passenger

19

Grade Very easy.

Abstract Young female with no fever, burning micturition, or high-colored urine has increased frequency of micturition.

Story You are on a flight from London to Delhi, and you figure you might try to while away the long hours by talking to the twenty something lady who has the window seat on your row.

"I'm Kartika," you introduce yourself.

"I'm Neha," the lady says tersely and pointedly looks back at her screen.

"Oh well, I tried." you tell yourself and browse through the inflight entertainment for something decent to watch. The stewardess hands out the warm nuts and cold drinks, and you settle yourself in to watch "Shrinking". Five minutes later, Neha taps you on your shoulder—you turn apologetically, thinking that maybe you were laughing too loudly.

"Sorry, I have to use the loo," she says, and you politely move aside so she can leave.

Over the next 2 h, you have to get up from your seat no less than six times because Neha needs to use the toilet.

"Excuse me—I couldn't help but notice that you are using the loo fairly frequently. I'm a doctor—may I help? Do you have any burning when you pass urine? Or fever? Or diabetes?"

"No!" she says rudely, turning back to the window.

"Would you like to sit near the aisle?" you ask her, exasperated, when she taps your shoulder yet again.

"No! I paid for a window seat." she says loudly, tossing back her glass of wine in one swallow.

S. Bhat, *Clinical Conundrums to Practice Diagnostic Reasoning*,
https://doi.org/10.1007/978-981-95-0636-1_19

You stare at your screen, counting to 10 and spend the rest of the journey moving out of the seat every time Neha needs to go to the loo.

After the journey from hell, you reach Delhi, get back to work, get over your jet lag. A couple of days later, you meet your friend for lunch. Over chole bhatura and cold beer, you talk about the journey to London, the fun you had while there and the nightmare trip back. You are walking back home in a blissful haze of good food and great conversation when—you cannot believe your eyes—you see the infamous Neha with the bladder that would not take a break. But then you catch sight of the clinic she is walking into and the name and the qualification on the sign above the clinic door—"Dr. A...consultant psychiatrist," and all becomes clear to you.

Questions What was the revelation that struck you? What might the connection be between a doctor's clinic and Neha's frequent urination?

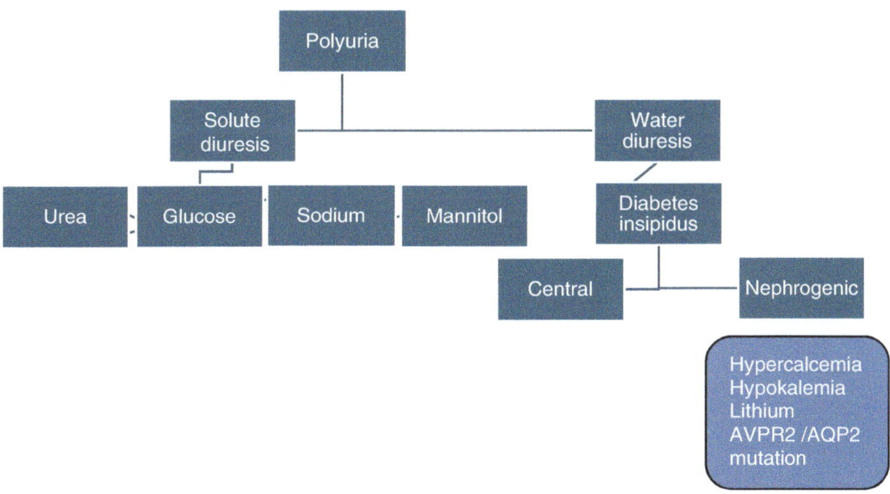

Fig. 19.1 Causes of polyuria

Analysis

This case boils down to an analysis of the causes of polyuria (Fig. 19.1).

There are some clues provided to narrow it down further.

It is unlikely to be a solute diuresis (Neha says she does not have diabetes, and the other causes are not likely). Of the various reasons of water diuresis, lithium is a more likely cause, as Neha is walking into a psychiatrist's clinic.

(a) Diabetes insipidus (DI) is a rare endocrine disorder characterized by the excretion of large volumes (exceeding 3 L per day) of hypotonic urine resulting from a deficiency in the secretion or action of arginine vasopressin (AVP). This leads to an inability to concentrate urine, causing excessive renal water losses and compensatory thirst [1].

Classification

DI is classified into four main types [2]:

(a) Central diabetes insipidus (CDI): Results from a deficiency in the release of AVP from the posterior pituitary gland or impaired synthesis of AVP in the hypothalamus
(b) Nephrogenic diabetes insipidus (NDI): Characterized by the resistance of the kidneys to AVP. This resistance occurs at the level of the distal convoluted tubule and collecting duct

(c) Dipsogenic diabetes insipidus: Involves an abnormally low thirst threshold, leading to excessive fluid intake
(d) Gestational diabetes insipidus: Occurs during pregnancy due to increased concentration of placental vasopressinase, which degrades vasopressin

Epidemiology

DI is a rare condition, affecting approximately 1 in 25,000 people worldwide [3]. It can manifest at any age, with hereditary forms developing earlier in life. The prevalence is similar among males and females.

Etiology

Central Diabetes Insipidus [4]

1. Tumors affecting the hypothalamus or pituitary gland
2. Trauma: Head injury or neurosurgical procedures (trans-sphenoidal or transcranial surgery for pituitary tumors can lead to acute CDI)
3. Autoimmune disorders: Lymphocytic infundibuloneurohypophysitis
4. Genetic mutations: Mutations in genes responsible for AVP synthesis and secretion

Nephrogenic Diabetes Insipidus

NDI can be congenital or acquired:

1. Genetic mutations: Mutations in the AVPR2 gene, encoding the arginine vasopressin receptor 2, or the AQP2 gene, encoding aquaporin
2. Drug-induced: Medications like lithium
3. Electrolyte imbalances: Hypercalcemia and hypokalemia
4. Renal diseases: Chronic renal failure and other conditions affecting tubular function

Dipsogenic Diabetes Insipidus

Excessive fluid intake: Abnormally low thirst threshold leading to increased fluid intake

Psychiatric disorders: Some psychiatric conditions are associated with excessive water drinking

Gestational Diabetes Insipidus

Placental vasopressinase: Increased levels of placental vasopressinase during pregnancy

Pathogenesis

Central Diabetes Insipidus

In CDI, damage or dysfunction of vasopressinergic neurons in the hypothalamus or posterior pituitary impair the synthesis and secretion of AVP3. The deficiency of AVP results in decreased water reabsorption in the collecting ducts, leading to the excretion of large volumes of dilute urine.

Nephrogenic Diabetes Insipidus [5]

NDI occurs due to renal AVP resistance. Mutations in the AVPR2 or AQP2 genes disrupt the normal signaling pathway, preventing AVP from increasing water permeability in the collecting ducts. Acquired forms of NDI may result from drug-induced interference with this pathway or from renal damage affecting tubular function.

Dipsogenic Diabetes Insipidus

Dipsogenic DI is characterized by an abnormally low thirst threshold, causing individuals to drink excessive amounts of water. This leads to suppression of AVP secretion and subsequent polyuria.

Gestational Diabetes Insipidus

During pregnancy, increased levels of placental vasopressinase degrade AVP, leading to DI. This condition typically resolves after delivery.

Clinical Features

The patient presents with polyuria, polydipsia, and nocturia. Patients often crave cold water and may exhibit signs of dehydration if fluid intake is insufficient to compensate for urinary losses. Polyuria may be dramatic, typically more than 3–3.5

litres in a 24 h period but in severe cases, as high as 12 L per day. Nocturia may disrupt sleep. Polydipsia and increased fluid intake may compensate for the water loss, but if not, hypovolemia may occur.

Hypernatremia is a result of salt-free water loss and may result in fatigue and weakness.

In patients with adipsic DI, there is an absence of thirst, which can lead to severe hypernatremia and associated complications.

Investigations

(a) Measurement of 24-h urine volume and urine osmolality.
(b) Measurement of plasma osmolality and sodium levels to assess water balance.
(c) Water deprivation test: Restricting fluid intake and monitoring urine output and plasma osmolality. This serves to differentiate CDI from NDI and primary polydipsia.
(d) Hypertonic saline infusion test: Measures AVP response to hypertonic saline infusion.
(e) Copeptin measurement: Copeptin, a surrogate marker for AVP, can be measured in response to osmotic or nonosmotic stimuli.
(f) Arginine stimulation test.
(g) Magnetic resonance imaging (MRI): To identify structural abnormalities such as pituitary tumors or infiltration.

Treatment

The primary goal of DI treatment is to maintain fluid balance and alleviate symptoms.

Central Diabetes Insipidus

Desmopressin (DDAVP): Synthetic AVP analogue used to replace deficient hormone. It is available in oral, intranasal, and injectable forms.

Fluid intake: Ensuring adequate fluid intake to match urinary losses.

Nephrogenic Diabetes Insipidus

Discontinuation of offending medications: If drug-induced, discontinuing the causative agent, such as lithium.

Dietary modifications: Low-sodium diet to reduce polyuria.

Thiazide diuretics: Thiazide diuretics can paradoxically reduce polyuria in NDI.

Amiloride: Potassium-sparing diuretic that can be used in conjunction with thiazides to prevent hypokalemia.

Adequate fluid intake: Ensuring sufficient fluid intake to prevent dehydration.

Monitoring: Close monitoring of fluid and electrolyte balance.

References

1. Robertson GL. Diabetes insipidus. Endocrinol Metab Clin N Am. 1995;24(3):549–72.
2. Christ-Crain MI, Winzeler B, Refardt J. Diagnosis and management of diabetes insipidus for the internist: an update. J Intern Med. 2021;290(1):73–87.
3. Fenske W, Allolio B. Current state and future perspectives in the diagnosis of diabetes insipidus: a clinical review. J Clin Endocrinol Metabol. 2012;97(10):3426–37.
4. Tomkins M, Lawless S, Martin-Grace J, Sherlock M, Thompson CJ. Diagnosis and management of central diabetes insipidus in adults. J Clin Endocrinol Metabol. 2022;107(10):2701–15.
5. Vaz de Castro PA, Bitencourt L, de Oliveira Campos JL, Fischer BL, Soares de Brito SB, Soares BS, Drummond JB, Simões e Silva AC. Nephrogenic diabetes insipidus: a comprehensive overview. J Pediatr Endocrinol Metab. 2022;35(4):421–34.

20 Disproportionate Fatigue and Abdominal Pain in an Adult Male with Cirrhosis and Portal Hypertension: Sometimes the Hoofbeats Are Zebras

Grade Difficult.

Abstract A known case of cirrhosis and portal hypertension presents with some symptoms that are not explained by this diagnosis—disabling fatigue, occasional difficulty in swallowing, and severe abdominal pain.

Story As you walk into your clinic, you notice that your clinic receptionist—Mrs Mehta—is in tears.

"What happened, Mrs Mehta? Is there anything I can do to help?"

"My husband is not keeping well doctor. I'm so worried. Please, can I bring him to see you?"

"Of course! Any time."

Mr. and Mrs. Mehta visit you the next evening. As they walk in, you note that, unfortunately, Mr. Mehta has all the stigmata of chronic ethanol use. His eyes are bloodshot, there is bilateral parotid enlargement, and he appears icteric.

"Please sit down. Tell me what's wrong."

"He's ruined his health with alcohol. I've tried so hard to make him stop but he hasn't! Alcohol is more important to him than his family!" Mrs. Mehta sobs.

"I keep telling you, it's not the alcohol! It's something different this time!" Mr. Mehta bursts out, exasperated. "If you give me a moment to tell the doctor what's happening, he can help me. But it's always the same. Once you start talking, it's like a runaway train. No one else can get a word in."

"Ok fine, you tell him then."

"Doctor, I agree I have been drinking a little more than is good for me."

"A little more?!" Mrs. Mehta expostulates. "He was diagnosed to have alcoholic liver disease last November, when he vomited blood. He had to undergo an endoscopic variceal ligation."

S. Bhat, *Clinical Conundrums to Practice Diagnostic Reasoning*,
https://doi.org/10.1007/978-981-95-0636-1_20

"I've cut down on drinking now—I just have a mug of beer once a week" says Mr. Mehta.

"Why can't you stop that?"

"Stop fussing, woman. Give the doctor a chance to think! It's not like it was last time. I feel different. It's no the alcohol. It's something else. It's something ELSE!!!"

"Please calm down Mr. Mehta. I will examine you in detail, and I'll find out what exactly is going on. But before that, can you tell me the issues that are troubling you now?"

"I've been feeling really tired all the time for the last 4–5 months. I have tummy pain once in a while, and it gets pretty severe sometimes. Sometimes I find it difficult to swallow."

"I can see how all this can be worrying."

"There's another problem doctor."

"What is that?"

"I've not been able to have marital relations with my wife for maybe 4–5 months."

"That's true" Mrs. Mehta nods sadly.

"One more thing, doctor. I visited another hospital a week ago. They said my iron levels were low, and they gave me what they said was an 'iron injection.'"

"OK..."

"But I became really sick after that injection. I think it worsened my jaundice, because my urine looked reddish after that. And now my acidity is worse, and my tummy seems bloated."

"I'm sorry to hear that. May I examine you?"

"Yes, doctor." He lies down.

You note that the patient is icteric. There is no clubbing. Pallor is present, but it does not seem to be severe enough to cause the disabling fatigue that is afflicting Mr. Mehta. There are blanching purpura present on both lower limbs.

The abdomen is distended and tense. Bowel sounds are present. Splenomegaly is present three finger breadths below the left costal margin.

Abdominal imaging picks up a portal vein thrombosis (Fig. 20.1).

Question Who was right? Mrs. or Mr. Mehta? Are all Mr. Mehta's complaints ascribable to ethanol alone or do the labs and clinical features point to something else?

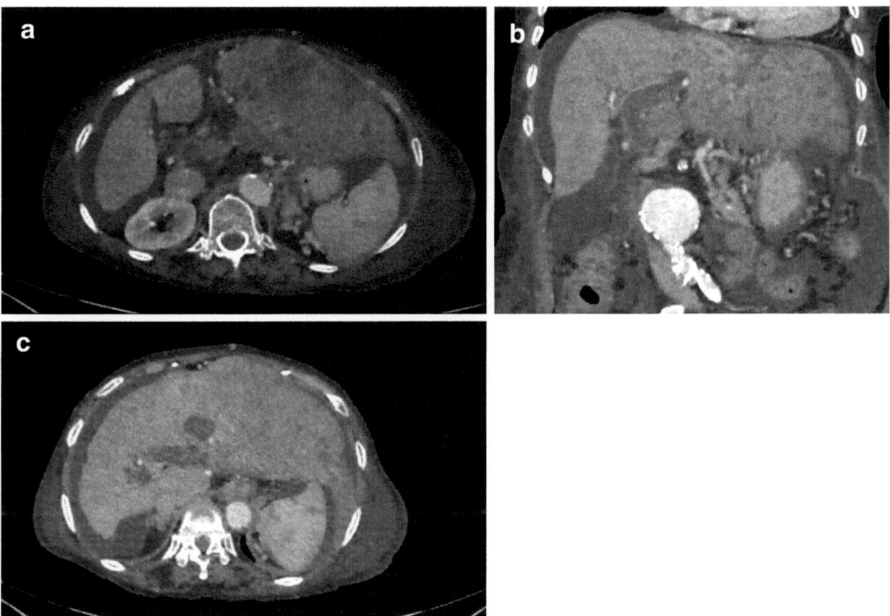

Fig. 20.1 (**a**–**c**) Portal vein thrombosis. (Images contributed by Dr. Ram Shenoy Basti, FMMC)

Analysis

This is a tricky case to analyze. At first look, it seems to be a straightforward case of alcoholic liver disease with cirrhosis and portal hypertension. However, some features are difficult to explain. Dysphagia is not a common feature of chronic liver disease. One might be tempted to consider an esophageal malignancy, but the dysphagia in esophageal cancer is unlikely to be intermittent. Abdominal pain is also not a common feature of cirrhosis (unless there is spontaneous bacterial peritonitis too). Another clue to a condition other than cirrhosis alone is the apparent worsening of the patient's condition (darkening of urine and exacerbation of symptoms) on being administered an iron infusion. This is suggestive of hemolysis. Thus, there is a combination of abdominal pain, intermittent dysphagia (unlikely to be mechanical—might be due to smooth muscle dystonia) and precipitation of hemolysis with iron infusion, along with portal vein thrombosis. Hemolysis, thrombosis, and smooth muscle spasm should prompt one to consider paroxysmal nocturnal hemoglobinuria (PNH).

Paroxysmal Nocturnal Hemoglobinuria

PNH is an acquired hemopoietic stem cell (HSC) disorder, where the absence of GPI-anchored proteins on the cell surface predispose to chronic intravascular hemolysis, venous thrombosis, and hypoplastic bone marrow. It affects males and females equally and is most common between the ages of 20 and 40 [1].

Etiopathogenesis

Complement inhibitors play a crucial role in blocking complement-mediated intravascular (CD59) and extravascular (CD55) hemolysis. They are anchored to the cell by the GPI anchor (Fig. 20.2) whose synthesis is directed by the PIGA gene in the X chromosome [2].

The initial event in PNH is an acquired mutation in the PIGA gene. The mutation may be due to excessive radiation, mutagenic chemotherapy, or autoimmune conditions. Once this occurs, the HSC carrying the PIGA gene mutation undergoes clonal expansion [3] or neutral evolution [4] (Fig. 20.2). Cells from this clone are unable to anchor complement inhibitors to the cell. The consequence is a chronic hemolysis interspersed with exacerbations. Free hemoglobin in the plasma causes renal injury, hypercoagulability, and increased smooth muscle tone (Fig. 20.3).

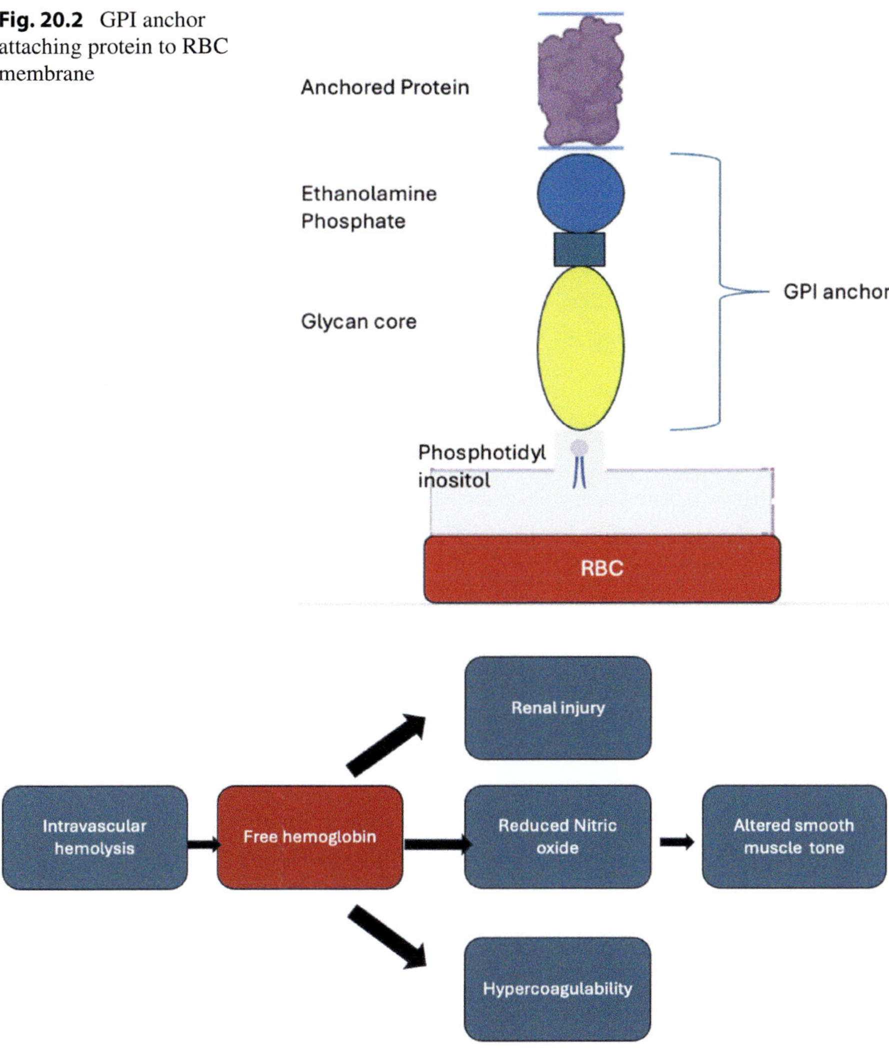

Fig. 20.2 GPI anchor attaching protein to RBC membrane

Fig. 20.3 Intravascular hemolysis and its consequences

Clinical Features

1. Due to hemolysis : Fatigue (out of proportion to the anemia), jaundice, hemoglobinuria(red or cola colored urine)

   Iron supplementation in these patients may worsen hemolysis (which is what happened in the case described).
2. Due to anemia: Fatigue, exertional breathlessness.
3. Thrombosis—especially intra-abdominal veins [5]—CT detected portal vein thrombosis in Mr. Mehta.

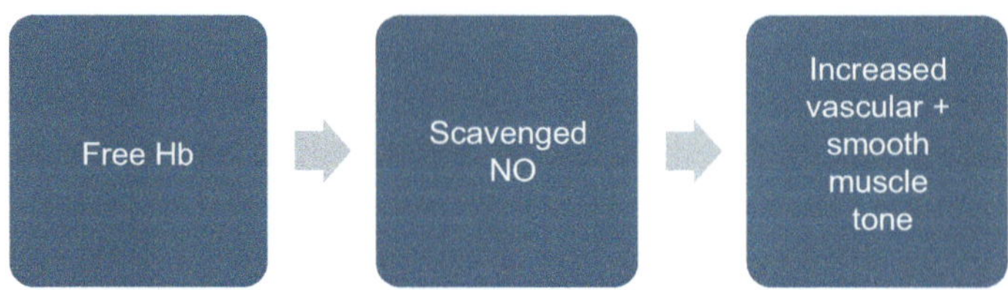

Fig. 20.4 Consequences of free hemoglobin

4. Due to reduced NO (Fig. 20.4):
   - Abdominal pain
   - Erectile dysfunction
   - Fatigue
   - Esophageal spasm
5. Bone marrow failure leading to pancytopenias.

Investigations

1. CBC, reticulocyte count, D dimer
2. Blood biochemistry
3. Flow cytometry
4. Bone marrow

Treatment [6, 7]

C5 inhibitors like Ravilizumab with/without immunosuppressant therapy
Alternative complement pathway inhibitors like pegcetacoplan [8]
Stem cell transplantation

Key Takeaway
Though we are taught in medical school that "when you hear hoofbeats, think of horses, not zebras," sometimes the hoofbeats are zebras. The importance of diagnosing a rare condition lies in the fact that specific, effective therapy may be available.

References

1. Jv D. Paroxysmal nocturnal haemoglobinuria: clinical manifestations, haematology, and nature of the disease. Ser Haematol. 1972;5(3):3–23.
2. Brodsky RA. Paroxysmal nocturnal hemoglobinuria. Blood, The Journal of the American Society of Hematology. 2014;124(18):2804–11.

3. Clemente MJ, Przychodzen B, Hirsch CM, Nagata Y, Bat T, Wlodarski MW, Radivoyevitch T, Makishima H, Maciejewski JP. Clonal PIGA mosaicism and dynamics in paroxysmal nocturnal hemoglobinuria. Leukemia. 2018;32(11):2507–11.
4. Dingli D, Luzzatto L, Pacheco JM. Neutral evolution in paroxysmal nocturnal hemoglobinuria. Proc Natl Acad Sci. 2008;105(47):18496–500.
5. Intagliata N, Caldwell S, Tripodi A. Diagnosis, development, and treatment of portal vein thrombosis in patients with and without cirrhosis. Gastroenterology. 2019;156(6):1582–99.
6. Parker CJ. Update on the diagnosis and management of paroxysmal nocturnal hemoglobinuria. Hematology 2014, the American Society of Hematology Education Program Book. 2016;2016(1):208–16.
7. Fattizzo B, Serpenti F, Giannotta JA, Barcellini W. Difficult cases of paroxysmal nocturnal hemoglobinuria: diagnosis and therapeutic novelties. J Clin Med. 2021;10(5):948.
8. Lee JW, Brodsky R, Nishimura J, Kulasekararaj A. The role of the alternative pathway in paroxysmal nocturnal hemoglobinuria and emerging treatments. Expert Rev Clin Pharmacol. 2022;15:851–61.

21 Subacute Onset of Apathy and Fatigue in a Previously Well Male: The Apathetic Attender

Grade Moderate.

Abstract A previously healthy adult male has disinterest, fatigue, and loss of libido.

Story Mrs. Kavita is attending your clinic for management of her diabetes.

She is accompanied by her husband Mr. Giri, who seems to be a quiet, thoughtful man. He sits expressionless, stolid, and silent as you examine Mrs. Kavita. His phone rings, and he stands to take the call outside the room. However, he sways a little bit and leans on your desk for support.

"Are you OK?" you ask concerned.

"Yes, yes. I'm okay—just a little lightheaded," he answers and walks out of the room to answer his phone.

"I hope everything is OK with your husband," you tell Mrs. Kavita.

"Doctor, I just can't figure it out," she responds. "He seems to live in a world of his own. He is not interested in what's happening at home, what our kids are up to. He looks tired all the time—he's so exhausted after he returns from work that he has a quick shower and goes to bed. To tell the truth, he is not interested in marital relations either."

"I am sorry to hear that," you reply. "I wonder if he is depressed. Do you think you should get a psychiatrist to see him?"

"I don't know what to do…" Mrs. Kavita responds sadly. "He was absolutely fine up till June last year. Unfortunately, while on a trek in the Western Ghats, he was bitten by a snake. I don't know if that is what affected his confidence. But things have gone downhill since then."

"May I examine him briefly?" you ask. Mrs. Kavita calls in her husband, and he returns to the room reluctantly.

S. Bhat, *Clinical Conundrums to Practice Diagnostic Reasoning*, https://doi.org/10.1007/978-981-95-0636-1_21

"I'm a little worried about your lightheadedness, Sir," you tell him and proceed to measure his blood pressure. It is 112/ 70 mm Hg supine and 90/60 mm Hg when he stands for 2 min. His heart rate is 60 beats per min. He looks sad, pale, and puffy.

Question What ails Mr. Giri? Is it a post-traumatic stress disorder after the snake bite? Or should you rule out something else?

Analysis

The key features here are apathy, significant postural fall in blood pressure, and bradycardia. The postural hypotension is a pointer toward hypocortisolism and the bradycardia a clue to hypothyroidism. Hypocortisolism and hypothyroidism, along with the history of lack and libido and the preceding history of snake bite should prompt you to consider hypopituitarism as a diagnosis. Hypopituitarism is a rare complication of snake bite, especially viper bite [1].

Hypopituitarism is an endocrine disorder characterized by diminished or absent secretion of one or more anterior pituitary hormones which can arise either due to pituitary disease itself (primary hypopituitarism) or from inadequate stimulation by hypothalamic releasing hormones (secondary hypopituitarism) [2]. The clinical features depend upon the rapidity of disease progression, the degree of hormonal deficit, and the multiplicity of hormonal axes involved. The estimated incidence of hypopituitarism is 4.2 cases per 100,000 individuals per year, with a prevalence of 45.5 cases per 100,000 [3].

Etiology

The etiology of hypopituitarism is multifarious. Key causes [4]:

Invasive: Space-occupying lesions, including pituitary adenomas, craniopharyngiomas, meningiomas, and metastatic neoplasms via direct compression or disruption of the hypothalamic–hypophysial portal system.

Infarction: Pituitary apoplexy (acute hemorrhage or infarction of the pituitary gland) and Sheehan's syndrome (postpartum pituitary necrosis secondary to hemorrhage).

Infiltrative: Sarcoidosis, Langerhans cell histiocytosis, hemochromatosis, and amyloidosis.

Injury: Traumatic brain injury (TBI), subarachnoid hemorrhage (SAH), neurosurgical interventions, and cranial irradiation.

Immunologic: Autoimmune hypophysitis, encompassing lymphocytic, granulomatous, and IgG4-related subtypes. Furthermore, immune checkpoint inhibitors can precipitate hypophysitis.

Iatrogenic: Pituitary surgery and radiation therapy.

Infectious: Infections, including pituitary abscess, meningitis, encephalitis, tuberculosis, and syphilis.

Pathogenesis of Hypopituitarism in Snake Bite [5]

The mechanism of pituitary apoplexy in snake bite and Russel viper envenomation is similar to what happens in postpartum hemorrhage and Sheehan's syndrome. Two conditions need to be fulfilled:

(a) Enlarged and engorged pituitary: Due to capillary leak syndrome following the snake bite. Additionally, the Russel viper venom causes stimulation and release of pituitary hormones GH, ACTH, and TSH.
(b) Compromised vascular supply to the pituitary due to hypotension, due to micro-thrombi deposition secondary to disseminated intravascular coagulation, and due to changes in intravascular pressure caused by capillary leak syndrome.

Clinical Features [6]

(a) Growth Hormone (GH) Deficiency

Paediatric population: Growth retardation, resulting in short stature.

Adult population: Manifestations include fatigue, reduced muscle mass and strength, increased adiposity, diminished bone mineral density, impaired quality of life, and elevated cardiovascular risk.

(b) Luteinizing Hormone (LH) and Follicle-Stimulating Hormone (FSH) Deficiency (Hypogonadotropic Hypogonadism) [7]

Female patients: Present with amenorrhea, oligomenorrhea, infertility, diminished libido, and vaginal dryness.

Male patients: Present with decreased libido, erectile dysfunction, infertility, reduced muscle mass and strength, and testicular atrophy.

(c) Thyroid-Stimulating Hormone (TSH) Deficiency (Central Hypothyroidism)

Fatigue, weight gain, constipation, cold intolerance, xeroderma, and cognitive dysfunction [8].

(d) Adrenocorticotropic Hormone (ACTH) Deficiency (Secondary Adrenal Insufficiency)

Fatigue, asthenia, anorexia, weight loss, nausea, emesis, hypotension, and hypoglycemia [9]. Notably, hyperpigmentation is absent, distinguishing it from primary adrenal insufficiency.

(e) Prolactin (PRL) Deficiency

Inability to initiate or sustain postpartum lactation [10].

(f) Diabetes Insipidus (DI)

Characterized by polyuria, polydipsia, and resultant hypernatremia. DI is more commonly associated with the compromise of the posterior pituitary or hypothalamus [11].

Investigations [12]

Basal Hormone Levels:

GH: Insulin-like growth factor 1 (IGF-1) levels are frequently diminished in GH deficiency, although normal levels do not preclude the diagnosis.

LH and FSH: Low or inappropriately normal levels in the context of hypogonadism are suggestive of hypogonadotropic hypogonadism.
TSH: Reduced or inappropriately normal TSH levels in conjunction with low free T4 are indicative of central hypothyroidism.
ACTH: Early morning cortisol levels are typically reduced in ACTH deficiency.
Prolactin: Reduced prolactin levels may signify pituitary damage; however, interpretation requires caution due to the multitude of factors influencing prolactin secretion

Dynamic Stimulation Tests [13]

(a) GH stimulation tests: Insulin tolerance test (ITT), glucagon stimulation test, or GHRH-arginine test may be performed. The macimorelin stimulation test may also be utilized [14].
(b) ACTH stimulation test: Short Synacthen test is used to evaluate adrenal function.
(c) TRH stimulation test: Assesses TSH and prolactin reserve.

Neuroradiologic Evaluation

MRI of the pituitary gland: Facilitates identification of structural anomalies, including pituitary adenomas, craniopharyngiomas, empty sella, and pituitary apoplexy (Fig. 21.1).

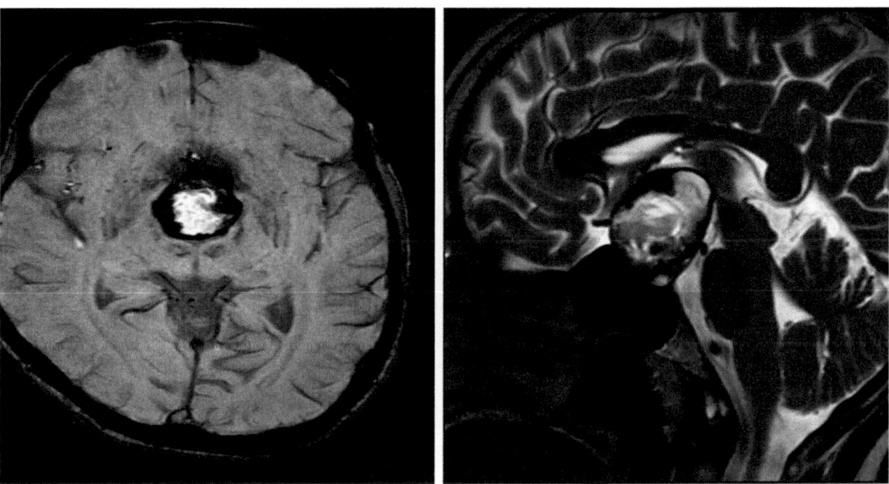

Fig. 21.1 Pituitary apoplexy.
(Image contributed by Dr. Ram Shenoy Basti, Department of Radiology, Father Muller Medical College)

Visual Field Testing

To check for visual field aberrations resulting from pituitary tumors with suprasellar extension.

Differential Diagnosis

(a) Primary endocrine disorders: Such as primary hypothyroidism, primary adrenal insufficiency, and primary hypogonadism
(b) Non-endocrine disorders: Including depression and chronic fatigue syndrome
(c) Genetic disorders: Congenital syndromes affecting pituitary development

Treatment

Hormone replacement therapy to restore physiological hormone levels [15].

(a) GH replacement: Recombinant human GH is indicated for GH deficiency in both pediatric and adult patients.
(b) Sex steroid replacement:
    (i) Female patients: Estrogen and progesterone replacement therapy is administered to restore menstrual cyclicity and prevent osteoporosis.
    (ii) Male patients: Testosterone replacement therapy is utilized to restore libido, muscle mass, and bone density.
    (iii) Thyroid hormone replacement: Levothyroxine is prescribed for central hypothyroidism, with dosage adjustments guided by clinical response and free T4 levels.
    (iv) Adrenal hormone replacement: Hydrocortisone or prednisone is administered for secondary adrenal insufficiency. Patients require education regarding stress-dose steroid administration during periods of illness or surgical procedure.
    (v) Desmopressin: For the management of diabetes insipidus.

Key Takeaway
Though hypopituitarism is a rare consequence of hemotoxic snake bite, the possibility should be kept in mind, and the physician must have a high index of suspicion to suspect and diagnose it.

References

1. Wolff H. Is it time to denominate hypopituitarism after snake bite?. QJM. 2013;106(4):390.
2. Schneider HJ, Aimaretti G, Kreitschmann-Andermahr I, Stalla GK, Ghigo E. Hypopituitarism. Lancet. 2007;369(9571):1461–70.

3. Krivosheeva YG, Ilovayskaya IA. The prevalence rate of hypopituitarism in patients with pituitary macroadenomas with various hormonal activities. Alm Clin Med. 2021;49(4):261–7.
4. Fleseriu M, Christ-Crain M, Langlois F, Gadelha M, Melmed S. Hypopituitarism. Lancet. 2024;403(10444):2632–48.
5. Bhattacharya S, Krishnamurthy A, Gopalakrishnan M, Kalra S, Kantroo V, Aggarwal S, Surana V. Endocrine and metabolic manifestations of snakebite envenoming. Am J Trop Med Hygiene. 2020;103(4):1388.
6. Hypopituitarism - Endotext - NCBI Bookshelf [Internet]. [cited 2025 Mar 22]. Available from: https://www.ncbi.nlm.nih.gov/sites/books/NBK278989/
7. Berger K, Souza H, Brito VN, d'Alva CB, Mendonca BB, Latronico AC. Clinical and hormonal features of selective follicle-stimulating hormone (FSH) deficiency due to FSH beta-subunit gene mutations in both sexes. Fertil Steril. 2005;83(2):466–70.
8. Jansen HI, Boelen A, Heijboer AC, Bruinstroop E, Fliers E. Hypothyroidism: the difficulty in attributing symptoms to their underlying cause. Front Endocrinol. 2023;14:1130661.
9. Cooper MS, Stewart PM. Diagnosis and treatment of ACTH deficiency. Rev Endocr Metab Disord. 2005;6(1):47.
10. Al-Chalabi M, Bass AN, Alsalman I. Physiology, Prolactin. In: StatPearls. Treasure Island: StatPearls Publishing; 2025. PMID: 29939606.
11. Tomkins M, Lawless S, Martin-Grace J, Sherlock M, Thompson CJ. Diagnosis and management of central diabetes insipidus in adults. J Clin Endocrinol Metabol. 2022;107(10):2701–15.
12. Schilbach K, Bidlingmaier M. Pitfalls in the lab assessment of hypopituitarism. Rev Endocr Metab Disord. 2024;25(3):457–65.
13. Adrogué HJ, Madias NE. Diagnosis and treatment of hyponatremia. Am J Kidney Dis. 2014;64(5):681–4.
14. Garcia JM, Biller BM, Korbonits M, Popovic V, Luger A, Strasburger CJ, Chanson P, Medic-Stojanoska M, Schopohl J, Zakrzewska A, Pekic S. Macimorelin as a diagnostic test for adult GH deficiency. J Clin Endocrinol Metabol. 2018;103(8):3083–93.
15. Smith JC. Hormone replacement therapy in hypopituitarism. Expert Opin Pharmacother. 2004;5(5):1023–31.

22 Hirsutism in Women: Hairy Harini

Grade Easy.

Abstract A young lady with symptoms and signs suggestive of polycystic ovarian syndrome improves with naturopathy but then relapses.

Story Harini was one of those girls who had been blessed by good angels. Beautiful, intelligent, hardworking, and kind, she was loved by her friends and family and seemed destined for a career in modeling or movies—she was that lovely. Unfortunately, things changed when she turned 19. She started gaining weight, her creamy complexion was ruined when she developed severe cystic acne, and she became quite hairy. When she returned home in tears after a bully in her class called her "big bear", her mother decided that something had to be done.

She brought her daughter to your outpatient clinic on a sunny Monday morning. You interviewed Harini and learned that her periods had become irregular for the last 4 months. There was no family history of autoimmune thyroid disease. Harini had a BMI of 32, was richly pimpled, and quite hirsute. The blood pressure was 130/80 mm Hg. You noted the presence of acanthosis nigricans. Physical examination was otherwise noncontributory.

You discussed the differential diagnosis with Harini and her mother and suggested blood tests and an ultrasound abdomen.

Harini's mother objected to the cost of the investigations and left the clinic, Harini in tow, muttering about how doctors demanded unnecessary investigations and saying "kickbacks" with a dark look in your direction.

The story continues:

Harini was then taken to a lady in the neighborhood with a reputation for providing natural remedies. "Polycystic", she pronounced and prescribed a dairy-free diet. She assured the mother and daughter that things would improve soon.

S. Bhat, *Clinical Conundrums to Practice Diagnostic Reasoning*,
https://doi.org/10.1007/978-981-95-0636-1_22

Funnily enough, they did. Harini's acne cleared, and she lost some weight (a strict diet and exercise regime may have had something to do with this).

Five months later, Harini's mother brought her to your clinic again. "She's grown fat again, doctor," the mother said despairingly. "She complains of heaviness of the head and is angry all the time."

You agree to examine the patient and magnanimously decide not to mention your advice the last time they visited.

You find that the blood pressure is a worrying 160/100 mm Hg.

You measure the weight and force yourself not to react when you see the frightening number on the scale. You request Harini to stand up so you can measure her height. She rises with reluctance and difficulty. You note down the height and weight and calculate the BMI to be 35. In fact, Harini has put on so much weight that she now has stretch marks on her abdomen.

Question What is the diagnosis? Are there supporting points for and against PCOS?

Analysis

The initial presentation was suggestive of insulin resistance.

(a) Obesity
(b) Acanthosis nigricans

The hirsutism and acne point to increased testosterone, and together, a diagnosis of PCOS is justified.

Investigations at that time may have included thyroid profile, blood glucose, lipid profile, and an ultrasonogram to demonstrate polycystic morphology.

The modified Rotterdam criteria to diagnose PCOs require that at least two of the following be present [1].

Modified Rotterdam Criteria

1. Biochemical hyperandrogenism (elevated total free testosterone or calculated indices of free testosterone).
2. Clinical hyperandrogenism: A modified Ferryman–Gallwey score of >4 to >8.
3. Oligo anovulation: Oligo-amenorrhea (cycles >35 days apart or less than eight menstrual cycles per year).
4. Polycystic ovarian morphology: > 20 follicles per ovary in either ovary or > 10 cm^3 ovarian volume.

At the second visit, there are some causes for concern.

The first is the high blood pressure; the second is the history suggestive of proximal muscle weakness (stands up from the chair reluctantly and with difficulty); and the third is the presence of abdominal striae. All of these are suggestive of Cushing's syndrome.

PCOS is the most common endocrine disorder in women of the reproductive age group, with the prevalence ranging from 5 to 20%. It is characterized by clinical or biochemical androgen excess, polycystic ovarian morphology, and oligo- or anovulation [2] [3].

Cushing's syndrome is a disease state with various causes (Fig. 22.1) produced by

(a) Chronic glucocorticoid excess
(b) Loss of diurnal variation of glucocorticoid secretion
(c) Loss of the feedback mechanism in the hypothalamo–pituitary–adrenal axis

It is relatively rare with an annual incidence of 2–3/million and a female-to-male ratio of 3:1 [4].

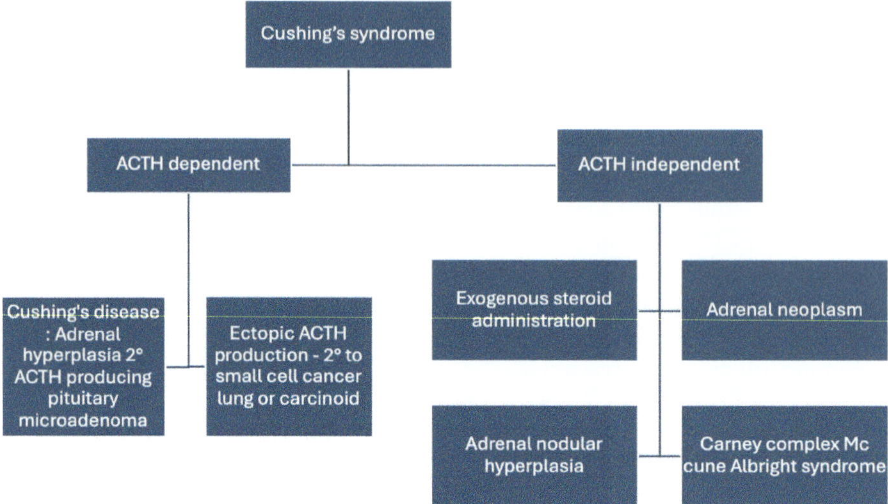

Fig. 22.1 Causes of Cushing's syndrome

Clinical Features [5]

Symptoms Irregular menstrual cycles, erectile dysfunction in males, decreased libido, weight gain, proximal muscle weakness, irritability, backache, recurrent infections, lethargy, and mood changes.

Signs Hypertension, obesity, acne, hirsutism, plethora, balding, moon face, buffalo hump, bruisability, purple abdominal striae, and muscle atrophy.

Lab Abnormalities

- Abnormal glucose tolerance
- ECG abnormalities

Diagnosis [6]

Step 1: Confirm hypercortisolism (Cushing's syndrome)

(a) Late-night salivary cortisol.
(b) 24 h urinary free cortisol.
(c) Low-dose dexamethasone suppression test: 1 mg dexamethasone is administered orally between 11 pm and midnight. Blood for serum cortisol is drawn between 8 and 9 am.

Reasoning When the hypothalamo–pituitary axis is intact, administration of dexamethasone will suppress ACTH and CRH. If serum cortisol > than 1.8 microgram/dL, then hypercortisolism is likely.

Step 2 [7]: Detect the source of hypercortisolism: ACTH must be estimated. If ACTH is low, this would indicate an ACTH-independent cause of Cushing's syndrome, as detailed in the figure above, and investigation must proceed accordingly. If ACTH is high, this would mean that the hypercortisolism is ACTH-dependent, either due to Cushing's disease (pituitary ACTH hypersecretion) or ectopic ACTH secretion.

To differentiate between these two, the- high dose dexamethasone secretion test (HDDST) is performed.

HDDST

Baseline morning cortisol is drawn, and 8 mg dexamethasone is administered orally between 11 pm and midnight. Serum cortisol is measured between 8 and 9 am the next morning.

Reasoning: The ACTH secretion in Cushing's disease (pituitary-dependent ACTH secretion) but not in ectopic ACTH secretion will be suppressed by high-dose dexamethasone.

Treatment [8]

1. Stop exogenous steroids. Keep in mind that many native medications actually contain fairly high doses of steroids; carefully elicit history regarding the same.
2. Trans-sphenoidal resection of pituitary adenoma.
3. If the cause of Cushing's syndrome is not detected and the patient continues to be symptomatic, bilateral adrenalectomy may be considered.
4. Adrenalectomy, followed by radiotherapy and mitotane if adrenal cancer present.
5. Ectopic ACTH secretion: Tumor excision. Ketoconazole or metyrapone may be used preoperatively.

PCOS

Polycystic ovary syndrome (PCOS) is a heterogeneous endocrine disorder characterized primarily by ovulatory dysfunction and hyperandrogenism. It is the most common cause of infertility in women, with manifestations frequently beginning during adolescence.

Internationally accepted diagnostic criteria for adults, primarily based on the Rotterdam consensus, involve combinations of unexplained hyperandrogenism, anovulation, and polycystic ovarian morphology.

PCOS affects a significant proportion of women of reproductive age, with estimates ranging from 6% to 20% depending on the diagnostic criteria applied [9].

The precise cause of PCOS remains unknown, but it is believed to arise from a complex interplay of heritable and nonheritable factors, including intrauterine and extrauterine influences. Functional ovarian hyperandrogenism is generally the main contributor to the androgen excess, leading to hirsutism, anovulation, and polycystic ovaries.

Hyperandrogenism Excessive androgen production from the ovaries is a hallmark of PCOS. This can manifest as hirsutism, acne, and menstrual irregularities.

Insulin resistance (IR) Hyperinsulinemia can exacerbate ovarian androgen secretion and decrease hepatic sex hormone-binding globulin (SHBG) synthesis, leading to increased circulating testosterone concentrations.

Ovarian dysfunction Characterized by abnormal steroidogenesis and folliculogenesis, leading to anovulation. There appears to be a constitutively increased androgen production and CYP17A1 expression in theca cells in PCOS ovaries.

Neuroendocrine disruption Alterations in the hypothalamic–pituitary–ovarian axis including increased LH pulse amplitude and frequency.

Epigenetic and environmental factors [10] Include stress, diet, and exposure to environmental toxins.

Gut microbiome Emerging evidence suggests a potential role of the gut microbiome in the pathogenesis of PCOS.

Clinical Features [11]

Adolescent and adult females with PCOS may present with various clinical features, including:

Menstrual irregularities: Oligomenorrhea (infrequent periods) or amenorrhea (absence of periods) is common.

Hirsutism: Excessive terminal hair growth in a male pattern distribution. This is one of the primary clinical signs of hyperandrogenism. The modified Ferriman–Gallwey scoring system is a common tool used to evaluate hirsutism.

Acne: Treatment-resistant acne and inflammatory acne may be present.

Obesity.

Acanthosis nigricans.

Investigations [12]

Androgens (such as testosterone and androstenedione) are elevated.
LH levels—increased.
Anti-Müllerian hormone (AMH) levels are often elevated, reflecting increased follicle numbers.
Transvaginal ultrasound (TVUS): To assess ovarian morphology and identify polycystic ovaries, which are defined as having 20 or more follicles in one or both.

Differential Diagnosis

Hyperprolactinemia
Hypothyroidism
Cushing's syndrome
Adrenal hyperplasia

Management [13]

Diet and exercise.
Combined oral contraceptive pills (COCPs): To regulate menstrual cycles and treat hyperandrogenism. May be used only after the assessment of risk for thromboembolism.
Metformin: Used to improve insulin sensitivity and weight loss.
Spironolactone: An anti-androgen used to manage symptoms of hyperandrogenism such as hirsutism.
Anti-androgen medications: Such as cyproterone acetate can be used to reduce androgenic effects.

Fascinating Factoid Social media-trolled American comedienne Amy Schumer for her increasing weight and moon-like face. She was diagnosed to have Cushing's syndrome and went public about her condition to increase awareness of the condition.

Take-Home
Cushing's syndrome, a dangerous disease which requires active intervention may be masked by more common conditions like PCOD and obesity.

1. Thin skin, purple stria, and muscle wasting would call for a diagnosis of PCOD in to doubt and mandate evaluation for Cushing's syndrome.
2. Even if the diagnosis were PCOS alone, it has implications for the patient's future health since PCOS is a harbinger of the metabolic syndrome and T2DM.

References

1. Al Wattar BH, Fisher M, Bevington L, Talaulikar V, Davies M, Conway G, Yasmin E. Clinical practice guidelines on the diagnosis and management of polycystic ovary syndrome: a systematic review and quality assessment study. J Clin Endocrinol Metabol. 2021;106(8):2436–46.
2. Teede HJ, Misso ML, Costello MF, Dokras A, Laven J, Moran L, Piltonen T, Norman RJ. Recommendations from the international evidence-based guideline for the assessment and management of polycystic ovary syndrome. Hum Reprod. 2018;33(9):1602–18.
3. Hoeger KM, Dokras A, Piltonen T. Update on PCOS: consequences, challenges, and guiding treatment. J Clin Endocrinol Metabol. 2021;106(3):e1071–83.
4. Steffensen C, Bak AM, Zøylner Rubeck K, Jørgensen JO. Epidemiology of Cushing's syndrome. Neuroendocrinology. 2010;92(Suppl. 1):1–5.
5. Castinetti F, Morange I, Conte-Devolx B, Brue T. Cushing's disease. Orphanet J Rare Dis. 2012;7:1–9.
6. Buliman A, Tataranu L, Paun D, Mirica A, Dumitrache C. Cushing's disease: a multidisciplinary overview of the clinical features, diagnosis, and treatment. J Med Life. 2016;9(1):12–8.
7. Savas M, Mehta S, Agrawal N, van Rossum EF, Feelders RA. Approach to the patient: diagnosis of Cushing syndrome. J Clin Endocrinol Metabol. 2022;107(11):3162–74.
8. Castinetti F. Pharmacological treatment of Cushing's syndrome. Arch Med Res. 2023;54(8):102908.
9. Deswal R, Narwal V, Dang A, Pundir CS. The prevalence of polycystic ovary syndrome: a brief systematic review. J Hum Reprod Sci. 2020;13(4):261–71.
10. Diamanti-Kandarakis E, Kandarakis H, Legro RS. The role of genes and environment in the etiology of PCOS. Endocrine. 2006;30:19–26.
11. Futterweit W, Diamanti-Kandarakis E, Azziz R. Clinical features of the polycystic ovary syndrome. In: Androgen excess disorders in women: polycystic ovary syndrome and other disorders; 2007. p. 155–67.
12. Spritzer PM, Marchesan LB, Santos BR, Fighera TM. Hirsutism, normal androgens and diagnosis of PCOS. Diagnostics. 2022;12(8):1922.
13. Papadakis G, Kandaraki EA, Garidou A, Koutsaki M, Papalou O, Diamanti-Kandarakis E, Peppa M. Tailoring treatment for PCOS phenotypes. Expert Rev Endocrinol Metab. 2021;16(1):9–18.

23 Commonly Missed Diagnoses in the Elderly: The Quiet Grandma

Grade Easy.

Abstract An elderly lady with no previous comorbidities is found unconscious with no lateralizing neurological signs. Heart sounds are slightly muffled and bronchial breath sounds are present below scapula.

Story You are glad to hear that Mrs. Dominique, your old school headmistress, has moved to your neighborhood. She was a taskmaster when she was your teacher, but she has metamorphosed into a gentle, affectionate, old lady. The hard lines of her countenance and her lean greyhound body have changed into a round, jolly face and a pleasantly plump form. You visit her one evening with a gift of macaroons and settle down for a nice long chat.

She draws her embroidered cashmere shawl around herself and asks you about your work.

You describe your colleagues, your students, and your patients while discreetly mopping at the sweat on your forehead.

"Sorry if the temperature is set too high for you, Sahana."

"No problem at all, Ma'am."

Mrs. D sits plump and placid, munching on the macaroons and says

"You'll have to speak louder, my dear." You repeat your tale in a much louder voice and then ask, "How has your health been, Ma'am?"

"Well, at my age, I can't complain. Though I do feel tired, and my legs tend to ache at the end of the day."

"Mrs. D, have you considered a lifestyle modification to try and lose some weight?" She laughs loudly and says, "Life is short, eat dessert first!" and munches on another couple of macaroons.

You're busy the next couple of months juggling work and home when Mrs. Dominique's daughter phones you and tells you that she walked into her mother's house to find her unconscious. You quickly call an ambulance and run to the house.

S. Bhat, *Clinical Conundrums to Practice Diagnostic Reasoning*, https://doi.org/10.1007/978-981-95-0636-1_23

You do a rapid assessment of Mrs. D while waiting for the ambulance to arrive. She is stuporous.

GCS: E2V2M5. No lateralizing neurological signs.

Her skin is cool and dry.

Pulse: 60 beats per minute, BP 110/80 mm Hg

SpO2: 98% on room air.

She looks a little bloated but not very different from when you saw her 2 months ago. Your quick examination of systems yields little, though you do find that the heart sounds are slightly muffled, and there are bronchial breath sounds auscultable below the left scapula. The ambulance arrives and you accompany Mrs. D and her daughter to the hospital, praying sincerely that she recovers soon.

Question

(a) Was it just old age that was causing Mrs. D's initial nonspecific complaints or was something else going on?
(b) What might be responsible for the coma with no lateralizing signs?

Analysis

The following are the pertinent points from history and examination.

(a) History suggestive of weight gain—"her lean body has become pleasantly plump."
(b) History suggestive of cold intolerance (she has the heat on high and is wearing a shawl in spite of the heat).
(c) History suggestive of difficulty in hearing—"You'll have to speak louder"
(d) Bradycardia

All these are suggestive of hypothyroidism. However, further information may be obtained from the auscultatory findings. The muffled heart sounds and the bronchial breath sounds in the left infrascapular area (Ewart's sign) are suggestive of a pericardial effusion which further strengthens the diagnosis of hypothyroidism. The diagnosis at the time of hospital admission is likely to be due to myxedema coma.

Hypothyroidism and Myxedema Coma

Primary hypothyroidism accounts for 95% of cases, while central (secondary/tertiary) hypothyroidism comprises the remainder. Myxedema coma, the most severe manifestation of hypothyroidism, is a rare but life-threatening emergency with mortality rates approaching 40% despite treatment [1].

The prevalence of overt hypothyroidism in developed nations is approximately 0.3–0.4%, while subclinical hypothyroidism affects 4.3–8.5% of the population [2]. Myxedema coma occurs predominantly in elderly females during winter months, with an estimated incidence of 0.22 per million people annually.

Etiopathogenesis

Primary hypothyroidism typically results from autoimmune thyroiditis (Hashimoto's disease), characterized by progressive thyroid destruction through cell-mediated immunity and autoantibody production [3]. Other causes include iatrogenic (post surgery, post radioactive iodine treatment, due to antithyroid drugs), iodine deficiency or excess, and infiltrative disorders.

The clinical features of hypothyroidism may be attributed to one of two basic pathophysiological mechanisms. The first is a slowing of almost all metabolic processes—this results in fatigue, constipation, somnolence, bradycardia, intolerance to cold, and weight gain.

The second is the accumulation of glycosaminoglycans in many tissues—resulting in the characteristic nonpitting edema, the hoarseness of voice, and macroglossia [4].

Myxedema coma develops when severe hypothyroidism is complicated by a precipitating factor that overwhelms the body's compensatory mechanisms. Common triggers include infections, medications (especially sedatives), cold exposure, trauma, or cardiovascular events [5].

Clinical Features [6]

(a) Weight gain, fatigue, somnolence, nonpitting pedal edema, periorbital edema, macroglossia.
(b) Sensorineural deafness, delayed relaxation of tendon jerks, and hoarseness of voice
(c) Pericardial effusion

Myxedema coma manifests with [7, 8]:

- Altered mental status—ranging from lethargy to coma
- Hypothermia (often <35 °C)
- Bradycardia and hypotension

Diagnosis: Labs reveal either

(a) High TSH, low T4—hypothyroidism
(b) High TSH, normal T4—subclinical hypothyroidism
(c) Low/normal TSH, low T4—secondary hypothyroidism

In myxedema coma [9]:

- Thyroid function tests: Elevated TSH with low free T4 in primary hypothyroidism
- Complete blood count: Normocytic anemia, possible leukopenia
- Basic metabolic panel: Hyponatremia, hypoglycemia
- Cortisol level: To rule out concurrent adrenal insufficiency
- Blood gases: Respiratory acidosis, hypoxemia
- Cardiac enzymes: To evaluate for precipitating cardiac event

Treatment [10]

Management of uncomplicated hypothyroidism involves oral levothyroxine replacement, starting at 25–50 mcg daily in elderly or cardiac patients and gradually increasing to achieve target TSH levels.

Myxedema coma requires aggressive intervention:

1. Thyroid hormone replacement:
    - IV levothyroxine: Loading dose 200–400 mcg, followed by 50–100 mcg daily.
    - Consider concurrent T3 supplementation in severe cases.
2. Supportive care:
    - Mechanical ventilation if needed
    - Careful fluid replacement
    - Passive rewarming
    - Treatment of precipitating factors
3. Stress-dose glucocorticoids until adrenal insufficiency is excluded

Key Takeaway
Hypothyroidism is difficult to diagnose in the elderly because of the comorbid illnesses which might mask the presentation, because many of the features of hypothyroidism mimic those of normal aging and because normal aging itself causes an upward shift in TSH levels.

References

1. Ono Y, Ono S, Yasunaga H, Matsui H, Fushimi K, Tanaka Y. Clinical characteristics and outcomes of myxedema coma: analysis of a national inpatient database in Japan. J Epidemiol. 2017;27(3):117–22.
2. Taylor PN, Albrecht D, Scholz A, Gutierrez-Buey G, Lazarus JH, Dayan CM, Okosieme OE. Global epidemiology of hyperthyroidism and hypothyroidism. Nat Rev Endocrinol. 2018;14(5):301–16.
3. Zamwar UM, Muneshwar KN. Epidemiology, types, causes, clinical presentation, diagnosis, and treatment of hypothyroidism. Cureus [Internet]. 2023 [cited 2025 Mar 19]. Available from: https://www.cureus.com/articles/175208-epidemiology-types-causes-clinical-presentation-diagnosis-and-treatment-of-hypothyroidism
4. Smith TJ, Bahn RS, Gorman CA. Connective tissue, glycosaminoglycans, and diseases the thyroid. Endocr Rev. 1989;10(3):366–91.
5. Wiersinga WM. Myxedema and coma (severe hypothyroidism). Endotext [Internet]. 2018 Apr 25.
6. Garber JR, Cobin RH, Gharib H, Hennessey JV, Klein I, Mechanick JI, Pessah-Pollack R, Singer PA, Woeber KA. Clinical practice guidelines for hypothyroidism in adults: cosponsored by the American Association of Clinical Endocrinologists and the American Thyroid Association. Endocr Pract. 2012;18(6):988–1028.
7. Tsai TY, Tu YK, Munir KM, Lin SM, Chang RH, Kao SL, Loh CH, Peng CC, Huang HK. Association of hypothyroidism and mortality in the elderly population: a systematic review and meta-analysis. J Clin Endocrinol Metabol. 2020;105(6):2068–80.
8. Chen DH, Hurtado CR, Chang P, Zakher M, Angell TE. Clinical features and outcomes of myxedema coma in patients hospitalized for hypothyroidism: analysis of the United States national inpatient sample. Thyroid. 2024;34(4):419–28.
9. Bourcier S, Coutrot M, Ferré A, Van Grunderbeeck N, Charpentier J, Hraiech S, Azoulay E, Nseir S, Aissaoui N, Messika J, Fillatre P. Persichini, R., Carreira, S., Lautrette, A., Delmas, C., Terzi, N., Mégarbane, B., Lascarrou, J. B., Razazi, K., Repessé, X., … Schmidt, M. Critically ill severe hypothyroidism: a retrospective multicenter cohort study. Annals of intensive care, 2023;13(1):15. https://doi.org/10.1186/s13613–023–01112–1
10. Wall CR. Myxedema coma: diagnosis and treatment. Am Fam Physician. 2000;62(11):2485–90.

24 Dizziness, Blurred Vison, and Slurred Speech: The Depressed Decorator

Grade Easy.

Abstract An adult male smoker presents with dizziness and dysarthria while at work. Neurological examination is normal.

Story Nag, your first patient on a winter Monday, is a quiet, sad-looking man. He allows his wife to describe his health issues, while he sits silent and pensive, gazing at the floor.

"I'm more than a little worried doctor," Mrs. Nag says. "Nag is just not himself these days. For the last month or so, he has been coming home early from work saying he is tired and unable to function. But yesterday was especially bad. His employee brought him home saying he was talking gibberish."

"What work do you do?" you ask Nag.

"I have my own interior decoration firm. I have 3 people working under me," he responds.

"Do you remember what happened yesterday?"

"Of course. I was hammering in some nails to hang a really large painting on the wall. As has been happening for the last couple of months, I started getting tired very soon. Still, I forced myself to continue. But then, I started feeling dizzy and I couldn't see clearly. Frightened, I called for help."

Mrs. Nag continues the tale.

"His employee said Nag was mumbling words that could not be understood. He brought him home immediately, but by then things had settled somewhat."

"Mr. Nag, you said you were feeling tired. Can you describe what exactly you mean?"

"I found it difficult to continue hammering the nails in—my arm, especially my left arm started cramping and hurting like crazy."

"Have there been any medical problems in the past?"

"No, I've been perfectly well."

S. Bhat, *Clinical Conundrums to Practice Diagnostic Reasoning*,
https://doi.org/10.1007/978-981-95-0636-1_24

"Any stressors?"

"Not really. I had really weird parents though—they thought that the fact that I used my left hand to write and paint was sinister, and they tried their best to change that. I'm happy to say that I resisted their efforts and I'm a proud lefty."

"We are facing some financial issues and Nag is losing his sleep over that doctor," Mrs. Nag confides.

"May I know whether you smoke, drink or use recreational drugs?"

"I don't drink or do drugs, but I smoke occasionally. "

Mrs. Nag snorts, "Occasionally?! He smokes at least one pack a day, doctor."

You proceed with a detailed neurological examination. Cranial nerves, including fundus are normal. You examine the extraocular movements and find they are full. Power and sensation are normal, deep tendon reflexes are preserved, and the plantar is down-going. In fact, apart from the nicotine stains on the fingers, an arcus lipemialis, and a slight discrepancy between the pulse volume in the upper limbs, you are surprised to find that the examination is essentially normal.

Questions What was wrong with Nag? Was it lack of sleep and stress? Or something else?

How would you like to proceed with investigations and diagnosis?

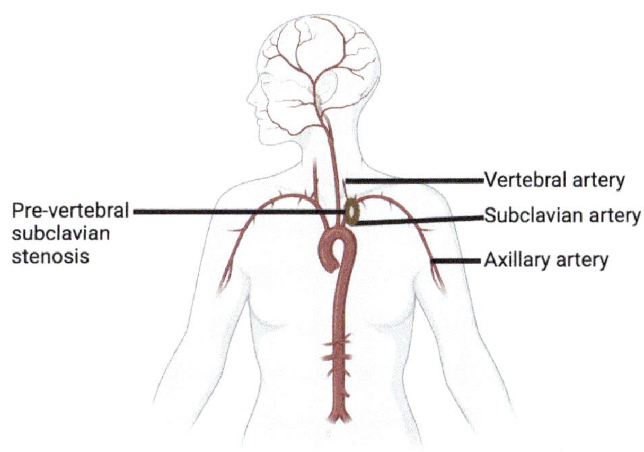

Fig. 24.1 Vertebral, subclavian, and axillary arteries. (Created in BioRender. Bhat, S. (2025) https://BioRender.com/i60h880)

Analysis

Here is an adult male with risk factors for atherosclerosis—smoking and dyslipidemia (the presence of arcus lipemialis is a clue). He gives a clear history of cramping and ache in the left upper limb on exertion which is suggestive of claudication pain. This would suggest vascular disease involving the axillary artery which supplies the upper limb. How do we connect this to his brainstem symptoms—dizziness, diplopia, and dysarthria? The answer lies in the anatomy of upper limb circulation (Fig. 24.1).

Occlusion of the subclavian artery proximal to the branching off of the vertebral artery results in a decrease in blood flow to the axillary artery, especially during exertion [1]. The lower pressure in the axillary artery may result in retrograde flow in the vertebral artery [2]. If the collateral circulation is not sufficiently well developed, then symptoms of brainstem ischemia may develop [3].

Subclavian steal syndrome is defined as vertebrobasilar insufficiency causing brainstem ischemia caused by prevertebral stenosis of the subclavian artery [4]. Vascular steal which remains asymptomatic is known as the subclavian steal *phenomenon* [5]. In some case series, subclavian steal syndrome is associated with 2.2% cases of acute ischemic stroke [6].

Etiopathogenesis

The main cause of subclavian steal syndrome is atherosclerosis [7]. Other causes include Takayasu arteritis, giant cell arteritis, and thoracic outlet syndrome.

The subclavian artery, after giving off branches including the vertebral artery, continues as the axillary artery which is the main blood supply to the upper limb. The vertebral arteries unite to form the basilar artery which connects through the circle of Willis to the carotid arterioles. When there is stenosis in the subclavian artery, blood supply to the affected arm is decreased, especially during exercise [8].

Hence, exertion is associated with cramping and pain in the upper limb. Retrograde flow from the vertebral artery to the subclavian may cause symptoms and signs of vertebrobasilar insufficiency.

Clinical Features [1, 9]

The following neurological symptoms may be precipitated by exercise of the ischemic arm:

(a) Dizziness
(b) Binocular diplopia
(c) Dysarthria
(d) Syncope
(e) Drop attacks
(f) Asymmetry between upper limb pulses and difference in blood pressure between the left and right upper limbs (more than 20 mm Hg)
(g) Supraclavicular / suboccipital thrills/bruits
(h) Atrophic nails

Diagnosis

1. Risk factor assessment: fasting blood sugar and lipid profile.
2. Duplex ultrasonography (US), computed tomography (CT) angiography (CTA), four-vessel cerebral arteriography, magnetic resonance angiography (MRA), and chest radiography.
3. MRA techniques like 2-D TOF MRI and phase contrast MRI can show flow reversal in the vertebral artery (VA).

Treatment [9]

1. Smoking cessation program
2. Risk factor assessment and management (blood sugar, lipid profile, hyperhomocysteinemia)
3. Antiplatelet agent if subclavian stenosis is due to atherosclerotic artery disease
4. Stenting or angioplasty of stenosed artery
5. Endarterectomy
6. Surgical by-pass
7. Stenting or angioplasty of stenosed artery

References

1. Osiro S, Zurada A, Gielecki J, Shoja MM, Tubbs RS, Loukas M. A review of subclavian steal syndrome with clinical correlation. Med Sci Monit. 2012;18(5):RA57–63.
2. Platz M. Doppler ultrasound studies of subclavian steal hemodynamics in subclavian stenosis. Thorac Cardiovasc Surg. 2008;27:404–7.
3. Marshall RJ, Mantini EL. Dynamics of the collateral circulation in patients with subclavian steal. Circulation. 1965;31(2):249–54.
4. Parrott JC. The subclavian steal syndrome. Arch Surg. 1964;88(4):661–5.
5. Toole JF, McGraw CP. The steal syndromes. Annu Rev Med. 1975;26:321–9.
6. Bajko Z, Motataianu A, Stoian A, Barcutean L, Andone S, Maier S, Drăghici IA, Cioban A, Balasa R. Prevalence and clinical characteristics of subclavian steal phenomenon/syndrome in patients with acute ischemic stroke. J Clin Med. 2021;10(22):5237.
7. Potter BJ, Pinto DS. Subclavian steal syndrome. Circulation. 2014;129(22):2320–3.
8. Saha T, Naqvi SY, Ayah OA, McCormick D, Goldberg S. Subclavian artery disease: diagnosis and therapy. Am J Med. 2017;130(4):409–16.
9. Fields WS. Neurovascular syndromes of the neck and shoulders. Semin Neurol. 2008;1:301–9.
10. Rafailidis V, Li X, Chryssogonidis I, Rengier F, Rajiah P, Wieker CM, Kalva S, Ganguli S, Partovi S. Multimodality imaging and endovascular treatment options of subclavian steal syndrome. Can Assoc Radiol J. 2018;69(4):493–507.

Middle-Aged Male with Burning Sensation at Fingertips and Rash: The Alpha Gal and Her Husband

25

Grade Moderate.

Abstract A middle-aged male presenting with history suggestive of transient ischemic attack and burning pain in his fingers.

Story Ms. J is the CEO of a company that makes pretty, yet practical shoes for women. She is a true Alpha Gal—a boss lady who is shining in her career, is known for her kindness and decisiveness, and is the mother of two wonderful kids. So, you have a bit of a fan girl moment when your secretary tells you that not only does Ms. J want to come to you for her annual health check, but she wants to bring her husband to you too!

Ms. J reaches your clinic at exactly the right time, greets you politely and introduces her husband Mr. J.

"Doctor, my annual health check is pending, but that can happen at any time. The main reason that I came here today is that I'm very concerned about J's health, and I heard that you are an expert diagnostician."

"I certainly will do my very best to help. Mr J, can you please sit down and let me know what exactly is going on?"

"There are lots of things—I've met so many doctors but after numerous tests they finally suggest that it's stress and it's all in my mind. But I'm sure it is not, doctor. I'm not stressed, and …"

"And he's certainly not the kind of person to have an imaginary illness," chimes in Ms. J. "If he says something is wrong, I believe him."

"So, Mr. J, what problem troubles you the most?"

"Well, I would say it's the burning pain in my fingers and toes. It is most unpleasant. It comes on once in a while, in waves. Some days, I'm absolutely fine and on some days the pain is disabling."

"I see. What else?"

S. Bhat, *Clinical Conundrums to Practice Diagnostic Reasoning*,
https://doi.org/10.1007/978-981-95-0636-1_25

"Doctor, one particular problem dates from my childhood. You know, I can't tolerate heat at all! Perhaps it is because I do not sweat much."

"That must be quite troublesome. Is there anything else?"

"I'm very sensitive to the environment and to what I eat and drink. Even a slight deviation from my usual diet means I start throwing up and have tummy pain and loose stools. But the reason that both my wife and I panicked is this: last night we were at a dinner honouring her and suddenly I couldn't move my right hand to use my knife … my speech didn't make sense. It didn't last more than a couple of minutes, but it was really frightening."

"Yes, it must have been," you say sympathetically.

"May I ask—do you have diabetes? Or do you consume a significant quantity of alcohol? Do you smoke?"

"No to all. I've been abstinent since the age of 20."

"How about your parents and siblings? How is their health?"

"I'm the only child. My parents are healthy. But my mother's 2 brothers passed away at a young age—one due to a stroke and one due to a heart attack."

"May I examine you?"

You look at Mr. J's face again and begin to notice that it actually is a little strange looking. His lips are full, almost like a woman's. However, this is counteracted by the prominence of his jaw, and the bushiness of his eyebrows. Further examination reveals a strange rash on his abdomen which you can't quite characterize.

The apex is forceful and palpable on the left 5th intercostal space half an inch lateral to the midclavicular line. The ankle jerk is absent bilaterally, but there are no other focal neurological deficits.

Questions In spite of what Mr. and Mrs. J believe, is this disparate set of symptoms and signs more functional than organic?

Analysis

The problem with rare diseases like this is they do not form part of the mental list of differential diagnoses that physicians have. However, there are certain clues to be discerned from the story:

(a) First, acroparesthesias—the burning pain in the fingers and toes. The causes of acroparesthesia are the Guillain–Barré syndrome or vasculitis (when acute in onset and rapid in progression). Chronic acroparesthesia may be due to diabetes, Vitamin B12 deficiency, monoclonal gammopathy of undetermined significance, or Fabry's disease [1]. Periodic crises of acroparesthesia are highly suggestive of Fabry's disease.
(b) The hypohidrosis and heat intolerance.
(c) The chronic pain in abdomen, vomiting, and loose stools.
(d) The history suggestive of a TIA.
(e) The rash.
(f) The family history of maternal uncles suffering from premature vascular disease suggesting X-linked inheritance.
(g) Finaly, there is the clue in the title—the Alpha Gal.

Thus, we have an X-linked disease which causes paroxysmal acroparesthesia, rash, transient ischemic attacks and left ventricular hypertrophy. Taken together, they are indicative of Fabry's disease.

Fabry's disease is an X-linked inborn error of metabolism which affects the functioning of the glycosphingolipid pathway and leads to the accumulation of globotriaosylceramide (Gb3) in various cells causing multisystem clinical manifestations [2].

Etiopathogenesis [3, 4]: The GLA gene is located on the long arm of the X chromosome (Xq22)4 and encodes the lysosomal hydrolase alpha-galactosidase A (alpha-Gal A). Alpha-Gal A catalyzes the hydrolytic cleavage of the terminal galactose from Gb32 (Fig. 25.1).

Deficiency of this hydrolase results in the accumulation of the incompletely degraded Gb3 substrate intracellularly, particularly in lysosomes [5]. The debris is

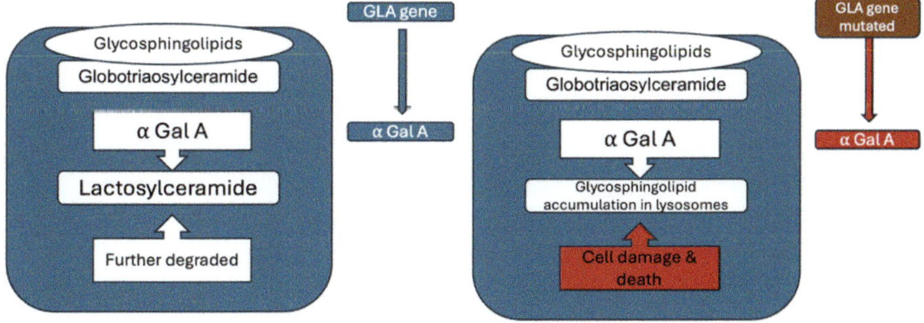

Fig 25.1 Pathogenesis of Fabry's disease

stored as intracytoplasmic masses and leads to cellular dysfunction or degeneration—it has cytotoxic, pro-inflammatory, and profibrotic effects.

Gb3 accumulates in the kidneys, heart, and CNS. In the heart, Gb3 leads to left ventricular hypertrophy (LVH), myocardial fibrosis, and arrhythmias. In the nervous system, it contributes to neuropathic pain, TIA, and stroke.

Being X-linked, males with a GLA mutation are typically more severely affected. Heterozygous females can exhibit a range of symptoms, from asymptomatic to severe.

Clinical Features [6]

(a) Hypohidrosis
(b) Angiokeratomas [7]
(c) Corneal opacities
(d) *Neurologic manifestations* [8]:
  (i) Neuropathic pain (acroparesthesia)
  (ii) TIA and stroke
  (iii) Autonomic dysfunction
  (iv) Aneurysms
  (v) White matter lesions
(e) *Cardiovascular system* [9]:
  (i) Angina, dyspnea
  (ii) Palpitations or syncope
  (iii) Unexplained LVH is typical of Fabry's cardiac disease
  (iv) Aortic and mitral regurgitation
  (v) Conduction defects and arrhythmias

GIT: Loose stools, vomiting, and abdominal pain [10]
Kidneys: Proteinuria, isosthenuria, polyuria, and polydipsia, CKD [11]

Investigations [12]

(a) Urinalysis and quantification of proteinuria.
(b) Electrocardiogram.
(c) Enzyme assay to measure alpha-Gal A activity in leukocytes / plasma.
(d) Molecular genetic testing to confirm the diagnosis.
(e) Tissue biopsy: Renal or endomyocardial biopsy, particularly in patients with newly described GLA variants of unknown significance.
(f) Imaging: Baseline magnetic resonance imaging (MRI) of the heart and brain may be performed, especially in females and patients with cardiac or neurologic manifestations.

Treatment [13, 14]

(a) Enzyme replacement therapy (ERT): Recombinant alpha-Gal A (agalsidase alfa and agalsidase beta) [15].
(b) Pharmacologic chaperone therapy: Migalastat hydrochloride is an oral chaperone that stabilizes mutated alpha-Gal A, improving its folding and trafficking [16, 17].
(c) Gabapentin, pregabalin, carbamazepine, or amitriptyline for the alleviation of neuropathic pain [18].
(d) Antiarrhythmic therapy and heart failure management.
(e) ACE inhibitors or ARBs to lower blood pressure and reduce proteinuria.
(f) Primary / secondary prevention of ischemic stroke with antiplatelet agents and statins.

Key Takeaway
A diagnosis of Fabry's disease must be considered in any patient who presents with neuropathic pain and early TIA/stroke.

References

1. Harzer K, Beck-Wödl S, Haack TB. Angiokeratoma corporis diffusum with severe acroparesthesia, an endothelial abnormality, and inconspicuous genetic findings. J Cutan Pathol. 2022;49(3):293–8.
2. Zarate YA, Hopkin RJ. Fabry's disease. Lancet. 2008;372(9647):1427–35.
3. Masson C, Cissé I, Simon V, Insalaco P, Audran M. Fabry disease: a review. Joint Bone Spine. 2004;71(5):381–3.
4. Kok K, Zwiers KC, Boot RG, Overkleeft HS, Aerts JMFG, Artola M. Fabry disease: molecular basis, pathophysiology, diagnostics and potential therapeutic directions. Biomolecules. 2021;11(2):271.
5. Li X, Ren X, Zhang Y, Ding L, Huo M, Li Q. Fabry disease: Mechanism and therapeutics strategies. Front Pharmacol [Internet]. 2022 [cited 2025 Mar 24];13. Available from: https://www.frontiersin.org/journals/pharmacology/articles/10.3389/fphar.2022.1025740/full
6. Brady RO, Schiffmann R. Clinical features of and recent advances in therapy for Fabry disease. JAMA. 2000;284(21):2771–5.
7. Al-Chaer RN, Folkmann M, Mårtensson NL, Feldt-Rasmussen U, Mogensen M. Cutaneous manifestations of Fabry disease: a systematic review. J Dermatol [Internet]. [cited 2025 Mar 24]. Available from: https://onlinelibrary.wiley.com/doi/abs/10.1111/1346-8138.17690
8. Møller AT, Jensen TS. Neurological manifestations in Fabry's disease. Nat Clin Pract Neurol. 2007;3(2):95–106.
9. Hung CL, Wu YW, Lin CC, Lai CH, Juang JJ, Chao TH, Kuo L, Sung KT, Wang CY, Wang CL, Chu CY. 2021 TSOC expert consensus on the clinical features, diagnosis, and clinical management of cardiac manifestations of Fabry disease. Acta Cardiologica Sinica. 2021;37(4):337.
10. Lenders M, Brand E. Fabry disease—a multisystemic disease with gastrointestinal manifestations. Gut Microbes. 2022;14(1):2027852.
11. Silva CAB, Moura-Neto JA, dos Reis MA, Vieira Neto OM, Barreto FC. Renal manifestations of Fabry disease: a narrative review. Can J Kidney Health Dis. 2021;(8):2054358120985627.

12. Michaud M, Mauhin W, Belmatoug N, Garnotel R, Bedreddine N, Catros F, Ancellin S, Lidove O, Gaches F. When and how to diagnose Fabry disease in clinical pratice. Am J Med Sci. 2020;360(6):641–9.
13. van der Veen SJ, Hollak CE, van Kuilenburg AB, Langeveld M. Developments in the treatment of Fabry disease. J Inherit Metab Dis. 2020;43(5):908–21.
14. Umer M, Kalra DK. Treatment of Fabry disease: established and emerging therapies. Pharmaceuticals. 2023;16(2):320.
15. Iacobucci I, Hay Mele B, Cozzolino F, Monaco V, Cimmaruta C, Monti M, Andreotti G, Monticelli M. Enzyme replacement therapy for FABRY disease: possible strategies to improve its efficacy. Int J Mol Sci. 2023;24(5):4548.
16. Nowicki M, Bazan-Socha S, Błażejewska-Hyżorek B, Kłopotowski MM, Komar M, Kusztal MA, et al. A review and recommendations for oral chaperone therapy in adult patients with Fabry disease. Orphanet J Rare Dis. 2024;19(1):16.
17. Lenders M, Nordbeck P, Kurschat C, Eveslage M, Karabul N, Kaufeld J, et al. Treatment of Fabry Disease management with migalastat—outcome from a prospective 24 months observational multicenter study (FAMOUS). Eur Heart J. 2022;8(3):272–81.
18. Burand AJJ, Stucky CL. Fabry disease pain: patient and preclinical parallels. Pain. 2021;162(5):1305.

26 Bone, Skin, and GI Symptoms in a Young Female: The Bachelorette Party

Grade Moderate.

Abstract A young female presenting with history suggestive of polyarthritis, abdominal pain, and fever.

Story Sampriti presents to your clinic one rainy Wednesday morning. She winces as she sits down, briefly leaning on the table for support. You open her file and note that that she is 26 years old and has no previous comorbidities.

"I'm feeling a little run down since last month when I returned from a trip that we had arranged as a bachelorette party for one of our friends," she says.

"Where did you travel?" you inquire politely.

"Koh Samui—3 days of sunshine, swimming, hot sun, and cold beer. I guess I'm paying for my sins now," she says ruefully. "It's not just this trip—I've been living dangerously for a while now," she smiles wanly—"Too much alcohol, too little sleep and…"

"And?"

"And nothing."

"I noticed—you seemed to be in pain."

"Yes, doctor. I thought it was because of too much dancing—my feet started hurting, then my left knee. But what's weird is now my right wrist hurts too and that doesn't make sense."

"Is there anything apart from the joint pain?"

"Not really—oh wait—I did have a little bit of a fever a week ago, just when we returned from our trip. And I'm not sure if this is important but I've had this rash on my hands for 2 days but then it disappeared."

"Is there anyone in the family who suffers from joint pain or rash? Anyone with lupus or rheumatoid arthritis?"

"No, doctor."

S. Bhat, *Clinical Conundrums to Practice Diagnostic Reasoning*,
https://doi.org/10.1007/978-981-95-0636-1_26

"You mentioned that you have been drinking a little too much lately—how much would you say is your average weekly consumption?"

"Oh, I don't know—may be a glass of wine or two everyday along with lunch or dinner. And then a nightcap—maybe a whiskey on the rocks. Cocktails when I go out with my gang, maybe a couple of times a week."

"Ok. May I ask—are you sexually active?"

"Yes, I have been since I was 17."

"And do you practice safe sex?"

"Usually, yes. Though when I don't, I am sure to use a douche."

"One more thing, doc—I've been having this pain here in my tummy for more than a couple of months now," she says, indicating her right hypochondrium.

You proceed to examine Sampriti and note the following:

Temperature: 38.5 degrees C. BP: 120/70 mm Hg.

There is no jaundice or anemia.

The patient's right wrist is tender, especially on the flexor aspect, and the index finger is swollen. The fingers of the right hand are slightly flexed when at rest, and passive extension is painful.

There is rebound tenderness in the right hypochondrium, but other systems are essentially normal, apart from a friction rub just below the right lung base.

You obtain consent to perform a pelvic examination and note that the uterus is tender on bimanual palpation.

Question Is there a unifying diagnosis for Sampriti's rash, joint pain, and abdominal pain?

Analysis

The crucial points to note here are a sexually active young female presenting with fever, polyarthritis, and a rash on the palms. Rash involving the palms and soles is not very common; some of the conditions with this pattern of rash include [1]:

(a) Dyshidrotic eczema
(b) Secondary syphilis.
(c) Rocky mountain spotted fever
(d) Gonorrhea
(e) Bacterial endocarditis
(f) Toxic shock syndrome

Of these, endocarditis and toxic shock syndrome are less likely given the history. Secondary syphilis is a possibility; however, arthritis is not often seen in syphilis. Rocky mountain spotted fever is still a possibility. The tenosynovitis, especially the painful passive extension on the background of the palmar rash [2], and the tender uterus on bimanual examination [3] narrow the diagnosis down to disseminated gonococcal infection.

Answer

Sampriti has disseminated gonococcal infection (DGI) along with the Fitz Hugh Curtis syndrome.

The constellation of signs and symptoms including tenosynovitis, arthritis, and skin lesions due to bacteremic spread of the sexually transmitted bacteria Neisseria gonorrhea is known as Disseminated Gonococcal Infection (DGI) [4].

The importance of timely diagnosis and treatment of gonorrhea lies in its propensity to cause pelvic inflammatory disease [5] as well as to facilitate the transmission of HIV [6]. The consequences of gonorrhea, especially in females, are long-lasting—tubal factor infertility, cervicitis, ectopic pregnancy, and chronic pelvic pain [7].

Epidemiology

Infection with Neisseria gonorrheae is quite common, especially in the African continent; DGI less so. DGI affects approximately 0.5–3% of patients with gonorrheal infections, predominantly impacting young, sexually active adults aged 15–35 [8].

Etiopathogenesis

Neisseria gonorrheae is a Gram-negative diplococcus.

Certain strains of N. gonorrheae are more likely to cause DGI [9].

These strains cause less complement activation and hence are able to evade host defenses and thrive in the joints, skin, and blood.

Fitz Hugh Curtis syndrome is due to the inflammation of Glisson's capsule of the liver and occurs with sexually transmitted illnesses including gonorrhea and chlamydia.

Risk Factors for DGI

- Menstruation [10].
- Pregnancy or postpartum period [11].
- Congenital or acquired complement deficiencies (C5, C6, C7, or C8).
- Systemic lupus erythematosus (SLE).
- Therapy with eculizumab.
- The use of a douche may predispose to gonorrhea and other pelvic inflammatory disease [12].

Clinical Features [13]

(a) Rash may occur either by direct inoculation or as one of the manifestation of DGI [14].
(b) Nonpruritic papules on palms, soles, and trunk.
(c) Abscesses, cellulitis, petechiae, purpuric macules, necrotizing fasciitis, and vasculitis [15].
(d) Polyarthralgia.
(e) Tenosynovitis [16].

Diagnosis

1. Culture of blood, synovial fluid, and specimens from genitourinary samples.
2. Gram stain or methylene blue stain of secretions will show the characteristic coffee bean diplococci.

To Note Even in patients with Fitz Hugh Curtis syndrome, though there is notable tender hepatomegaly, liver function is frequently normal.

Treatment

Patients with DGI require hospitalization for intravenous antibiotics [17].

Antibiotic resistant strains are increasing; effective antibiotics include ceftriaxone, tigecycline, and ertapenem. Doxycycline may be added if chlamydia is suspected, and pregnancy has been excluded.

Prevention

At present, no effective vaccine for gonorrhea exists, though some evidence from real-world experience shows that meningococcal vaccine may decrease the incidence and severity of gonorrhea.

Fascinating Factoid The colloquial term for gonorrhea "the clap" probably originates from the French red-light district of Les Clapiers.

Key Takeaway
Suspect DGI in a sexually active adult presenting with asymmetrical oligoarthritis +/− rash and systemic symptoms.

References

1. Wright K, Valley V. Clinical Pearls Palmar Rash. Acad Emerg Med. 2001;8(12):1178–86.
2. Jain N, Saadat S, Goldberg M. Flexor Tenosynovitis caused by Neisseria gonorrhea infection: case series, literature review, and treatment recommendations. Arch Plast Surg. 2023;50:216–9.
3. Comkornruecha M. Gonococcal infections. Pediatr Rev. 2013;34(5):228–34.
4. Rice PA. Gonococcal Arthritis (Disseminated Gonococcal Infection). Infect Dis Clin. 2005;19(4):853–61.
5. Sexually transmitted disease surveillance 2018 [Internet] [cited 2025 Jan 24]. Available from: https://stacks.cdc.gov/view/cdc/79370
6. Bowen VB, Braxton J, Davis DW, Flagg EW, Grey J, Grier L, Harvey A, Kidd S, Kreisel K, Llata E, Mauk K. Sexually transmitted disease surveillance. 2018.
7. Mårdh PA. Complications and long-term sequelae of infections by Neisseria gonorrhoeae. In: Sequelae and long-term consequences of infectious diseases [Internet]. John Wiley & Sons, Ltd; 2009 [cited 2025 Mar 26]. p. 169–85. Available from: https://onlinelibrary.wiley.com/doi/abs/10.1128/9781555815486.ch9
8. Noble RC, Reyes RR, Parekh MC, Haley JV. Incidence of disseminated gonococcal infection correlated with the presence of AHU auxotype of Neisseria gonorrhoeae in a community. Sex Transm Dis. 1984;11(2):68–71.
9. Unemo M, Dillon JA. Review and international recommendation of methods for typing Neisseria gonorrhoeae isolates and their implications for improved knowledge of gonococcal epidemiology, treatment, and biology. Clin Microbiol Rev. 2011;24(3):447–58.
10. Britigan BE, Cohen MS, Sparling PF. Gonococcal infection: a model of molecular pathogenesis. N Engl J Med. 1985;312(26):1683–94.
11. El Mezouar I, Tahiri L, Lazrak F, Berrada K, Harzy T. Gonococcal polyarthritis with sternoclavicular joint involvement in pregnant woman: a case report. Pan Afr Med J. 2014;17:242.

12. Ness RB, Hillier SL, Kip KE, Richter HE, Soper DE, Stamm CA, McGregor JA, Bass DC, Rice P, Sweet RL. Douching, pelvic inflammatory disease, and incident gonococcal and chlamydial genital infection in a cohort of high-risk women. Am J Epidemiol. 2005;161(2):186–95.
13. Bleich AT, Sheffield JS, Wendel GD Jr, Sigman A, Cunningham FG. Disseminated gonococcal infection in women. Obstetr Gynecol. 2012;119(3):597–602.
14. Scott MJ. Primary cutaneous Neisseria gonorrhoeae infections. Arch Dermatol. 1982;118(5):351–2.
15. Beatrous SV, Grisoli SB, Riahi RR, Matherne RJ. Cutaneous manifestations of disseminated gonococcemia. Dermatol Online J [Internet]. 2017 [cited 2025 Mar 26];23(1). Available from: https://escholarship.org/uc/item/33b24006.
16. García-De La Torre I, Nava-Zavala A. Gonococcal and nongonococcal arthritis. Rheum Dis Clin N Am. 2009;35(1):63–73.
17. Ruiz García Y, Marrazzo J, Martinón-Torres F, Workowski K, Giordano G, Pizza M, Sohn WY. Urgent need to understand and prevent gonococcal infection: from the laboratory to real-world context. J Infect Dis. 2024;230(4):e758–67.

Fever and Rash in a Traveller: The Catastrophic Rash

27

Grade Very easy.

Abstract A traveller to the Middle East presenting with complaints of sore throat, body ache, headache, and fever.

Story Manad returns from Haj tired but happy. He assumes it is the exertion and excitement of the journey which is exhausting him. Four days later, however, he is feeling worse and calls his boss at the taxi service to ask for some days off.

He looks a little ill when he comes to your clinic for a consult.

"What seems to be the problem?" you ask.

"It began with a sore throat after I got back from my trip, but I managed with hot tea and saltwater gargles—I thought it would get better soon. However, it didn't. I started developing severe body ache, doctor—maybe because of the strain of the distance I have travelled over the last week."

"Anything apart from these problems?"

"My head hurts too, and I couldn't keep down my breakfast this morning."

"Ok, can you lie down please, let me examine you."

You perform a detailed physical examination, but apart from a temperature of 100 degree, you find nothing abnormal. You prescribe an antipyretic and bed rest and tell Manad to review if he is not feeling better in the next couple of days.

The next morning, you get a call from the emergency department saying that Manad has just presented with a very severe headache, and he is quite sick. You rush down to the ED and realize that the casualty medical officer was not exaggerating. The hapless patient's heart rate is 100/min, and BP is 96/60 mm Hg. He is sweating profusely. You note that there is a faint ecchymotic rash at the waistline which Manad ascribes to the new tight belt that he is wearing. Kernig's sign and Brudzinski's head and neck sign are positive.

S. Bhat, *Clinical Conundrums to Practice Diagnostic Reasoning*,
https://doi.org/10.1007/978-981-95-0636-1_27

You shift the patient to the intensive care unit and order appropriate investigations and treatment. Nurse calls you to say that there is significant oozing from intravenous access and venipuncture sites.

Question What is happening to Manad? Is it the seasonal flu or something worse? How would you manage him?

Analysis

The clues:

(a) Return from Haj [1, 2]
(b) Headache, rash, and severe muscle ache

All these together go in favor of meningococcal meningitis. It is important to remember that the *absence of signs of meningeal irritation does not rule out meningeal infection, as these are not invariably present*. The severe muscle ache and headache along with the travel history is a strong pointer to meningitis. The rash, low blood pressure, and tachycardia are warning signs that the patient may be going in for further complications—septic shock or disseminated intravascular coagulation (DIC).

Definition

Neisseria meningitides is a common etiology of bacterial meningitis, and mortality rates are high, ranging from 13% in high-income countries to 54% in low-income countries. Meningococcal septicemia may be associated with the production of endotoxin which activates the coagulation cascade, suppresses fibrinolysis, and results in disseminated intravascular coagulation (Fig. 27.1).

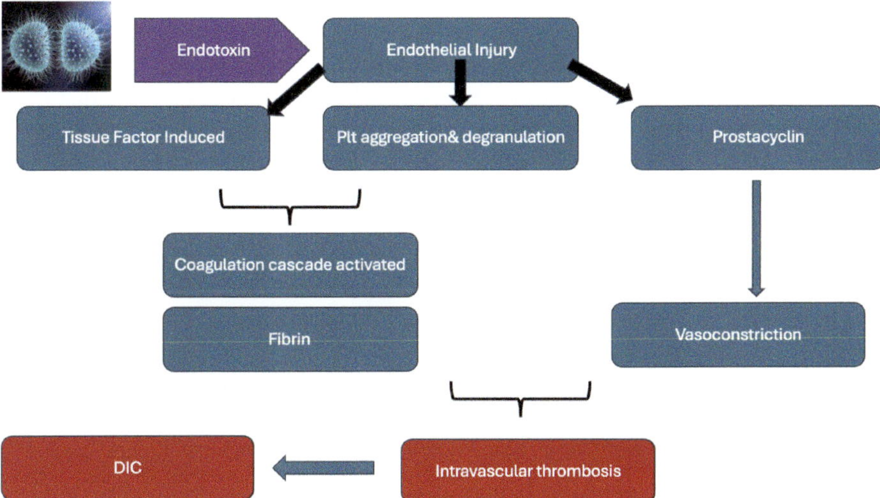

Fig. 27.1 Pathogenesis of DIC in meningococcemia

Etiopathogenesis

Meningococcemia is caused by *Neisseria meningitidis*, a Gram-negative diplococcus. Meningococcal endotoxin is the initiating factor for intravascular thrombosis and consumption coagulopathy [3] (Fig. 27.1).

Clinical Features [4]

History

Sudden onset of cold hands and feet, headache, fever, seizures, myalgia, photophobia, delirium.

Examination

Hypotension
Tachycardia
Diaphoresis
Pallor
Rash—petechial or ecchymotic
Neck stiffness, Kerning's sign, and Brudzinski's sign

Purpura fulminans can occur in 20% of patients with meningococcemia [5]. DIC and intravascular thrombosis may occur which result in skin necrosis. The course of the disease may be complicated by adrenal hemorrhage, which results in catastrophic hypoadrenalism and shock, known as Waterhouse Friedrichsen syndrome [6].

Other systems may be involved—up to 50% patients may have myocarditis ranging from mild to severe. Pericarditis [7] and arthritis [8] may occur due to immune complex deposition during convalescence. Sequelae may include deafness, memory loss, and cranial neuropathies [9].

Diagnosis

N. meningitidis is a fastidious organism, hence CSF specimens must be processed rapidly and sent for analysis. Neuroimaging must be done prior to lumbar puncture. The following features are suggestive of bacterial meningitis [10]:

TC > 10,000/dL
CSF TC > 2000/microliter
CSF neutrophils >1180/microliter
CSF protein >22 mg%
CSF glucose <34 mg %

Complications and Sequelae

Hearing loss, memory loss, hemiparesis, and cranial neuropathies [11].

Treatment

Treatment of bacterial meningitis, particularly meningococcal meningitis is time-sensitive. Increased bacterial loads correlate with increased mortality rates, and given the high rate of division of meningococcus, early administration of antibiotics is crucial [12].

Ceftriaxone 2 gm iv BD for 4–7 days in adults is recommended. In patients who cannot be given beta-lactams, chloramphenicol is a viable alternative. The role of dexamethasone is controversial—it is indicated in pneumococcal meningitis, and some guidelines recommend discontinuing dexamethasone once meningococcal meningitis is confirmed [13].

Protein C concentrate may be tried in patients with purpura fulminans on a background of meningococcal sepsis [14].

Glucocorticoids may be required in the Waterhouse Friderichsen syndrome [15].

Prevention

Meningococcal vaccine [16] is available in polysaccharide and conjugate vaccine formulations. At present, the vaccine is recommended [17] for individuals travelling to Haj [18, 19], those with high-risk medical conditions including asplenia, HIV and complement deficiency, military recruits, and those who might be exposed in laboratories to the bacterium.

Take-Home

The presentation of meningococcal meningitis varies and may not include the triad of fever, neck stiffness, and altered sensorium. Hence, it is essential to maintain a high index of suspicion for accurate diagnosis and timely management.

References

1. Al-Abri SS, Abuhasan MY, Albayat SS, Bai X, Bastaki H, Borrow R, Caugant DA, Dbaibo G, Deghmane AE, Dinleyici EC, Ghuneim N. Meningococcal disease in the Middle East: a report from the Global Meningococcal Initiative. J Infect. 2024;88(2):71–6.
2. Hoang VT, Gautret P. Infectious diseases and mass gatherings. Curr Infect Dis Rep. 2018;20:1–2.
3. Boeddha NP, Bycroft T, Nadel S, Hazelzet JA. The inflammatory and hemostatic response in sepsis and meningococcemia. Crit Care Clin. 2020;36(2):391–9.
4. Heckenberg SG, de Gans J, Brouwer MC, Weisfelt M, Piet JR, Spanjaard L, van der Ende A, van de Beek D. Clinical features, outcome, and meningococcal genotype in 258 adults with meningococcal meningitis: a prospective cohort study. Medicine. 2008;87(4):185–92.

5. Barret AS, Parent du Châtelet I, Taha M, Maine C, Fonteneau L, Lepoutre A. Les infections invasives à méningocoques en France en 2012: principales caractéristiques épidémiologiques. Bulletin épidémiologique hebdomadaire. 2014;2014(1–2):25–31.
6. Rijal R, Kandel K, Aryal BB, Asija A, Shrestha DB, Sedhai YR. Waterhouse–Friderichsen syndrome, septic adrenal apoplexy. Vitam Horm. 2024;124:449–61.
7. Singh A. Meningococcal disease presenting with acute myopericarditis and concurrent acute meningitis. Emerg Care Med. 2024;1(2):95–102.
8. Kelley J, Vempati A. Meningococcal meningitis with Waterhouse-Friderichsen syndrome. J Educ Teach Emerg Med. 2021;6(3):S1.
9. Schiess N, Groce NE, Dua T. The impact and burden of neurological sequelae following bacterial meningitis: a narrative review. Microorganisms. 2021;9(5):900.
10. Deghmane AE, Taha S, Taha MK. Global epidemiology and changing clinical presentations of invasive meningococcal disease: a narrative review. Infect Dis. 2022;54(1):1–7.
11. Hasbun R. Progress and challenges in bacterial meningitis: a review. JAMA. 2022;328(21):2147–54.
12. van de Beek D, Brouwer MC, Koedel U, Wall EC. Community-acquired bacterial meningitis. Lancet. 2021;398(10306):1171–83.
13. Dujari S, Gummidipundi S, He Z, Gold CA. Administration of Dexamethasone for bacterial meningitis: An unreliable quality measure. Neurohospitalist. 2021;11(2):101–6.
14. Clarke RC, Johnston JR, Mayne EE. Meningococcal septicaemia: treatment with protein C concentrate. Intensive Care Med. 2000;26:471–3.
15. Karki BR, Sedhai YR, Bokhari SR. Waterhouse-Friderichsen syndrome. In: StatPearls [Internet] 2023 Jun 26. StatPearls Publishing.
16. Herrera-Restrepo O, Kwiatkowska M, Huse S, Ndegwa N, Kocaata Z, Ganz ML. Meningococcal vaccination disparities in the United States (2010–2021): Findings from the National Immunization Survey-Teen and a commercial insurance database. Hum Vaccin Immunother. 2025;21(1):2479338.
17. Dutta AK, Swaminathan S, Abitbol V, Kolhapure S, Sathyanarayanan S. A comprehensive review of meningococcal disease burden in India. Infect Dis Ther. 2020;9:537–59.
18. Badur S, Khalaf M, Öztürk S, Al-Raddadi R, Amir A, Farahat F, Shibl A. Meningococcal disease and immunization activities in Hajj and Umrah pilgrimage: a review. Infect Dis Ther. 2022;11(4):1343–69.
19. Yezli S, Gautret P, Assiri AM, Gessner BD, Alotaibi B. Prevention of meningococcal disease at mass gatherings: lessons from the Hajj and Umrah. Vaccine. 2018;36(31):4603–9.v

28 Loose Stools, Breathlessness, and Blurring of Vision in a Previously Healthy Person: The Girl Who Felt Guilty

Grade Moderate.

Abstract An elderly lady presenting with loose stools, blurred vision, and breathlessness.

Story Your last patient in the evening clinic is Mrs. Iyengar, accompanied by her daughter, Revathi.

"Please sit down," you tell them.

"Thank you, doctor," says Revathi. Both Revathi and her mother are tearing. Revathi wipes her eyes and says "Doctor, I'm a little bit worried about my mother's health. I'm afraid I am to blame."

"I'm sure that's not true," you tell her gently. "Can you tell me what happened?"

"I stay with my elderly parents to take care of them, Doctor. I try to do most of my work from home. However, there was a business meeting that I just could not get out of, so I had to go out of town for five days. I came back to find my mother like this."

"She takes very good care of me, doctor. We're very lucky to have a daughter who is so concerned about our well-being," Mrs. Iyengar says.

"Can you tell me what exactly is going on with you?"

"I've not been feeling that good for the last two days. I had loose motions 4 or 5 times."

"Did you eat outside home? In a not so hygienic place?"

"No, no it's all home cooked food. I rarely eat out. I've been coughing since yesterday, there's some breathlessness too, and somehow I can't see very clearly. Everything looks slightly blurred."

"Was there any fever?"

"No, doctor."

S. Bhat, *Clinical Conundrums to Practice Diagnostic Reasoning*,
https://doi.org/10.1007/978-981-95-0636-1_28

"What about your past medical history? Are you on any regular treatment for maybe diabetes, hypertension anything like that?"

"No doctor, by God's grace, I'm quite healthy. I take calcium and vitamins daily."

"Is there any family history of any illness that I should know about?"

"Not really, but my husband has some muscle weakness and he is taking treatment for that."

"So, you mentioned that you had loose motions. Is there any problem with passing urine?"

"I think I'm passing urine more frequently."

"Is there anything else?"

"I feel a little restless and twitchy."

"Can you see well? Hear well?"

"My hearing is absolutely fine, I don't need a hearing aid. I can see ok with my glasses, but I lost them the day Revathi went for her trip and I have been unable to replace them."

"It's all my fault," says Revathi miserably.

"No Reva, it's not. You take such good care of us—your papa and I understand that your work is important." Mrs. Iyengar wipes her tears yet again.

"Can you please lie down?" you tell Mrs. Iyengar and proceed to examine her.

You note that her heart rate is 52 per minute, blood pressure is 100 / 60 mm Hg. You auscultate extensive bilateral crackles and wheeze. Oxygen saturation at room air is 90%. The pupils are constricted, reactive normally to light and accommodation.

Your findings concern you a bit; you draw Revathi aside and tell her:

"Please don't take this the wrong way, but is there a possibility that your mother might have overdosed on anything? Taken something toxic deliberately?"

"Of course not, Doctor! How can you suggest such a thing? I'm already feeling guilty. This is so unkind of you."

"I didn't mean anything by it. I'm sorry. I'm just trying to figure out what is wrong."

Question What is happening with Mrs. Iyengar? How would you manage her? Is your suspicion of deliberate self-harm by overdose or consumption justified? Or are there subtle clues in the history and examination findings which might indicate something else?

Analysis

The loose stools, breathlessness, constricted pupils, bradycardia, and extensive crackles are what make you consider consumption—perhaps organophosphorus—poisoning because of the multitude of cholinergic effects. However, there is no characteristic kerosene odor, besides which Revathi strongly denies this possibility.

Keeping in mind the signs and symptoms of cholinergic excess, is there some other way we can explain this? Yes, if you are astute enough to put certain points together.

First, the fact that Mrs. Iyengar's glasses are lost, thus compromising her vision—maybe causing an error in the medications she is consuming. The second is that her husband is taking some medicines for muscle weakness.

Combining all of these would lead to a diagnosis of cholinergic crisis, secondary to an accidental consumption of her husband's treatment for muscle weakness (likely to be myasthenia gravis).

A cholinergic crisis is a clinical condition that results from the overstimulation of nicotinic and muscarinic receptors at neuromuscular junctions and synapses (Fig. 28.1) due to excessive acetylcholine (ACh) [1]. This overstimulation is caused by the inactivation or inhibition of acetylcholinesterase (AChE), the enzyme responsible for the degradation of Ach [2].

The resulting accumulation of ACh at the neuromuscular junctions and synapses leads to symptoms of both muscarinic and nicotinic toxicity [3].

A cholinergic crisis is caused by the overstimulation of the postsynaptic membrane by ACh [4]. ACh is synthesized at the nerve terminal from acetyl coenzyme A (acetyl CoA) and choline, a reaction catalyzed by choline acetyltransferase (CAT). ACh is then packaged in vesicles and released upon stimulation. The action of ACh

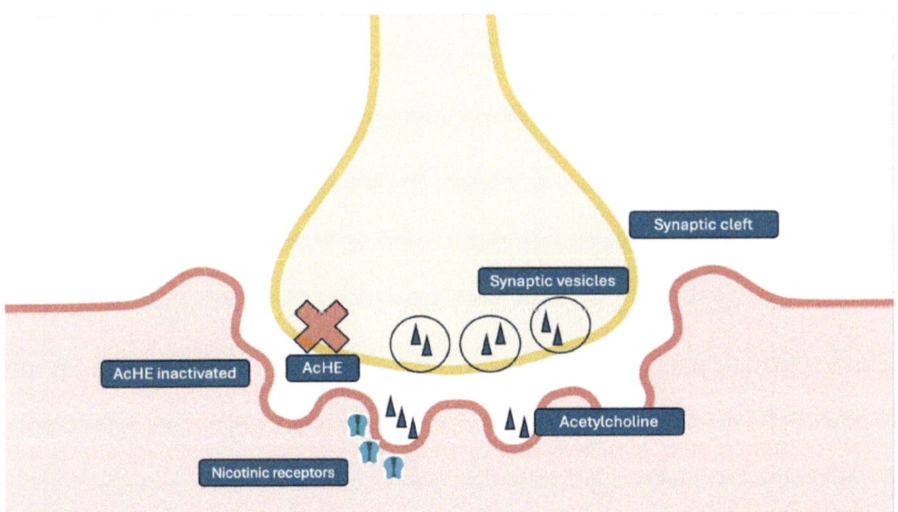

Fig. 28.1 Accumulation of acetylcholine at synapse due to inactivation of acetylcholinesterase

is terminated by AChE, which hydrolyzes ACh into choline and acetate [4]. The inhibition or inactivation of AChE leads to an excessive accumulation of ACh at the neuromuscular junction, causing overstimulation of muscarinic and nicotinic receptors. This results in the characteristic signs and symptoms of cholinergic toxicity [3].

Data on the epidemiology of cholinergic crises is limited. However, it is known that cholinergic crises are more commonly seen in the pediatric population and in patients with myasthenia gravis (MG). In children, cholinergic crisis is often due to accidental contact with or ingestion of organophosphates. Globally, approximately three million people are exposed to organophosphate poisoning annually, with around 300,000 deaths [5]. A cholinergic crisis may also be caused by accidental ingestion or overdose of cholinesterase inhibitors [2].

The clinical features of cholinergic crisis result from excessive stimulation of muscarinic and nicotinic receptors. Symptoms and signs include diarrhea, urination, miosis, bronchospasm, emesis, lacrimation, and salivation [6]. Other symptoms are muscular weakness, paralysis, muscular fasciculation, and blurred vision. Respiratory distress, including increased bronchial secretions, and respiratory muscle paralysis may occur. Bradycardia and hypotension are common.

Treatment

Antidotes: Atropine is an effective antidote for the muscarinic effects, competitively binding to postsynaptic muscarinic receptors [7].

Key Takeaway

In puzzling presentations of possible drug toxicity, information of prescription medications of family members may be of assistance.

References

1. Lott EL, Jones EB. Cholinergic toxicity. In: StatPearls [Internet] 2022 Dec 5. StatPearls Publishing.
2. Ohbe H, Jo T, Matsui H, Fushimi K, Yasunaga H. Cholinergic crisis caused by cholinesterase inhibitors: a retrospective nationwide database study. J Med Toxicol. 2018;14:237–41.
3. Colovic MB, Krstic DZ, Lazarevic-Pasti TD, Bondzic AM, Vasic VM. Acetylcholinesterase inhibitors: pharmacology and toxicology. Curr Neuropharmacol. 2013;11(3):315–35.
4. Adeyinka A, Kondamudi NP. Cholinergic Crisis. In: StatPearls. Treasure Island: StatPearls Publishing; 2025. PMID: 29494040.
5. Sinha PK, Sharma A. Organophosphate poisoning: a review. Med J Indonesia. 2003;12(2):120–6.
6. Mew EJ, Padmanathan P, Konradsen F, Eddleston M, Chang SS, Phillips MR, Gunnell D. The global burden of fatal self-poisoning with pesticides 2006-15: systematic review. J Affect Disord. 2017;219:93–104.
7. Patel A, Chavan G, Nagpal AK. Navigating the neurological abyss: a comprehensive review of organophosphate poisoning complications. Cureus. 2024;16(2).

Face Swelling and Abdominal Pain in a Young Female: Anagha's Absenteeism

29

Grade Moderate.

Abstract A young lady with episodes of severe abdominal pain and attacks of swelling of the face and lips.

Story You are more than a little worried about Anagha, your employee. When you interviewed her for the position of your clinic practice manager, you were quite impressed with her resume, her analytical skills, and her enthusiasm. She settled into her job nicely; however, for the last month, she seems to be absenting herself frequently from work.

You request her to join you for lunch at the hospital cafeteria.

"Anagha, I hope you are comfortable in the office."

"Yes, ma'am. I am learning a lot and my colleagues are so helpful!"

"I couldn't help but notice that you have taken quite a few days off over the last month. I hope all is well…."

"Yes, of course, ma'am. Everything is okay. It's just that my husband and I are settling into this new city."

"Is he happy in his new job?"

"He seems okay, but he is also getting used to the new place."

"Anyway, Anagha, you know I'm always available if you have a problem and you want to discuss it."

This talk with Anagha unfortunately does not seem to have had much of an effect because she is absent again for the next 2 days.

"I've got a bad tummy ache," she says.

You resolve to have talk with human resources the next day, asking them to give a pre-termination warning to Anagha, but something happens the next day that makes you change your mind. You go to the neighborhood sweet shop to pick up dessert, and you spot Anagha on the same mission.

S. Bhat, *Clinical Conundrums to Practice Diagnostic Reasoning*,
https://doi.org/10.1007/978-981-95-0636-1_29

You say sarcastically, "I see your stomach is better, Anagha." but when she whirls around, you are shocked. The whole of the left half of her face is swollen.

"Oh my God! Who did this to you?"

"No one, I swear it was no one, but my face and hand, my lips sometimes are swelling up these days that's why I am absent so much."

"Is there any problem apart from the swelling? Itching or pain?"

"No, Ma'am."

"Did you hurt yourself or has anyone hurt you?"

"No, I swear no, Ma'am."

"What about your tummy ache? What did that turn out to be?"

"It subsided on its own. The ultrasonogram was normal."

"I think it's something in the family. My mom used to have these attacks of swelling too. Her mother too."

Question Do you think Anagha is malingering to avoid work? On the other hand, is it something more sinister like domestic violence? Or is this an illness which can be diagnosed and treated? Is the abdominal pain part of the clinical picture?

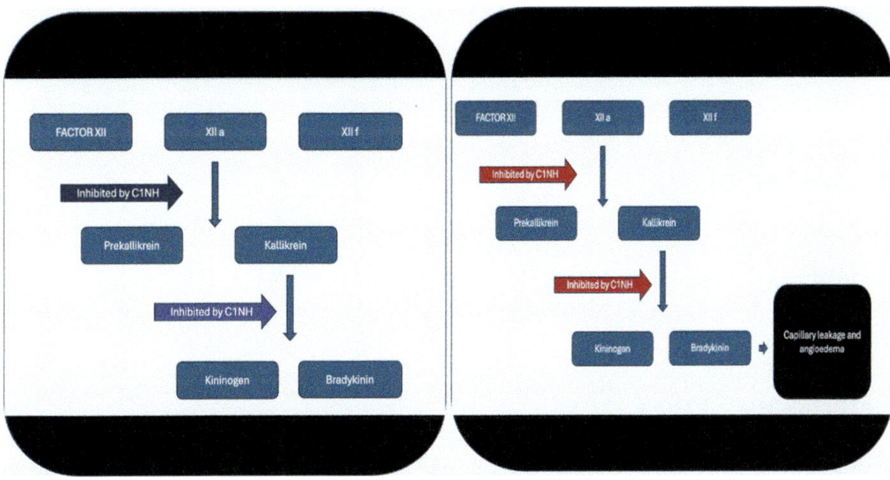

Fig. 29.1 Action of C1NH (panel 1); unchecked production of kallikrein and bradykinin when C1NH is absent (panel 2)

Analysis

If you trust Anagha (and you should), she has attacks of swelling of different parts of the body, with no identifiable precipitating factors and no associated symptoms. Additionally, it seems to be an autosomal dominant condition considering that her mother and grandmother both had it.

Putting all these together, Anagha seems to have C1 esterase inhibitor deficiency causing hereditary angioedema.

Hereditary angioedema is an autosomal dominant disorder characterized by angioedema without urticaria, causing swelling of areas of skin, the respiratory system, and the gastrointestinal tract. It has a global prevalence of around 1 per 500,000 [1].

Pathogenesis: C1 esterase inhibitor (C1NH) regulates the production of bradykinin, and in its absence, bradykinin production continues, unchecked [2]. Bradykinin promotes capillary leakage and angioedema [3] (Fig. 29.1).

Clinical Features [4]

(a) Swelling of extremities, face, tongue, lips, and genitals
(b) Bowel wall edema: Edema resulting in attacks of colicky abdominal pain
(c) Laryngeal edema which can be life-threatening

Labs [5]

Measurement of C4, C1NH, and C1NH function

Treatment [6]

1. Human plasma-derived C1INH concentrate
2. Icatibant, a bradykinin B2-receptor antagonist
3. Ecallantide, a kallikrein inhibitor

References

1. Schöffl C, Wiednig M, Koch L, Blagojevic D, Duschet P, Hawranek T, et al. Hereditary angioedema in Austria: prevalence and regional peculiarities. JDDG. 2019;17(4):416–23.
2. Cugno M, Zanichelli A, Foieni F, Caccia S, Cicardi M. C1-inhibitor deficiency and angioedema: molecular mechanisms and clinical progress. Trends Mol Med. 2009;15(2):69–78.
3. Björkqvist J, Sala-Cunill A, Renné T. Hereditary angioedema: a bradykinin-mediated swelling disorder. Thromb Haemost. 2017;109:368–74.
4. Gompels MM, Lock RJ, Abinun M, Bethune CA, Davies G, Grattan C, et al. C1 inhibitor deficiency: consensus document. Clin Exp Immunol. 2005;139(3):379–94.
5. Sinnathamby ES, Issa PP, Roberts L, Norwood H, Malone K, Vemulapalli H, et al. Hereditary angioedema: diagnosis, clinical implications, and pathophysiology. Adv Ther. 2023;40(3):814–27.
6. Treatment of Hereditary Angioedema | AAAAI [Internet]. [cited 2025 Mar 29]. Available from: https://www.aaaai.org/tools-for-the-public/drug-guide/immunomodulator-medications

Family Clustering of Vague Symptoms and Neurological Signs: The Depressed Worker

30

Grade Moderate.

Abstract A migrant laborer complains of body ache, polyuria, loose stools, and vomiting. He reports various health issues in his children as well.

Story You play golf on Sunday mornings with Naveen, boss of a flourishing construction business. As you walk to the clubhouse for a post-play mug of beer, Naveen says, "Doc, if you don't mind, I'd like to pick your brain for a moment." Having scored a birdie on the last hole, you are in an expansive mood and say "Certainly. What's up?"

"Well, I'm a little worried about one of my employees. His name is Denon, he's from Andra Pradesh, and his work is just not up to the mark. Initially, I thought it was just homesickness which would soon get better. But it's been 3 months now and he really isn't pulling his weight. I'm a little concerned that it is his health which is hampering his performance."

"Why don't you tell him to pop into my clinic tomorrow? Let me have a look and see if there's something that we can do to make him feel better."

Denon reports to your clinic the next evening, looking quite unhappy. You tell him to sit down and encourage him to explain what is going on with him.

"I feel tired all the time and my whole body aches. My back and my fingers are stiff. I get breathless when I walk fast or climb stairs. When I tell my friends, they say it is because I am missing my hometown. But how can it be? Does homesickness cause vomiting and loose motions? Also, I've had this same problem for the last year, even when I was in Andhra Pradesh. I met many doctors who checked me and found absolutely nothing wrong with me!"

"Is there anything else apart from the tiredness and aches and pains?"

"One minute, doctor, I need to use the bathroom." He returns and says that he feels thirsty all the time and he is passing urine frequently.

S. Bhat, *Clinical Conundrums to Practice Diagnostic Reasoning*,
https://doi.org/10.1007/978-981-95-0636-1_30

"Apart from the tiredness and aches and pains, I feel my hands are getting small, and my legs feel tight when I am walking."

"Is there anything else that concerns you?"

"I am a little worried about my 2 children back in my village. Both of them need to visit a dentist often because their teeth are getting yellow in color. My daughter has started getting her periods at age 10 and her mother is quite concerned about this."

You proceed with the examination and note the following:

Heart rate: 58/min.

Pallor present. No thyroid swelling or lymphadenopathy.

While examining the motor system, you note that he is unable to touch his toes without bending his knees. He cannot flex his neck till his chin touches his chest and is unable to join his hands together at the back of his head.

The tone is increased in both lower limbs, deep tendon reflexes are exaggerated, and plantar is upgoing bilaterally. There seems to be small muscle wasting in both hands.

Question What's going on with Denon? It definitely is something more than simple homesickness. What should you consider? Please note that his blood sugar and thyroid function are normal.

Analysis

These are the undebatable features:

(a) Myelopathy
(b) Diminished ability to flex neck and back
(c) Polyuria and polydipsia
(d) Loose stools and vomiting
(e) Early menarche in his daughter

Answer: Unfortunately, Denon is in phase 3 of endemic fluorosis.

Endemic skeletal fluorosis is a debilitating metabolic bone disorder caused by chronic excessive fluoride exposure and accumulation of fluoride in soft tissues and bones, primarily through contaminated water sources in specific geographic regions.

Epidemiology

It is common in India, China, Kenya, and Tanzania. Within India, the states of Andhra Pradesh, Gujarat, Rajasthan, and Telangana are most affected [1]. It is estimated that around six million people in India are affected by endemic fluorosis, and the number is similarly high in many countries in Asia and Africa [2].

Etiopathogenesis

A safe limit for fluoride consumption is 6 mg/day or 1.5 mg/L [3].

Humans acquire fluoride through diet, water, and fluoride-containing products [4]. Fluoride in the human skeleton has a half-life of 7 years. It increases osteoblast activity and causes bone remodeling.

Fluoride accumulation begins with the initial absorption in the gastrointestinal tract, where it rapidly enters the bloodstream. Once circulating, fluoride ions demonstrate a high affinity for calcified tissues, particularly bone mineral matrix. The primary pathological mechanism involves direct replacement of hydroxyl groups in hydroxyapatite crystals, forming fluorapatite—a more stable but less flexible crystalline structure.

Multiple deleterious mechanisms are at play at the cellular level [5]:

- Osteoblast dysfunction, with impaired collagen synthesis and mineralization
- Increased osteoclastic activity leading to abnormal bone remodeling
- Oxidative stress induction through mitochondrial disruption
- Inflammatory cascades triggered by fluoride-induced cellular damage

Chronic fluoride exposure progressively alters bone microarchitecture, resulting in characteristic radiographic findings: increased bone density, calcification of ligaments, and progressive skeletal deformities [6]. Metabolic alterations include impaired vitamin D utilization and altered calcium metabolism.

Genetic susceptibility and nutritional status significantly modulate individual fluorosis progression. Calcium- and protein-deficient individuals demonstrate accelerated pathological changes.

Glycosaminoglycans in the bones get converted to their sulfated isomers dermatan sulfate in the presence of excess fluoride [7]. Fluorosis results in osteophyte formation and ligament ossification which cause a compressive myeloradiculopathy. Direct neurotoxicity due to fluorosis has not been reported [8]. The disappearance of the normally present dermatan sulfate from nonmineralized soft tissue promotes ectopic calcification.

Anemia in fluorosis occurs as fluoride inhibits the ability of the body to absorb iron from iron-rich food sources. The consequences of anemia are especially harmful in the population which fluorosis affects (lower socioeconomic status and borderline malnutrition) as it significantly increases maternal mortality when it occurs in pregnant women. Deposition of fluoride in the pituitary gland may be associated with early menarche in females [9]. Diminished testosterone secretion has been reported in males affected by fluorosis [10]. Accumulation of fluoride in the pineal gland impairs melatonin secretion [11].

Clinical Features

Risk Factors [7]

(a) High ambient temperature
(b) Vigorous physical activity (both a and b increase water consumption)
(c) Renal insufficiency
(d) Malnutrition

Fluorosis causes tooth discoloration only if the exposure occurs during the development of teeth. Hence, discoloration of teeth in children is an important epidemiologic indicator of endemic fluorosis [12]. Pitting of the teeth is also seen. Persistent exposure (more than 10 years) to excessive levels of fluoride results in skeletal fluorosis too. Diagnosis of skeletal fluorosis requires a high degree of clinical suspicion as the initial features are nonspecific.

The initial symptoms of fluorosis include gastrointestinal symptoms like loose stools and vomiting. Fatigue, joint pains, polyuria, and polydipsia may also occur [7].

Specific clinical features of fluorosis depend on the phase of the disease:

Presymptomatic phase: X-rays may reveal increased bone density.
Phase 1: Joint stiffness and episodes of joint pain.

Phase 2: Continuous joint pain and osteoporosis.
Phase 3: Limitation of movement, signs and symptoms of compressive myelopathy, and fixed deformities.

A patient at phase 3 of the disease will have severely restricted movement of large joints and features of compressive myelopathy, including small muscle wasting of the hands, hypertonia, and brisk reflexes in the lower limbs along with the upgoing plantar [13]. Fluorosis may also cause anemia and hypothyroidism. Accumulation of fluoride in the pituitary gland may lead to precocious puberty [14].

As the disease advances, the patient may have a "poker back spine"—kyphotic spine with severely restricted mobility.

Diagnosis

(a) Osteoporotic spine and fusion of vertebrae [15]
(b) 24-h urine fluoride levels
(c) Estimation of fluoride in water supply (should be less than 1 ppm)
(d) Increased glycosaminoglycans and decreased sialic acid in the blood.
(e) Diffuse osteosclerosis, osteopenia, and calcification of muscles and ligaments

Treatment

Though controlling fluorosis is a public health measure—defluoridation of water and provision of safe drinking water resources [16]—some nutritional interventions may be of benefit. For example, a diet rich in vitamin C, E, and antioxidants may decrease the progression of fluorosis [17].

Calcium and Vitamin D supplementation may also help [18].

Once phase 3 develops, management is directed to symptom relief, physiotherapy, and avoidance of further exposure to fluoride.

References

1. Fluorosis: an ongoing challenge for India – The Lancet Planetary Health [Internet]. [cited 2025 Mar 20]. Available from: https://www.thelancet.com/journals/lanplh/article/PIIS2542-5196(20)30060-7/fulltext.
2. Prevention & control of fluorosis & linked disorders: developments in the 21st century – reaching out to patients in the community & hospital settings for recovery – PubMed [Internet]. [cited 2025 Feb 6]. Available from: https://pubmed.ncbi.nlm.nih.gov/30666981/.
3. FLUORIDES (EHC 227, 2002) [Internet]. [cited 2025 Feb 6]. Available from: https://www.inchem.org/documents/ehc/ehc/ehc227.htm.
4. Fluoride in drinking water and skeletal fluorosis: a review of the global impact | Curr Environ Health Rep [Internet]. [cited 2025 Mar 20]. Available from: https://link.springer.com/article/10.1007/s40572-020-00270-9.

5. Wei W, Pang S, Sun D. The pathogenesis of endemic fluorosis: research progress in the last 5 years. J Cell Mol Med. 2019;23(4):2333–42.
6. Choubisa S. A brief review of fluoride-induced bone disease skeletal fluorosis in humans and its prevention. J Pharm Pharmacol Res. 2024;7:1–7.
7. Aswin PS, Vandana KL. A comparative assessment of clinical parameters, sialic acid, and glycosaminoglycans levels in periodontitis patients with and without dental fluorosis: a clinical and biochemical study. J Indian Soc Periodontol. 2020;24(3):237.
8. Neurology India [Internet]. [cited 2025 Feb 6]. Available from: https://journals.lww.com/neur/fulltext/2009/57010/neurology_of_endemic_skeletal_fluorosis.4.aspx#O3-4-2.
9. Effect of fluoride on endocrine tissues and their secretory functions – review – ScienceDirect [Internet]. [cited 2025 Feb 6]. Available from: https://www.sciencedirect.com/science/article/abs/pii/S0045653520317604.
10. Fluoride exposure and pubertal development in children living in Mexico City – PMC [Internet]. [cited 2025 Feb 6]. Available from: https://pmc.ncbi.nlm.nih.gov/articles/PMC6439980/.
11. Fluoride and Pineal Gland [Internet]. [cited 2025 Feb 6]. Available from: https://www.mdpi.com/2076-3417/10/8/2885.
12. Dental Fluorosis: the Risk of Misdiagnosis—a Review | Biological Trace Element Research [Internet]. [cited 2025 Mar 20]. Available from: https://link.springer.com/article/10.1007/s12011-020-02296-4.
13. The continuing crippling challenge of skeletal fluorosis – Case series and review of literature – ScienceDirect [Internet]. [cited 2025 Mar 20]. Available from: https://www.sciencedirect.com/science/article/pii/S2214624522000089.
14. Fluoride exposure and pubertal development in children living in Mexico City | Environmental Health [Internet]. [cited 2025 Mar 20]. Available from: https://link.springer.com/article/10.1186/s12940-019-0465-7.
15. Skeletal fluorosis: don't miss the diagnosis! – PubMed [Internet]. [cited 2025 Feb 6]. Available from: https://pubmed.ncbi.nlm.nih.gov/31501957/.
16. Mitigation of Fluorosis – A Review – PMC [Internet]. [cited 2025 Mar 20]. Available from: https://pmc.ncbi.nlm.nih.gov/articles/PMC4525626/.
17. The fluorosis conundrum: bridging the gap between science and public health: toxicology mechanisms and methods: Vol 34, No 2 [Internet]. [cited 2025 Mar 20]. Available from: https://www.tandfonline.com/doi/abs/10.1080/15376516.2023.2268722.
18. Yang C, Wang Y, Xu H, Yang C, Wang Y, Xu H. Treatment and prevention of skeletal fluorosis [Internet]. Biomed Environ Sci. 2017 [cited 2025 Mar 20]. Available from: https://html.rhhz.net/SWYXYHJKX/html/t20170313_138964.htm.

31 Blurring of Vision and Eye Pain in A Young Male: The Man from Myanmar

Grade Moderate.

Abstract A young immigrant builder presents with blurring of vision and blind spots, posing a risk to his safety at his workplace.

Story Win Thaw has been in your country for a month now and has obtained employment as a laborer on a construction site. He visits your clinic for a consultation. You have an interpreter to assist you, but Win Thaw speaks English tolerably well

"Good morning. How may I help you today?"

"I am working as a bricklayer for the construction of a hotel on the main street."

"Yes..."

"I'm experiencing some discomfort because of the sun."

"Discomfort? In the sense?"

"My eyes become red and hurt quite a bit."

" But can you see well?"

"Unfortunately, no. This difficulty in seeing clearly is actually pretty dangerous at a building site and that's why my foreman insisted that I meet a doctor."

"Can you tell me what you mean when you say you can't see well?"

"It's difficult to describe, doctor. It's like sometimes some spots are floating in front of my eyes."

"Well, Mr. Win, those spots are called floaters and they're actually harmless."

"Really?" Win says doubtfully. "But sometimes these spots seem to be dancing, sometimes they look like flashes of light and things look blurred."

"That's a little worrying," you concede.

"Doctor, what's worse is this. Yesterday, a block of wood fell down from a higher floor—just to my right. I really don't know why I couldn't see it. If the foreman hadn't pulled me out of harm's way, I could have been badly hurt."

"That must have been frightening...." you say sympathetically.

S. Bhat, *Clinical Conundrums to Practice Diagnostic Reasoning*,
https://doi.org/10.1007/978-981-95-0636-1_31

"Are there are any other medical conditions I should be aware of? Anything that happened before you came to this country?"

"No. Nothing." Mr Win says with a slightly shifty look in his face that you can't figure out. Is he malingering? Is he trying to get out of work?

You proceed with the physical examination.

Win Thaw is conscious, oriented, afebrile. His BMI is 18. Physical examination is remarkable for generalized lymph node enlargement.

The eyes appear normal—the pupils are reactive, and extra-ocular movements are full. There are no focal neurological deficits. You send a consult to ophthalmology for a detailed ophthalmoscopic examination with a dilated pupil. Visual acuity is 20/60, and dilated fundoscopy reveals inflammation in both the anterior chambers and the vitreous humor.

Questions What ails Mr. Win Thaw? Is there something happening apart from homesickness and loneliness?

Analysis

The plain language summary is this: A young male with low BMI and generalized lymphadenopathy has ocular symptoms in the form of floaters, photopsia, scotomata, and blurring of vision. This suggests HIV-AIDS with either CMV retinitis or IRU (immune reconstitution uveitis). However, the ophthalmoscopic appearance is more suggestive of IRU. The evasiveness with which Win Thaw answered your question about a pre-existing medical condition is perhaps an indicator that he has already been diagnosed with HIV AIDS and has been started on highly active antiretroviral therapy (HAART)

Diagnosis

HIV-AIDS with CMV retinitis and immune reconstitution uveitis (IRU). IRU is part of a broader syndrome—immune reconstitution inflammatory syndrome (IRIS.)

IRIS is defined as a paradoxical worsening of a pre-existing infection due to inflammation and is commonly seen in patients with HIV-AIDS when HAART is commenced [1]. It can also occur in non-HIV settings like the treatment of extrapulmonary tuberculosis [2].

The prevalence of CMV retinitis is in 10% of HIV-AIDS patients in South East Asia [3].

IRIS may either be

(a) Paradoxical IRIS—worsening of an already diagnosed infection
(b) Unmasking IRIS—manifestation of a hitherto undiagnosed infection [4]

The risk of IRIS is related to two factors (Fig. 31.1).

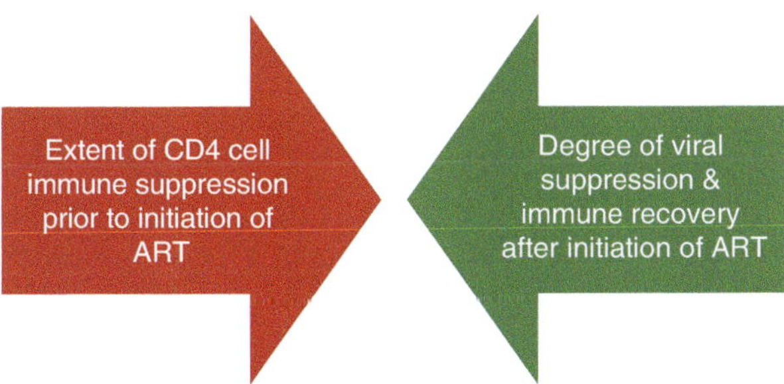

Fig. 31.1 Risk of IRIS

Clinical Features

Most patients develop IRIS within a few months of commencement of ART. Many cases of IRIS are mild and may be managed symptomatically. However, severe IRIS may require interruption of ART, which can increase the risk of opportunistic infections and drug resistance.

Some evidence shows that critical IRIS may be linked to more severe opportunistic infection (OI), perhaps because of the higher antigenic load [5].

Risk Factors [6]

(a) Lower CD4 count
(b) Higher HIV viral load
(c) Fungal infections
(d) High response to ART

The following infectious agents have been linked to IRIS [7]:

- Mycobacterium tuberculosis
- CMV
- Cryptococcus neoformans
- Pneumocystis jirovecii

Systemic Manifestations of IRIS Are as Follows

Neurological IRIS [8]:
- Cryptococcal meningitis reactivation
- Tuberculous meningitis exacerbation
- Focal neurological deficits
- Increased intracranial pressure

Pulmonary IRIS [9]:
- Tuberculous pneumonitis reactivation
- Paradoxical lung infiltrates
- Lymph node enlargement
- Pleural effusions

Cutaneous IRIS [10]:
- Rapid progression of pre-existing dermatological conditions

Diagnosis

The following criteria may be used to diagnose IRIS [11]:

Major Criteria

1. Atypical presentation of OI or tumors in patients responding to antiretroviral therapy.
2. Decrease in plasma HIV RNA level by at least 1 $\log_{10}$ copies/mL.

Minor Criteria

1. Increased blood CD4+ T-cell count after HAART.
2. Increase in immune response specific to the relevant pathogen, e.g., DTH response to mycobacterial antigens.
3. Spontaneous resolution of disease without specific antimicrobial therapy or tumor chemotherapy with the continuation of antiretroviral therapy.

Treatment

1. Continuation of ART (may be commenced 2 weeks after starting treatment for CMV retinitis).
2. Treatment of OI.
3. Glucocorticoids may be required.

Treatment of CMV Retinitis [12]

1. For severe retinitis, intravitreal ganciclovir or foscarnet plus systemic therapy
2. For retinitis which does not threaten sight, oral valganciclovir

Prevention of IRIS [13]

1. HAART should be commenced within 2 weeks after starting treatment of OI. IRIS must be anticipated and looked for in patients with CD4 count less than 50.

Key Takeaway
IRIS is just one of several causes of worsening in clinical and lab parameters after commencement of HAART. One should also consider progression of the opportunistic infection due to drug resistance or adverse effects of the drugs used in treatment.

In cases other than tuberculous meningitis and cryptococcosis, the benefits of instituting ART outweigh the risks of IRIS.

References

1. Shelburne Iii SA, Hamill RJ, Rodriguez-Barradas MC, Greenberg SB, Atmar RL, Musher DM, Gathe JC Jr, Visnegarwala F, Trautner BW. Immune reconstitution inflammatory syndrome: emergence of a unique syndrome during highly active antiretroviral therapy. Medicine. 2002;81(3):213–27.
2. Hawkey CR, Yap T, Pereira J, Moore DA, Davidson RN, Pasvol G, Kon OM, Wall RA, Wilkinson RJ. Characterization and management of paradoxical upgrading reactions in HIV-uninfected patients with lymph node tuberculosis. Clin Infect Dis. 2005;40(9):1368-71.c.
3. Ocieczek P, Barnacle JR, Gumulira J, Phiri S, Heller T, Grabska-Liberek I. Cytomegalovirus retinitis screening and treatment in human immunodeficiency virus patients in Malawi: a feasibility study. Open Forum Infect Dis. 2019;6(11):ofz439. US: Oxford University Press.
4. Haddow LJ, Easterbrook PJ, Mosam A, Khanyile NG, Parboosing R, Moodley P, Moosa MY. Defining immune reconstitution inflammatory syndrome: evaluation of expert opinion versus 2 case definitions in a South African cohort. Clin Infect Dis. 2009;49(9):1424–32.
5. Shelburne SA, Visnegarwala F, Darcourt J, Graviss EA, Giordano TP, White AC Jr, Hamill RJ. Incidence and risk factors for immune reconstitution inflammatory syndrome during highly active antiretroviral therapy. AIDS. 2005;19(4):399–406.
6. Sharma SK, Soneja M. HIV & immune reconstitution inflammatory syndrome (IRIS). Indian J Med Res. 2011;134(6):866.
7. Gupta S, Mathur P, Maskey D, Wig N, Singh S. Immune restoration syndrome with disseminated Penicillium marneffei and cytomegalovirus co-infections in an AIDS patient. AIDS Res Ther. 2007;4:1–4.8.
8. Johnson T, Nath A. Neurological complications of immune reconstitution in HIV-infected populations. Ann NY Acad Sci. 2010;1184(1):106–20.
9. Crothers K, Huang L. Pulmonary complications of immune reconstitution inflammatory syndromes in HIV-infected patients. Respirology. 2009;14(4):486–94.
10. Górecka A, Majewski S, Szymańska E, Walecka I. Skin and mucosal manifestations of immune reconstitution inflammatory syndrome in people living with HIV: a review. Int J Dermatol. 2024;63(7):852–7.
11. French MA, Price P, Stone SF. Immune restoration disease after antiretroviral therapy. AIDS [Internet]. 2004;18(12). Available from: https://journals.lww.com/aidsonline/fulltext/2004/08200/immune_restoration_disease_after_antiretroviral.2.aspx.
12. Jacobson MA. Treatment of cytomegalovirus retinitis in patients with the acquired immunodeficiency syndrome. N Engl J Med. 1997;337(2):105–14.
13. Brust JCM, McGowan JP, Fine SM, Merrick ST, Radix AE, Vail RM, et al. Management of IRIS [Internet]. Baltimore: Johns Hopkins University; 2024. [cited 2025 Mar 26]. (New York State Department of Health AIDS Institute Clinical Guidelines). Available from: http://www.ncbi.nlm.nih.gov/books/NBK570544/.

32 Loose Stools and Constipation in a Stressed Executive—Cut It Out

Grade Easy.

Abstract A stressed executive with alternating constipation and diarrhea now complains of weight loss and rash.

Story Vijay was the typical Type A personality. Driven at work, aggressive at play—he had made his accounting firm one of the top businesses in the city by the time he was 40. Not just that, he had won his club badminton trophy for the past 5 years. This does not mean he compromised on family—oh no, does not. He ensured he was on time for every PTA meeting, every school game, and every time his kids were on stage.

Maybe it was his lack of sleep and his slight addiction to caffeine which wreaked havoc with his gut. Physicians all over town began to dread his visits where he demanded a cure! Immediately! Hesitant suggestions that he should eat healthier and sleep more fell on deaf ears.

The day comes when Vijay darkens your doorway.

"Let me start by telling you, doc. I don't have irritable bowel syndrome. I read it up—and regardless of what your colleagues have told me, I do not have irritable bowel syndrome."

"Ok, ok," you say, trying to pacify him. "Why don't you tell me what exactly has been going on and we shall take it from there."

"I just have a sensitive stomach. Either I'm constipated or I'm having loose motions. I've told my wife time and time again to make her food a little blander and more gut-friendly, but she's just so stubborn. She refuses to change."

"This sounds like irritable bowel syndrome to me," you tell yourself.

"Ok—is there anything else apart from your constipation and diarrhea? Any blood in the stools? Loss of weight?"

"No blood in the stools. I have lost some weight, which is crazy since I also feel bloated all the time."

S. Bhat, *Clinical Conundrums to Practice Diagnostic Reasoning*,
https://doi.org/10.1007/978-981-95-0636-1_32

"Ok, may I examine you?" As Vijay walks to the examination couch, you notice that he sways a little. You examine him. Your findings make you doubt your initial impression of irritable bowel syndrome (IBS). You observe that Vijay is pale, and he has atrophic glossitis. Additionally, he has a rash on his elbows and his knees which he scratches at continuously.

Questions Is Vijay just a stressed executive who does not want to take ownership of his health issues and goes doctor shopping instead of making changes in his lifestyle? Or does he warrant further investigation? What tests would you do?

Analysis

While Vijay does fulfil some of the criteria of IBS, the anemia, the ataxia, and the rash are not typical; hence, he needs further tests.

The striking points in the history and physical examination are as follows:

(a) Altered bowel habit
(b) Loss of weight
(c) Anemia
(d) Atrophic glossitis
(e) Rash
(f) Ataxia

The anemia and atrophic glossitis suggest micronutrient deficiency—since in a man like Vijay, it is unlikely to be due to dietary deficiencies, the possibility of malabsorption arises—this would also yield a possible explanation for the ataxia—namely B12 deficiency and sensory ataxia. The extremely pruritic rash on extensor surfaces—elbows and knees—is what should alert one to the possibility of celiac disease.

Celiac disease (CD), also known as gluten-sensitive enteropathy or celiac sprue, is a chronic, immune-mediated inflammatory disorder of the small intestine triggered by dietary gluten in genetically predisposed individuals [1].

Classification [2]

(a) Responding: Responds within 3 months to gluten-free diet (GFD)
(b) Resistant: Recurrence of symptoms after remission even with GFD
(c) Refractory: No response to GFD—persistent gastrointestinal symptoms despite adherence to a GFD for more than 12 months
(d) Silent: Histology not typical
(e) Latent: Attenuated and nuanced symptoms
(f) Potential CD: Defined by positive serological and genetic markers (HLA-DQ2/DQ8) with a normal intestinal mucosa

Epidemiology [3]

The estimated global prevalence is approximately 1% with potential peaks of onset shortly after weaning with gluten in the first 2 years of life and in the second or third decades. It is more common in women, more common in Europe and the United States.

Asymptomatic first-degree relatives of patients with confirmed celiac disease are at higher risk, and screening should be considered in these individuals

Etiology

Gluten, a protein found in wheat, barley, and rye, damages the small intestinal mucosa resulting in villous atrophy, crypt hyperplasia, and infiltration of the lamina propria by immune cells. The development of celiac disease is multifactorial and requires a combination of genetic predisposition, exposure to dietary gluten, and environmental triggers [4].

Genetic Predisposition

Individuals with celiac disease have HLA-DQ2 and HLA-DQ87 haplotypes [4]. However, these haplotypes are carried by around 30% of the population, and only 1% develop celiac disease.

Dietary gluten is the primary environmental trigger for celiac disease. Gluten, found in wheat (gliadin), barley (hordein), and rye (secalin), contains peptides that are resistant to complete digestion in the upper gastrointestinal tract. In susceptible individuals, these peptides trigger an inappropriate immune response in the small intestine.

Viral infections and alterations in the gut microbiota may precipitate celiac disease in those who are genetically prone.

Pathogenesis [5]

Digestion of gluten results in the formation of gliadin peptides which may be resistant to complete proteolysis. These peptides can cross the intestinal epithelium due to increased intestinal permeability.

(a) Activation of innate immunity: Gliadin peptides can activate the innate immune system by binding to Toll-like receptor 4 (TLR4). This leads to the release of proinflammatory cytokines, such as interleukin-15 (IL-15), which causes activation and proliferation of intraepithelial lymphocytes (IELs).
(b) Activation of adaptive immunity: In genetically susceptible individuals with HLA-DQ2 or HLA-DQ8, gliadin peptides are deamidated by the enzyme tissue transglutaminase (tTG). Deamidated gliadin peptides have a higher affinity for HLA-DQ2/DQ8 molecules on antigen-presenting cells (APCs). These APCs present the deamidated gliadin peptides to CD4+ T helper cells in the lamina propria.
(c) T-cell response: The presented gliadin peptides activate gluten-specific CD4+ T cells, leading to the release of proinflammatory cytokines such as interferon-gamma (IFN-γ), tumor necrosis factor-alpha (TNF-α), and interleukin-21 (IL-21).
(d) B cell response and autoantibody production: Activated CD4+ T cells lead to the production of autoantibodies, including anti-tissue transglutaminase (anti-

tTG) IgA, anti-endomysial antibodies (EMA), and antibodies to deamidated gliadin peptides (DGP).

(e) Intestinal mucosal damage: The chronic inflammation mediated by T cells and cytokines leads to the characteristic villous atrophy and crypt hyperplasia in the small intestinal mucosa. The loss of villi reduces the absorptive surface area, resulting in the malabsorption of nutrients.

Clinical Features

(i) Gastrointestinal Symptoms:

- (a) Diarrhoea
- (b) Abdominal discomfort/pain
- (c) Bloating and distension
- (d) Constipation
- (e) Weight loss
- (f) Nausea and vomiting
- (g) Anorexia

Atypical presentations: An (IBS)-like presentation with constipation or alternating bowel habits and dyspepsia-like symptoms may be seen.

(ii) Extra-Intestinal Manifestations

- (a) Anemia: Either iron deficiency anemia or macrocytic anemia due to folate and/or vitamin B12 deficiency
- (b) Bone disease: Osteopenia and osteoporosis
- (c) Neurological manifestations: Peripheral neuropathy (gluten neuropathy), gluten ataxia, and cognitive impairment
- (d) Dermatitis herpetiformis: A chronic, intensely pruritic, papulovesicular skin rash typically located on extensor surfaces (elbows, knees, and buttocks)
- (e) Oral manifestations: Recurrent aphthous stomatitis and atrophic glossitis
- (f) Liver: Transaminitis and increased prevalence of NAFLD
- (g) Reproductive system: Late menarche, amenorrhea, recurrent miscarriages, premature birth, low birth weight offspring, reduced fertility, and poor sperm quality

Complications

- (a) Enteropathy-associated T-cell lymphoma (EATL)
- (b) Small intestinal adenocarcinoma
- (c) Hyposplenism

Investigations [6]

(a) Serological testing: Anti-tissue transglutaminase (tTG).
(b) Small intestinal biopsy: A small intestinal biopsy, obtained via esophagogastroduodenoscopy (EGD), is often required to confirm the diagnosis and assess the extent of mucosa.
(c) Genetic testing (HLA typing): Testing for HLA-DQ2 and HLA-DQ8 can be useful to support the diagnosis, especially in seronegative cases.

Treatment [7]

(a) Gluten-free diet:

Comprehensive education from a skilled dietitian, focusing on identifying gluten-containing foods, reading food labels carefully, and preventing cross-contamination during food preparation.

While a threshold for safe gluten contamination in gluten-free products has been established (typically <20 parts per million), strict avoidance is crucial for symptom resolution and mucosal healing.

(b) Appropriate supplementation (e.g., iron, folate, vitamin D, and calcium)
(c) Latiglutenase
(d) Tofacitinib

Note: Patients with celiac disease have an increased risk of other autoimmune diseases: Type 1 diabetes mellitus and autoimmune thyroid disease.

References

1. Rodrigo L. Celiac disease. World J Gastroenterol WJG. 2006;12(41):6577–84.
2. Perrotta G, Guerrieri E, Perrotta G, Guerrieri E. Celiac disease: definition, classification, historical and epistemological profiles, anatomopathological aspects, clinical signs, differential diagnosis, treatments and prognosis. Proposed diagnostic scheme for celiac disease (DSCNC)? Arch Clin Gastroenterol. 2022;8(1):008–19.
3. Lebwohl B, Rubio-Tapia A. Epidemiology, presentation, and diagnosis of celiac disease. Gastroenterology. 2021;160(1):63–75.
4. Kaur A, Shimoni O, Wallach M. Celiac disease: from etiological factors to evolving diagnostic approaches. J Gastroenterol. 2017;52(9):1001–12.
5. Wolters VM, Wijmenga C. Genetic background of celiac disease and its clinical implications. Off J Am Coll Gastroenterol ACG. 2008;103(1):190.
6. Lebwohl B, Rubio-Tapia A, Assiri A, Newland C, Guandalini S. Diagnosis of celiac disease. Gastrointest Endosc Clin N Am. 2012;22(4):661–77.
7. Machado MV. New developments in celiac disease treatment. Int J Mol Sci. 2023;24(2):945.

33 Daytime Sleepiness, Anemia, and Hepatomegaly in a Middle-Aged Female: Shauli's Somnolence

Grade Easy.

Abstract A middle-aged female presents with fatigue and somnolence and is noted to have anemia, bruising, and hepatomegaly.

Story Mrs. Shauli is accompanied by her sister Shupta when she visits you. You ask them to sit down and ask what brings them to your clinic.

"Shauli has been neglecting her health for a while, doctor. She's so busy at work (she's a school principal) and at home and she just doesn't have time to take care of herself."

It is true that Mrs. Shauli looks stressed and hassled. She blinks repeatedly, scratches her forearms compulsively, and looks quite miserable.

"I just feel so sleepy and tired all the time, doctor. I don't know what's wrong with me. Sometimes I fall asleep when I'm chairing meetings—it's quite embarrassing. And even when I am awake, I feel that my mind isn't functioning at 100%."

"She used to be a gold medalist at school, a debater at college, and till recently won the teachers chess championship every year," Shupta says.

"Not for the last 4 years," Shauli mumbles sadly, rubbing her tummy.

"Does your tummy hurt?" you ask her.

"It doesn't hurt that much—but there's this vague discomfort on the right side," she says dully.

"Do you think you have lost weight?"

"I haven't measured my weight, but my clothes have become a little loose, which is surprising considering I'm not eating less or exercising more than usual."

"Are there any health issues in your family members?"

" My mother, and her 3 sisters—all of them passed away before the age of 45 because of heart attacks. I believe there was a family tendency to high cholesterol."

S. Bhat, *Clinical Conundrums to Practice Diagnostic Reasoning*,
https://doi.org/10.1007/978-981-95-0636-1_33

"I'm sorry to hear that. Will you lie down on the examination couch so I can examine you?"

As she lies down, Shauli whispers to you—"For the last year or so, my poop is difficult to flush, doctor."

You observe that Shauli is pale. There is glossitis and cheilitis and a mild scleral icterus as well. Worryingly, considering the family history suggestive of hypercholesterolemia, there are xanthelasma on both lower eyelids.

Shauli's blood pressure is 130/80 mm Hg, but you note that her right hand goes into an uncomfortable looking spasm while you are measuring the pressure. You are concerned to note that there is a fair amount of bruising on her arms and legs. Other systemic examination is essentially normal, apart from a fairly large palpable liver. There is no splenomegaly and no free fluid in the abdomen.

Questions Is there a single diagnosis which can explain the diverse signs and symptoms? What investigations would you like to order?

Analysis

This is an interesting case—not only because it is rare, and requires a high index of suspicion to spot, but also because early diagnosis and treatment can improve outcomes significantly.

The key features here are as follows:

(a) Fatigue and daytime somnolence
(b) Pruritus and dry eyes—"She's blinking repeatedly, scratching her forearms compulsively and looking quite miserable."
(c) Vitamin and micronutrient deficiency—Bruising (Vitamin K), glossitis and cheilitis (Vitamin B), Trousseau's sign—carpopedal spasm on inflating BP cuff (Vitamin D), and pallor (iron)
(d) Xanthelasma (the family history of dyslipidemia is a red herring)
(e) Hepatomegaly

The vitamin deficiency along with the history of stools that are difficult to flush should lead one to suspect malabsorption; this, in conjunction with the xanthelasma, the pruritus, and the hepatomegaly point to a diagnosis of primary biliary cholangitis.

Primary biliary cholangitis (PBC) is a chronic, progressive, immune-mediated cholestatic liver disease characterized by the destruction of small- and medium-sized intrahepatic bile ducts, leading to cholestasis, inflammation, and fibrosis, leading to biliary cirrhosis and hepatic failure [1].

Epidemiology [2]

PBC exhibits a marked female predominance, with a reported female-to-male ratio ranging from 9:1 to 10:1. The prevalence varies geographically, with higher rates observed in Northern Europe and North America.

Etiology

Though the precise etiology of PBC is not completely known, it is thought to be an autoimmune disorder targeting the epithelium of small intrahepatic bile ducts. A combination of genetic susceptibility (certain HLA haplotypes) and environmental triggers is hypothesized to initiate and perpetuate the autoimmune response. Molecular mimicry, xenobiotics, and infectious agents have been implicated, though no definitive causal link has been established.

Pathogenesis [3]

The pathogenesis of PBC is characterized by an interplay of immune and inflammatory processes leading to the destruction of cholangiocytes. This involves:

(a) Loss of tolerance to mitochondrial autoantigens, especially the E2 subunit of pyruvate dehydrogenase complex (PDC-E2), resulting in the production of antimitochondrial antibodies (AMA).
(b) Infiltration of the portal tracts by lymphocytes (predominantly T cells, including CD4+ and CD8+ cells), macrophages, and plasma cells, leading to chronic inflammation.
(c) Activation of proinflammatory cytokines and chemokines that worsen the inflammatory cascade and contribute to cholangiocyte apoptosis and necrosis.
(d) Progressive fibrosis, initially in the portal areas and extending to form bridging fibrosis and ultimately cirrhosis. Ductopenia, the loss of small intrahepatic bile ducts, is associated with disease progression.
(e) The biliary bicarbonate umbrella is a protective mechanism against bile acid-induced injury in cholangiocytes, and this malfunctions in PBC.
(f) Alterations in bile acid metabolism and signaling contribute to cholangiocyte injury and fibrosis.

Hypercholesterolemia in PBC is multifactorial:

(a) Increased levels of lipoprotein-X (Lp-X) accumulates due to impaired biliary excretion of lipids.
(b) Decreased expression and function of hepatic LDL receptors in the setting of cholestasis impair the clearance of circulating LDL.

Clinical Features [4]

Common symptoms include:

(a) Pruritus, often generalized and worse at night
(b) Fatigue, which can be debilitating and is not always correlated with the degree of hepatic damage
(c) Icterus, high-colored urine, and clay-colored stools
(d) Hepatomegaly and, in advanced disease, splenomegaly.

Investigations [5]

(a) Liver enzymes: Cholestatic pattern with elevated alkaline phosphatase (ALP) and gamma-glutamyl transferase (GGT) out of proportion to transaminase elevation (AST and ALT). Serum bilirubin increases with the disease progression.
(b) Serology: Antimitochondrial antibodies (AMA), detected by indirect immunofluorescence or enzyme-linked immunosorbent assay (ELISA), are positive in over 90% of patients and are highly specific for PBC.
(c) Lipid profile: Typically reveals hypercholesterolemia, often with elevated HDL cholesterol in early stages and increasing triglycerides later. The presence of Lp-X can be confirmed with specific assays.
(d) Liver biopsy: While not always required for diagnosis in patients with characteristic biochemistry and positive AMA, liver biopsy is valuable for:
   - Confirming the diagnosis
   - Staging the disease according to histological classifications
   - Excluding other causes of liver disease
   - Identifying features suggestive of overlap with autoimmune hepatitis (AIH)

Imaging

1. Abdominal ultrasound
2. Magnetic resonance cholangiopancreatography (MRCP)

Differential Diagnosis

(a) Primary sclerosing cholangitis
(b) Autoimmune hepatitis
(c) Secondary biliary cholangitis
(d) Drug-induced liver injury
(e) Vanishing bile duct syndrome
(f) IgG4-related sclerosing cholangitis

Treatment [6]

The primary goals of PBC treatment are to slow disease progression, manage symptoms, and prevent complications.

(a) Ursodeoxycholic acid (UDCA): UDCA (13–15 mg/kg/day) is the first-line therapy for PBC. It is a hydrophilic bile acid that displaces more toxic endogenous bile acids, reduces cholestasis, and has demonstrated improved biochemical markers and prolonged transplant-free survival in responders [7].
(b) Obeticholic acid (OCA): A farnesoid X receptor (FXR) agonist approved for PBC patients who are either intolerant or have an inadequate response to UDCA. It improves biochemical markers but requires careful monitoring for potential side effects like pruritus.
(c) Fibrates: Bezafibrate and fenofibrate [8].

Symptomatic Management

(a) Pruritus: Managed with cholestyramine, colesevelam, rifampicin, and naltrexone [9]. Obeticholic acid may paradoxically worsen pruritus initially [10].
(b) Hyperlipidemia: Stains and fibrates.
(c) Fat-soluble vitamin deficiency (A, D, E, K): Should be monitored and supplemented as needed.
(d) Osteoporosis: Screening and supplementation of calcium, vitamin D, and bisphosphonates.

New treatment options for PBC are being studied, especially for patients who do not respond to UDCA or who are intolerant to current second-line treatments. Immunomodulatory drugs, selective bile acid transporter inhibitors, and peroxisome proliferator-activated receptor (PPAR) agonists like elafibrinor are examples of emerging treatments. Patients at higher risk of progression who might benefit from more aggressive or combination therapies are increasingly identified using the GLOBE and UK-PBC risk scores. Normalizing or significantly lowering bilirubin and alkaline phosphatase levels is an important therapeutic target. For patients with end-stage PBC who experience cirrhosis complications (variceal bleeding, ascites, and encephalopathy), intractable pruritus, or recurrent cholangitis in spite of receiving the most effective medical treatment, liver transplantation is still the only option. Post-transplantation survival rates are typically good. Although it usually happens slowly, PBC recurrence in the graft is possible [11]. Patients who showed a positive biochemical response to UDCA prior to transplantation have better outcomes.

References

1. Trivella J, Levy C. Primary biliary cholangitis. In: Hepatology. Academic; 2025. p. 483–530.
2. Colapietro F, Bertazzoni A, Lleo A. Contemporary epidemiology of primary biliary cholangitis. Clin Liver Dis. 2022;26(4):555–70.
3. Park JW, Kim JH, Kim SE, Jung JH, Jang MK, Park SH, Lee MS, Kim HS, Suk KT, Kim DJ. Primary biliary cholangitis and primary sclerosing cholangitis: current knowledge of pathogenesis and therapeutics. Biomedicines. 2022;10(6):1288.
4. Purohit T, Cappell MS. Primary biliary cirrhosis: pathophysiology, clinical presentation and therapy. World J Hepatol. 2015;7(7):926.
5. Shah RA, Kowdley KV. Current and potential treatments for primary biliary cholangitis. Lancet Gastroenterol Hepatol. 2020;5(3):306–15.
6. Assis DN. Advancing second-line treatment for primary biliary cholangitis. N Engl J Med. 2024;390(9):853–4.
7. Örnolfsson KT, Lund SH, Olafsson S, Bergmann OM, Björnsson ES. Biochemical response to ursodeoxycholic acid among PBC patients: a nationwide population-based study. Scand J Gastroenterol. 2019;54(5):609–16.
8. Zhang H, Li S, Feng Y, Zhang Q, Xie B. Efficacy of fibrates in the treatment of primary biliary cholangitis: a meta-analysis. Clin Exp Med. 2023;23(5):1741–9.
9. Düll MM, Kremer AE. Evaluation and management of pruritus in primary biliary cholangitis. Clin Liver Dis. 2022;26(4):727–45.
10. Zhao J, Li B, Zhang K, Zhu Z. The effect and safety of obeticholic acid for patients with nonalcoholic steatohepatitis: a systematic review and meta-analysis of randomized controlled trials. Medicine (Baltimore). 2024;103(7):e37271.
11. Mijic M, Saric I, Delija B, Lalovac M, Sobocan N, Radetic E, Martincevic D, Filipec Kanizaj T. Pretransplant evaluation and liver transplantation outcome in PBC patients. Can J Gastroenterol Hepatol. 2022;2022(1):7831165.

Loss of Libido in a Previously Healthy Male: The Unfulfilled Wife

34

Grade Easy.

Abstract A previously healthy male presents with loss of libido, backache, and hand pain.

Story Mr Stanley runs a bakery at the corner where his pastries are sought after by all. You too, are a fan of his delicious products and are quite concerned when he shows up at your clinic with his wife one fine Tuesday morning. You greet them both. Fittingly for a baker, Stanley's hands feel like unbaked bread dough. You disengage your fingers from his sweaty hand and surreptitiously try to wipe your palms on your pants.

"What seems to be the problem?" you enquire.

"Problem?! There's no problem with me! It's this woman. She's not happy with me—with anything I can do or say!" Stanley says, aggressively gesturing toward his wife.

You turn to her.

"He doesn't love me anymore," she says tearfully.

"Why do you think so?"

"He isn't interested in me as a woman anymore. All he does is fall into bed and snore like a plane taking off."

"Well, pardon me for working so hard to provide for the family, that I am exhausted when I get back home," Stanley growls.

"Is it the fatigue that made you take off your wedding ring? He must be having an affair, doctor." Mrs Stanley mutters, looking toward you for support.

"Let me hear your side of the story." you tell Stanley. "Please let me know if anything is troubling you."

"Nothing much to say, doctor. It's just that long days standing at the oven make my back hurt quite a bit. And maybe it's the continuous kneading of dough that makes my hands pain too, especially at night."

S. Bhat, *Clinical Conundrums to Practice Diagnostic Reasoning*,
https://doi.org/10.1007/978-981-95-0636-1_34

"I'm sorry to hear that. May I examine you?"

"Yes," says Stanley lumbering off to the examination couch, bumping against a shelf on his way there. You observe that he has kyphosis.

You note that his blood pressure is 170/100 mm Hg. The thyroid appears enlarged.

The apex is in the 5th intercostal space, laterally displaced an inch outside the midclavicular line.

Stanley has already met his primary care physician who has ordered some basic tests. You check the reports and note that the thyroid function is normal, and fasting blood sugar is 120 mg%.

Triglycerides are elevated, as is serum phosphate.

Question What is the story here? Is Stanley guilty of neglecting his better half? Or is there some way you might be able to help?

Analysis

The trick, in this question, as in the clinic while taking a history, is to glean the important points from the mass of information that is being presented to you.

These are the salient points:

(a) Doughy, sweaty hands
(b) Fatigue
(c) Loss of libido
(d) Removal of wedding ring—fingers becoming thicker?
(e) Snoring
(f) Kyphosis
(g) Hypertension
(h) Left ventricular hypertrophy
(i) Impaired fasting glucose
(j) Thyromegaly
(k) Hyperphosphatemia

The ring size increase is probably the most direct clue to the patient's underlying illness, i.e., acromegaly.

The fact that he bumped on the edge of the shelf is concerning—it implies he has a visual field defect—which could mean that he has a pituitary tumor.

Acromegaly is caused by excessive growth hormone (GH) secretion, usually from a benign pituitary adenoma [1]. This results in excessive insulin-like growth factor 1 (IGF-1) from the liver, which impacts different organs and tissues. The face, jaw, hands, and feet are disproportionately enlarged in adults. Growth hormone hypersecretion prior to fusion of epiphyseal plates results in gigantism.

Epidemiology

Acromegaly is a rare disease, with an estimated incidence of 2.8–13.7 cases per million per year and a prevalence of 40–130 cases per million [2]. The typical age of diagnosis is between 40 and 45 years, though the condition often develops slowly over years before detection. There is no clear gender predisposition.

Etiology [3]

(a) Pituitary adenomas: Account for more than 95% of cases. Adenomas are typically benign, slow-growing tumors.
(b) Ectopic GH-secreting tumors.
(c) Ectopic GHRH-secreting tumors: Extremely rare tumors that secrete growth hormone-releasing hormone (GHRH), leading to pituitary GH hypersecretion. Bronchial carcinoid tumors can ectopically secrete growth hormone-releasing hormone.

Pathogenesis [4]

1. *Excess GH secretion*:
    - Pituitary adenomas lead to autonomous and unregulated GH secretion.
    - Elevated GH levels circulate in the bloodstream, affecting various target tissues.
2. *IGF-1 Overproduction*:
    - GH stimulates the liver to produce IGF-1, a key mediator of GH effects.
    - IGF-1 promotes proliferation, growth, and survival of cells in various tissues. It stimulates chondrogenesis and bone formation, leading to acral enlargement and increased height if the epiphyses are not fused.
    - Soft tissue growth: IGF-1 induces proliferation of soft tissues, causing enlargement of the tongue, skin thickening, and organomegaly.
3. *Metabolic Disturbances*
    - IGF-1 affects glucose metabolism, leading to insulin resistance and increased risk of Type 2 diabetes mellitus. Dyslipidemia may occur, as well.

Clinical Features [5]

The clinical manifestations of acromegaly are diverse and affect multiple organ systems. The insidious onset and subtle progression often results in delayed diagnosis. Key clinical features include:

1. Acral enlargement:
    (a) Enlarged hands and feet: Patients often notice an increase in ring and shoe size.
    (b) Coarsening of facial features: Prominent brow, enlarged nose, and thickened lips.
    (c) Prognathism: Enlargement and protrusion of the lower jaw.
2. Soft tissue changes:
    (a) Skin thickening and increased sweating.
    (b) Macroglossia: This may lead to sleep apnea.
    (c) Deepening of the voice due to laryngeal hypertrophy.
3. Skeletal changes
    (a) Arthralgia and arthritis
    (b) Carpal tunnel syndrome
    (c) Kyphosis
4. Metabolic disturbances:
    (a) Insulin resistance and impaired glucose tolerance
    (b) Hyperlipidemia

5. Cardiovascular manifestations:
   (a) Cardiomyopathy
   (b) Hypertension
   (c) Arrhythmias
6. Neurological manifestations:
   (a) Headaches: Often severe and persistent
   (b) Visual field defects: Bitemporal hemianopia due to compression of the optic chiasm by the pituitary adenoma.
   (c) Peripheral neuropathy and entrapment neuropathies: Presenting with numbness, tingling, and pain in the extremities
7. Other manifestations:
   (a) Sleep apnea: Due to macroglossia and upper airway obstruction
   (b) Goitre
   (c) Increased risk of colon polyps and colorectal cancer
   (d) Galactorrhea and menstrual irregularities (in women) due to prolactin co-secretion
   (e) Erectile dysfunction in men

Investigations [6]

1. Hormonal assays:
   (a) IGF-1 level: This is the initial screening test. Elevated IGF-1 levels, adjusted for age and sex, are suggestive of acromegaly.
   (b) Growth hormone (GH):
      (i) Oral glucose tolerance test (OGTT): The gold standard for confirming GH excess. GH levels should be suppressed to less than 1 ng/mL after glucose ingestion in healthy individuals. Failure to suppress confirms acromegaly.
      (ii) Random GH Levels: Less reliable due to the pulsatile nature of GH secretion.
      (iii) Measurement of prolactin, TSH, LH, FSH, and ACTH to assess for co-secretion or pituitary dysfunction.
2. Imaging studies:
   (a) Pituitary MRI: The primary imaging modality to visualize the pituitary gland and identify adenomas. MRI can determine the size, location, and extension of the tumor (Fig. 34.1).

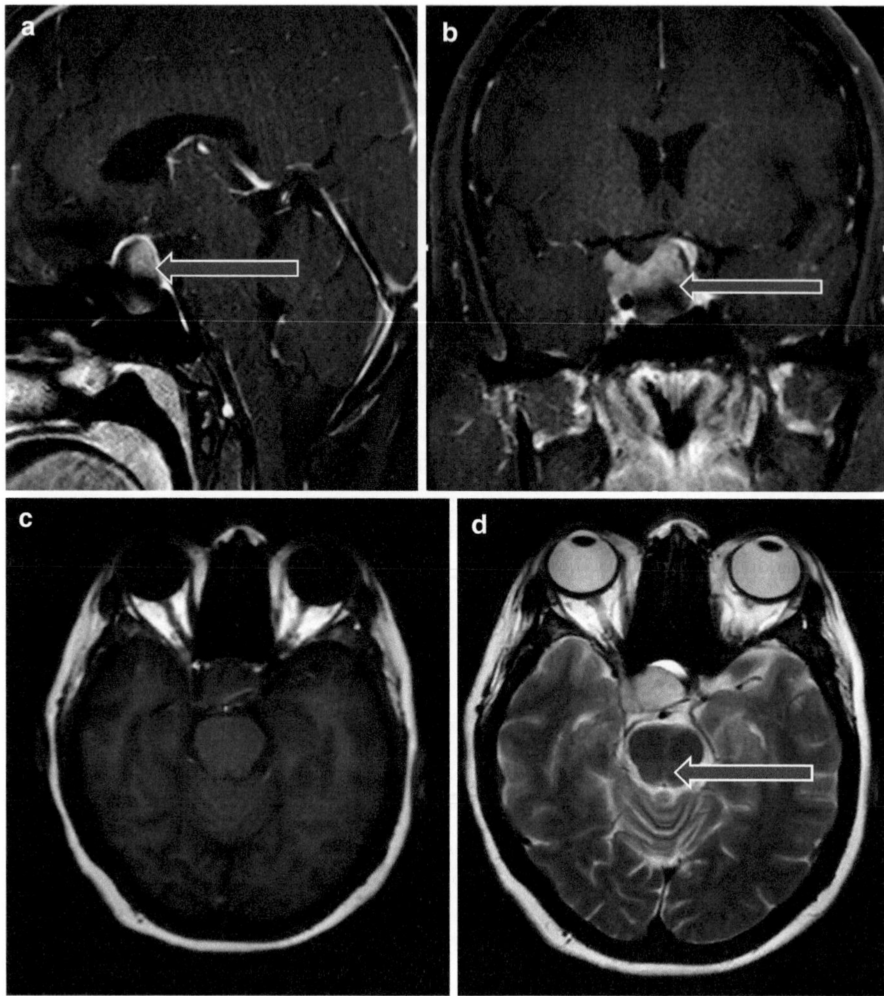

Fig. 34.1 (**a**–**d**) Pituitary macroadenoma (blue arrow). (Images contributed by Dr. Ram Shenoy Basti, FMMC)

Treatment

The goals of acromegaly treatment are to:

- Normalize GH and IGF-1 levels
- Remove or control the pituitary tumor
- Alleviate symptoms and prevent complications

Treatment modalities are as follows:

1. Surgery: Trans-sphenoidal surgery is the first-line treatment for most patients with pituitary adenomas [7]. This is a minimally invasive procedure. Surgical success depends on the size and location of the tumor and the surgeon's experience.
2. Medical therapy [8]:
   (a) Somatostatin analogs (SSAs): Octreotide and lanreotide—These mimic the effects of somatostatin, inhibiting GH secretion. They are administered via intramuscular injections and are effective in reducing GH and IGF-1 levels.
   (b) Growth hormone receptor antagonist: Pegvisomant—This blocks the action of GH at its receptor, reducing IGF-1 levels. It is particularly useful in patients who do not achieve adequate control with SSAs.
   (c) Dopamine agonists: Cabergoline and bromocriptine—These drugs can reduce GH and prolactin secretion, particularly in patients with mixed GH/prolactin-secreting tumors. Their efficacy in reducing GH levels is generally lower compared to SSAs and pegvisomant.
3. Radiation therapy [9]:
   (a) Stereotactic radiosurgery (SRS).
   (b) Gamma knife: Used when surgery and medical therapy are insufficient or not feasible. SRS delivers a high dose of radiation to the tumor while sparing surrounding tissues. However, it may take several years to achieve maximal effect, and the risk of hypopituitarism following the procedure is significant.
   (c) External beam radiation therapy (EBRT): Less commonly used due to a higher risk of hypopituitarism.

References

1. Giustina A, Biermasz N, Casanueva FF, Fleseriu M, Mortini P, Strasburger C, van der Lely AJ, Wass J, Melmed S. Consensus on criteria for acromegaly diagnosis and remission. Pituitary. 2024;27(1):7–22.
2. Lavrentaki A, Paluzzi A, Wass JA, Karavitaki N. Epidemiology of acromegaly: review of population studies. Pituitary. 2017;20:4–9.
3. Colao A, Pivonello C, Grasso LF, Pirchio R. Acromegaly. In: Endocrine pathology. Cham: Springer International Publishing; 2022. p. 9–11.
4. Fleseriu M, Langlois F, Lim DS, Varlamov EV, Melmed S. Acromegaly: pathogenesis, diagnosis, and management. Lancet Diabetes Endocrinol. 2022;10(11):804–26.
5. Slagboom TNA, van Bunderen CC, De Vries R, Bisschop PH, Drent ML. Prevalence of clinical signs, symptoms and comorbidities at diagnosis of acromegaly: a systematic review in accordance with PRISMA guidelines. Pituitary. 2023;26(4):319–32.
6. Akirov A, Masri-Iraqi H, Dotan I, Shimon I. The biochemical diagnosis of acromegaly. J Clin Med. 2021;10(5):1147.
7. Bray DP, Mannam S, Rindler RS, Quillin JW, Oyesiku NM. Surgery for acromegaly: indications and goals. Front Endocrinol. 2022;13:924589.

8. Giustina A, Uygur MM, Frara S, Barkan A, Biermasz NR, Chanson P, Freda P, Gadelha M, Haberbosch L, Kaiser UB, Lamberts S. Standards of care for medical management of acromegaly in pituitary tumor centers of excellence (PTCOE). Pituitary. 2024;27(4):381–8.
9. Bunevicius A, Trifiletti D, Sheehan J. Stereotactic radiosurgery and radiation therapy for acromegaly. In: Acromegaly: a guide to diagnosis and treatment. Cham: Springer International Publishing; 2022. p. 185–206.

Elderly Male with Backache and Restricted Movement: The Security Guard Who Always Stood Straight

35

Grade Difficult.

Abstract An elderly male with backache and stiffness later develops difficulty in swallowing and hoarseness of voice.

Story Karukappa has been the front gate security at your apartment complex for years now. He always stands straight; he always has a smile and a chocolate for the little ones. The only change is that his hair is white, and he seems a little weary at the end of the day.

He knows you are a doctor, and one day he approaches you as you are parking and says "Doctor, can you give me something for my back pain? It is becoming a little difficult to complete my duty hours."

You have a soft corner for Karukappa, and you accompany him to the guardhouse and ask him exactly what is going on. He says that his back and neck tend to ache toward the end of the day. Worse, he finds it quite difficult to bend to tie his shoelaces or tilt his neck to read a book.

On questioning, he says that he has never smoked, does not consume ethanol, and has neither lost nor gained weight. His appetite is normal, and he has no urinary symptoms after prostate surgery a year ago.

You examine him and note that his BMI is 30 and BP is 140/90 mm Hg. Acanthosis nigricans is present. You find that there is no vertebral tenderness, no limb weakness, and his plantar is down going bilaterally. He does, however, have significantly limited spinal movement, especially that of lateral thoracic flexion. There are some tiny nodular swellings on his elbow and fingers, but they do not seem significant.

You advise some blood tests and imaging of the spine, but he is very reluctant, and after a great deal of persuasion consents only for some basic blood investigations. Lab reports show impaired fasting glucose and mild dyslipidemia—you counsel him about his diet and ask him to repeat the lipid profile in 3 months' time. His

S. Bhat, *Clinical Conundrums to Practice Diagnostic Reasoning*,
https://doi.org/10.1007/978-981-95-0636-1_35

Hb is 15 and ESR is 4. Counts are normal. Only marginally reassured, you prescribe a pain-relieving gel for application and admonish Karukappa to review with you if the pain does not get better.

It is more than a month later that Karukappa—stooping and moving with difficulty—diffidently approaches you on your way to the elevator and says, "The pain is a little worse, doctor."

"Oh no, is there anything else troubling you?"

"I'm finding it a little difficult to swallow." You are extremely concerned now, considering Karukappa's age, dysphagia, back pain, and the fact that his voice as he volunteers the history sounds a little hoarse. Though the history is not typical, you are considering GI malignancy with spinal metastasis.

Question Are you right about poor Karukappa? Is metastatic malignancy the only possible diagnosis or would you like to consider a less sinister possibility?

Analysis

This is a slightly tricky question. The back pain along with the stiffness and limitation of movement might prompt you to consider a diagnosis of ankylosing spondylitis (AS); however, the fact that the symptoms are localized mainly to the cervical and thoracic involvement rather than lumbar region goes against AS. There are clear indicators of insulin resistance (increased BMI and impaired fasting glucose), and this, along with the history of limitation of thoracic movement, dysphagia, and hoarseness of voice, raises a possibility other than metastatic malignancy. This constellation of complaints and physical findings can be seen in Diffuse Idiopathic Skeletal Hyperostosis (DISH) [1, 2].

DISH (also called Forestier disease) is a proliferative musculoskeletal disease due to the ossification and calcification of spinal ligaments that causes in back pain, neck pain, and characteristic radiological changes [3]. Diffuse idiopathic skeletal *hyperostosis* (DISH) is characterized by the presence of at least three bony bridges at the anterolateral spine opposite to the aorta [4]. It is associated with constitutional and metabolic abnormalities [5].

DISH is more common in males, and the prevalence increases with age [6]. Interestingly, the skeletons of four pharaohs Amenhotep III (18th Dynasty), Ramesses II, his son Merenptah, and Ramesses III all show some signs of DISH [7].

Etiopathogenesis

Genetic, environmental, dietary, and mechanical factors have all been implicated in the key etiopathogenetic feature of DISH, viz. abnormal osteoblastic differentiation. Many of the symptoms of DISH can be ascribed to osteophyte formation [8].

Risk Factors [9]

(a) Male sex
(b) Age greater than 50 years
(c) Obesity, high waist-to-hip circumference ratio
(d) Dyslipidemia, hypertension, glucose intolerance, Type 2 diabetes, hyperuricemia, hyperinsulinemia, and possibly elevated growth hormone and insulin-like growth factor [10]
(e) Perhaps higher levels of vitamin A

Table 35.1 Distinguishing features between DISH and ankylosing spondylitis [12]

	DISH	Ankylosing spondylitis
Thoracic spine	Involved early	Involved late
Intervertebral disc height	Maintained	Reduced
Main pathology	Enthesis	Cartilage of intervertebral disc
Osteophytes	Vertical and bridging	Transverse

Clinical Features [11]

Neck pain, back pain, *limitation in thoracic flexion*, dysphagia because of esophageal compression by large cervical osteophytes, and hoarseness of voice. Palpable bony spurs at elbow and knee may be present. DISH can be differentiated from ankylosing spondylitis by certain features (Table 35.1).

Complications

Dysphagia, myelopathy, aspiration pneumonia, esophageal obstruction, stridor, hoarseness, and thoracic outlet syndrome

Diagnosis

Imaging reveals linear calcification and hyperostosis of the vertebral bodies. Bone density is increased, and bony excrescences may be present (Fig. 35.1). ESR, complete blood count, serum protein electrophoresis, calcium, and parathormone are *characteristically normal*. Unlike in ankylosing spondylitis, HLA B27 is not commonly associated with DISH.

Differential Diagnosis

The stooped posture of DISH is similar to that of ankylosing spondylitis, and the two must be distinguished.

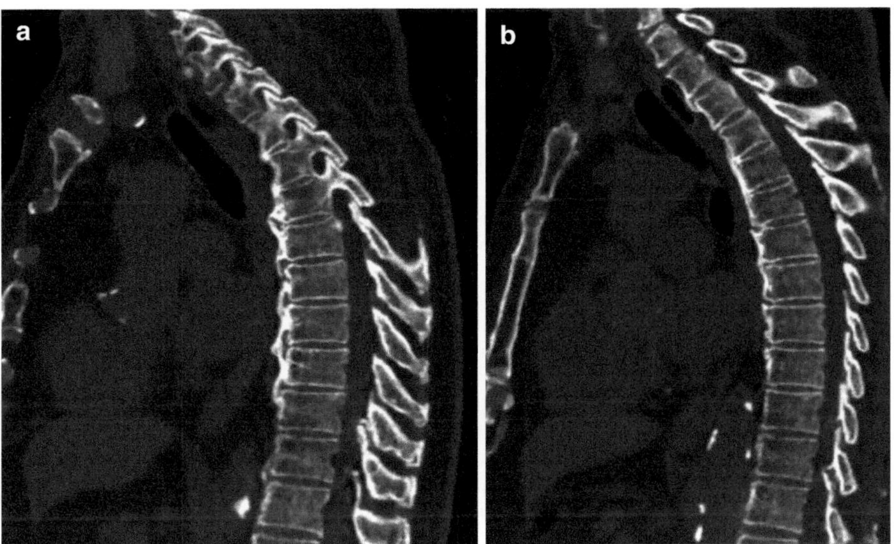

Fig. 35.1 DISH. (Image contributed by Dr. Ram Shenoy Basti, FMMC)

Treatment [13]

(a) Lifestyle management: Diet and exercise.
(b) Weight loss.
(c) Physiotherapy.
(d) Paracetamol, NSAIDS, and local glucocorticoid injections.
(e) Surgery may be required to remove bony spurs which are causing dysphagia.

Avoid thiazide diuretics and beta-blockers (since they increase insulin resistance).

Key Takeaway
DISH can be a marker for carotid atherosclerosis and metabolic syndrome; additionally, it is a risk factor for complicated spinal fractures.

Endotracheal intubation and endoscopy are difficult in these patients.

Though DISH is not immediately life-threatening, the possibility of spinal cord compression in patients with ossification of the posterior longitudinal ligament (OPLL)

must be kept in mind, especially when there are warning signs like sharp pain in the neck, unsteady gait, or brisk reflexes.

References

1. Foshang TH, Mestan MA, Riggs LJ. Diffuse idiopathic skeletal hyperostosis: a case of dysphagia. J Manipulative Physiol Ther. 2002;25(1):71–6.
2. Kuperus JS, Mohamed Hoesein FAA, de Jong PA, Verlaan JJ. Diffuse idiopathic skeletal hyperostosis: etiology and clinical relevance. Best Pract Res Clin Rheumatol. 2020;34(3):101527.
3. Diffuse idiopathic skeletal hyperostosis (DISH) with ossification of the posterior longitudinal ligament (OPLL) in the cervical spine without neurological deficit – A Case report – PMC [Internet]. [cited 2025 Feb 4]. Available from: https://pmc.ncbi.nlm.nih.gov/articles/PMC7680695/.
4. Utsinger PD. 7 – Diffuse Idiopathic Skeletal Hyperostosis. Clin Rheum Dis. 1985;11(2):325–51.
5. Diffuse Idiopathic Skeletal Hyperostosis of the Spine: Pathophysiology, Diagnosis, and Management – PubMed [Internet]. [cited 2025 Feb 4]. Available from: https://pubmed.ncbi.nlm.nih.gov/34559699/.
6. Prevalence of diffuse idiopathic skeletal hyperostosis (DISH) assessed with whole-spine computed tomography in 1479 subjects – PubMed [Internet]. [cited 2025 Feb 4]. Available from: https://pubmed.ncbi.nlm.nih.gov/29848322/.
7. Saleem SN, Hawass Z. Ankylosing spondylitis or diffuse idiopathic skeletal hyperostosis in royal Egyptian mummies of 18th–20th Dynasties? CT and archaeology studies. Arthritis Rheumatol Hoboken NJ. 2014;66(12):3311–6.
8. Mader R, Verlaan JJ, Buskila D. Diffuse idiopathic skeletal hyperostosis: clinical features and pathogenic mechanisms. Nat Rev Rheumatol. 2013;9(12):741–50.
9. Mader R, Lavi I. Diabetes mellitus and hypertension as risk factors for early diffuse idiopathic skeletal hyperostosis (DISH). Osteoarthr Cartil. 2009;17(6):825–8.
10. Sencan D, Elden H, Nacitarhan V, Sencan M, Kaptanoglu E. The prevalence of diffuse idiopathic skeletal hyperostosis in patients with diabetes mellitus. Rheumatol Int. 2005;25(7):518–21.
11. Clinical manifestations of diffuse idiopathic skeletal hyperostosis of the cervical spine – ScienceDirect [Internet]. [cited 2025 Feb 4]. Available from: https://www.sciencedirect.com/science/article/abs/pii/S0049017202000604.
12. Olivieri I, D'Angelo S, Palazzi C, Padula A, Mader R, Khan MA. Diffuse idiopathic skeletal hyperostosis: differentiation from ankylosing spondylitis. Curr Rheumatol Rep. 2009;11(5):321–8.
13. Mader R, Verlaan JJ, Eshed I, Jacome BA, Puttini PS, Atzeni F, et al. Diffuse idiopathic skeletal hyperostosis (DISH): where we are now and where to go next. RMD Open. 2017;3(1):rmdopen-2017-000472.

36 Polydipsia, Polyuria, and Pruritus—The Paan-Chewing Babu

Grade Moderate.

Abstract Polydipsia, polyuria, and pruritus in a middle-aged male with no known comorbidities.

Story You have to sort out an error that has been made in your property tax, and you walk into the District Commissioner's office, sighing at the thought of the tedious afternoon that awaits you. You walk up to the table of the concerned section. A hirsute government employee, Babu, sits at the table like a king on a throne and snaps at you "What?"

With extreme politeness and an assumed air of diffidence, you begin to describe the problem that you are facing. You quite admire yourself for maintaining your calm, though you are distracted by Babu chewing his paan and betel nut vigorously and expectorating noisily.

"What do you expect me to do?" Babu grunts, alternating between scratching his left forearm and right axilla.

"I wonder if you could help, sir," you mumble.

"Help??! He wants me to help!" Babu smirks at his colleagues, and they all laugh sycophantically. You, however, do not see the joke.

"Please, sir, I am a busy doctor. I would really appreciate it if you could help me."

"You are a doctor, is it? You have a clinic? OK, I will come and meet you to discuss my health issues."

"But can you help me with the taxation error?" you timidly ask.

"Wait!" he barks "I have to visit the bathroom. God only knows what is wrong. I drink water, pass urine, drink water again, pass urine again. I am only 59 but my muscles hurt as though I am 95. Plus, my previous doctor said my kidneys are delicate."

S. Bhat, *Clinical Conundrums to Practice Diagnostic Reasoning*,
https://doi.org/10.1007/978-981-95-0636-1_36

He returns and says "Ok, you please complete the necessary documentation and meet me in a week, I will see what I can do to help."

"Yes, of course, thank you, sir," you say.

As you bend forward to pick up your papers from the table, you catch his eye and are disconcerted to note that there is a kind of white patch on his left cornea. You are surprised that you had not noticed it earlier—perhaps it was the toxic environment of the government office that had put you off your game.

You walk back to your clinic, asking yourself if there is something really wrong with Babu, or was he like almost everyone else you meet—trying to cadge a free consultation.

Question What do you think? Was there anything wrong with Babu apart from a sedentary lifestyle and sketchy hygiene practices?

Analysis

The clues are as follows:

(a) Pruritus—“scratching his axilla and forearm”
(b) Polydipsia and polyuria—“drink water go to the bathroom, drink water go to the bathroom”
(c) Myalgia—“my muscles hurt as though I am 95”
(d) Band keratopathy—white patch on cornea

The important causes of polyuria are [1]

(a) Diabetes mellitus
(b) Diabetes insipidus
(c) Hypokalemia
(d) Hypercalcemia
(e) Drugs like diuretics
(f) Early chronic kidney disease
(g) Diuretic phase of recovery from acute tubular necrosis
(h) Inability to concentrate urine: Sickle cell anemia and chronic pyelonephritis
(i) Anxiety
(j) Psychogenic polydipsia
(k) Post-TURP

The polyuria along with the pruritus, betel nut chewing, and the final clue of the white patch on the cornea, i.e., band keratopathy, taken as a whole, point to hypercalcemia—perhaps secondary to milk alkali syndrome because of the excessive betel nut chewing [2]. The paste applied to the betel leaf is usually composed of ground oyster shells and contains a significant amount of calcium carbonate. The paste is alkaline, adding to the risk of milk alkali syndrome.

Definition: The milk alkali syndrome [3] comprises the triad of

(a) Hypercalcemia
(b) Metabolic alkalosis
(c) Kidney injury

Etiopathogenesis

Historically, milk alkali syndrome was due to the ingestion of Sippy’s mixture (milk and cream combined with an absorbable alkali such as magnesium oxide, sodium bicarbonate, or bismuth subcarbonate) for the treatment of peptic ulcer disease [4]. However, presently, it is due to increased ingestion of calcium either as

A. Excessive over-the-counter supplements, especially in postmenopausal women
B. Calcium carbonate given in the management of chronic kidney disease to prevent secondary hyperparathyroidism
C. Nicotine substitute chewing gum
D. Betel nut chewing

Pathogenesis [5] (Fig. 36.1)

The initial hypercalcemia due to increased ingestion contributes to volume depletion.

Volume depletion activates the renin angiotensin aldosterone axis resulting in (Fig. 36.2)

(a) Increased sodium reabsorption in exchange for H+ excretion
(b) Indirectly, increased bicarbonate reabsorption

Net increased bicarbonate reabsorption results in metabolic alkalosis, which in turn further exacerbates hypercalcemia. Individuals with decreased bone buffering capacity (e.g., the elderly) and those with impaired ability to suppress calcitriol when calcium levels rise are at increased risk for milk alkali syndrome.

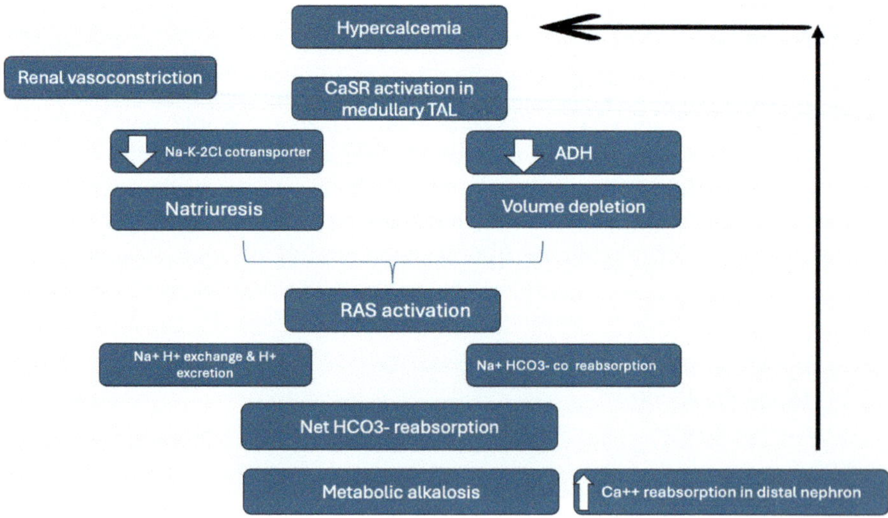

Fig. 36.1 Calcium reabsorption in the kidney. CaSR calcium sensing receptor, TAL thick ascending loop

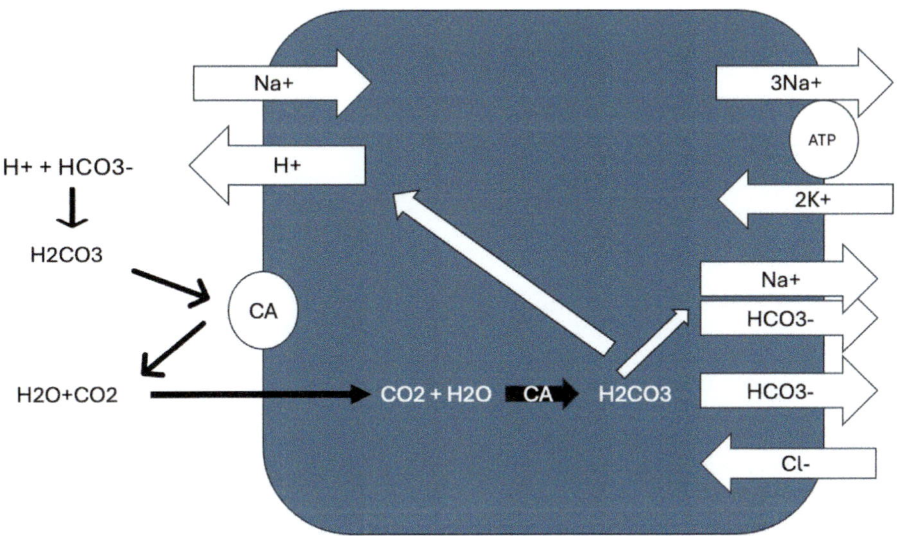

Fig. 36.2 Increased bicarbonate reabsorption

Clinical Features [6]

- Nausea and vomiting
- Altered sensorium
- Pruritus
- Polydipsia
- Polyuria
- Myalgia
- Band keratopathy

Diagnosis [7]

In patients with hypercalcemia, alkalosis, and renal impairment, other causes of hypercalcemia must be excluded, and a history of excessive consumption of calcium may be elicited. Lab investigations reveal hypomagnesemia and

hypophosphatemia in addition to hypercalcemia. Importantly, parathormone levels are suppressed in milk alkali syndrome, unlike in primary hyperparathyroidism.

Treatment [8]

1. Cessation of calcium supplements
2. Administration of isotonic saline
3. Furosemide

References

1. Ramírez-Guerrero G, Müller-Ortiz H, Pedreros-Rosales C. Polyuria in adults. A diagnostic approach based on pathophysiology. Revista Clínica Española (English Edition). 2022;222(5):301–8.
2. Lin SH, Lin YF, Cheema-Dhadli S, Davids MR, Halperin ML. Hypercalcaemia and metabolic alkalosis with betel nut chewing: emphasis on its integrative pathophysiology. Nephrol Dial Transplant. 2002;17(5):708–14.
3. Dorsch TR. The milk-alkali syndrome, vitamin D, and parathyroid hormone. Ann Intern Med. 1986;105(5):800–1.
4. He J, Morton A. Milk-alkali syndrome. Aust J Gen Pract. 2024;53(4):187–8.
5. Felsenfeld AJ, Levine BS. Milk alkali syndrome and the dynamics of calcium homeostasis. Clin J Am Soc Nephrol. 2006;1(4):641–54.
6. Zayed RF, Millhouse PW, Kamyab F, Ortiz JF, Atoot A. Calcium-alkali syndrome: historical review, pathophysiology and post-modern update. Cureus. 2021;13(2)
7. Picolos MK, Lavis VR, Orlander PR. Milk–alkali syndrome is a major cause of hypercalcaemia among non-end-stage renal disease (non-ESRD) inpatients. Clin Endocrinol. 2005;63(5):566–76.
8. Hossain MS, Azad MA, Rahaman MF, Aftab KA, Rahman IB, Monira S. A case of Milk Alkali syndrome: the forgotten diagnosis of generalized weakness and altered consciousness. J Med. 2024;25(2):184–6.

37 Gum Bleeding, Tinnitus, and Fatigue: The Bloody Apple

Grade Moderate.

Abstract An adult male with nonspecific symptoms of fatigue and loss of weight along with gum bleeding and tinnitus.

Story "Ah, the first apple of autumn!" You tell your school friend Gokul, handing him one as you sit in the park, reminiscing about the past.

"Yum!" He says taking a huge bite.

"Hey, hold it, hold it," you say, "there's some blood on this."

"Oh yes, just a little. I've been noticing it for a while. No big deal."

"It actually is a big deal. When did you first notice this?""This continuous oozing of my gums? I don't know exactly—maybe the last couple of months—But I don't think it's a big deal. We're both growing old, pal."

"60 years is not old! We are in the prime of life! Are there any problems apart from the oozing?"

"Well, I've been trying to eat clean—I guess that's why I have lost some weight and am feeling tired all the time."

"The last I heard eating clean does not cause fatigue," you scoff.

"Agreed, agreed. But I wonder does it cause this buzzing in my ears?"

"No, no it doesn't. Brother, come and meet me in hospital this week. Let's get a basic checkup. What's the point in having a medico friend if you are going to neglect your health?"

You notice, disturbed, that his flip flops tend to slip off as he walks to his car.

Gokul shows up for his checkup, and you switch from friend mode to doctor mode. You take the history again—one extra point that comes up is that Gokul has been treated for Hepatitis C 2 years ago and was declared to be cured. As you proceed with the examination, you get more and more worried.

S. Bhat, *Clinical Conundrums to Practice Diagnostic Reasoning*, https://doi.org/10.1007/978-981-95-0636-1_37

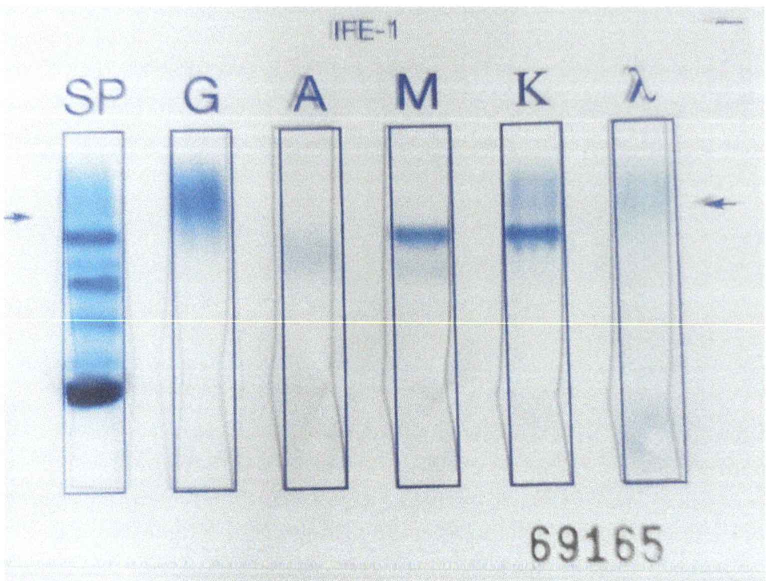

Fig. 37.1 Serum electrophoresis showing M band and IgM kappa. (Contributed by Dr. Shivashankara AR, FMCI)

You note that Gokul is pale, his BMI is 18, and there is a continuous ooze from the gums. He has hepatosplenomegaly and cervical lymphadenopathy. There is a glove and stocking sensory loss, and the ankle jerk is absent bilaterally. You check the optic fundus, and you are a little puzzled as you have not seen this particular appearance before—the retinal veins look stretched and segmented—with a weird resemblance to sausage links—and you order an ophthalmology consult since you have no clue what you are looking at.

Labs reveal anemia, an ESR of 100, and proteinuria. The peripheral smear demonstrates rouleaux formation. In light of this, you ask for a serum protein electrophoresis, which shows a monoclonal spike (Fig. 37.1).

Your colleague tells you that the IgM monoclonal spike is 4.5 gm and asks you to test the viscosity—it turns out that the viscosity is a worrying 4 centipoise.

Questions Putting all these together, what might be the likely diagnosis in the unfortunate Gokul? How do you confirm the diagnosis and proceed with treatment?

Analysis

The main symptoms here are

(a) Gum bleeding;
(b) Tinnitus;
(c) Fatigue;
(d) Loss of weight

The signs are hepatosplenomegaly, lymphadenopathy, and findings suggestive of a peripheral neuropathy.

The tinnitus and fatigue point toward anemia, and the gum bleeding is a clue toward a hematological malignancy. Anemia and peripheral neuropathy may be due to Vitamin B12 deficiency; however, the ESR of 100, the proteinuria, and the rouleaux formation lead one toward a diagnosis of a lymphoproliferative disorder or plasma cell dyscrasia. The specific pointer toward Waldenström's macroglobulinemia (WM) is the past history of Hepatitis C, the sausage link-like appearance in the fundus, and the very high viscosity.

Waldenström's macroglobulinemia is an IgM monoclonal gammopathy secondary to a lymphoplasmacytic lymphoma.

Etiopathogenesis (Fig. 37.2)

There is a higher than unexpected rate of 6q21e23 in patients with WM [1].

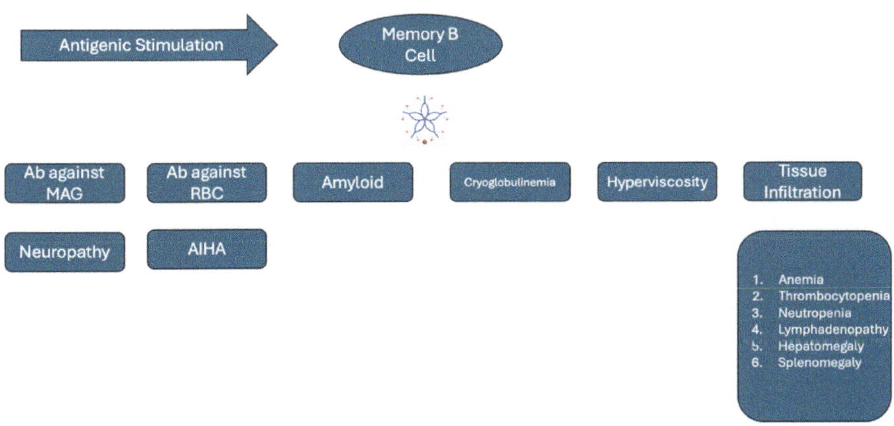

Fig. 37.2 Pathogenesis of WM. AIHA: Autoimmune hemolytic anemia. MAG : myelin associated glycoprotein

Clinical Features [8]

(i) Increased serum viscosity is a characteristic feature of Waldenström's macroglobulinemia [2]. Symptoms due to hyperviscosity: Headache, dizziness, blurring of vision, nystagmus, diplopia, tinnitus, ataxia, and oronasal bleeding. Confusion and focal neurological deficits can occur too [3].

(ii) Due to autoantibodies: Peripheral neuropathy, cranial neuropathy, and mononeuritis multiplex [4].

(iii) Due to cryoglobulinemia: Raynaud's phenomenon, acral cyanosis [5], immune-mediated glomerulonephritis.

(iv) Due to lymphocyte infiltration of central nervous system: Bing Neel syndrome [5]

(v) Due to AL amyloidosis: Nephrotic syndrome, axonal neuropathy, intestinal dysmotility, purpura, and macroglossia [7].

Investigations

CBC
Coagulation parameters
Serum protein electrophoresis
Bone marrow biopsy
Measurement of viscosity

Diagnosis is made by [6]

A. Presence of IgM monoclonal band
B. > 10% lymphoplasmacytic cells in bone marrow biopsy
C. Typical immunophenotype

Differential Diagnosis [9]

1. IgM monoclonal gammopathy of undetermined significance
2. Multiple myeloma
3. Chronic lymphocytic leukemia
4. Marginal zone lymphoma
5. Mantle cell lymphoma

Treatment

Patients must be staged as per the Modified Staging System for Waldenstrom macroglobulinemia [7].

Not all patients with Waldenström macroglobulinemia need to be treated. Indications for treatment [10] [11]:

(a) B symptoms
(b) Complications of hyperviscosity
(c) Symptomatic lymphadenopathy or organomegaly
(d) Autoimmune hemolytic anemia
(e) Nephropathy
(f) Amyloid

Symptomatic hyperviscosity is a medical emergency and will require plasmapheresis on an emergent basis [12].

Treatment regimens include

(a) Rituximab [13]
(b) BTK inhibitors
(c) Dexamethasone, rituximab, and cyclophosphamide (DRC)
(d) Bortezomib plus rituximab with or without dexamethasone (BDR) [14]

References

1. Schop RF, Kuehl WM, Van Wier SA, Ahmann GJ, Price-Troska T, Bailey RJ, Jalal SM, Qi Y, Kyle RA, Greipp PR, Fonseca R. Waldenstrom macroglobulinemia neoplastic cells lack immunoglobulin heavy chain locus translocations but have frequent 6q deletions. Blood J Am Soc Hematol. 2002;100(8):2996–3001.
2. Gertz MA, Kyle RA. Hyperviscosity syndrome. J Intensive Care Med. 1995;10(3):128–41. https://doi.org/10.1177/088506669501000304. PMID: 10155178.
3. Waldenstrom J. Zwei interessante syndrome mit hyperglobulinamie (purpura hyperglobulinaemica und makroglobulinamie). Schweiz Med Wschr. 1948;78:927–8.
4. Stone MJ, Merlini G, Pascual V. Autoantibody activity in Waldenström's Macroglobulinemia. Clin Lymphoma. 2005;5(4):225–9.
5. Stone MJ. Waldenström's Macroglobulinemia: hyperviscosity syndrome and Cryoglobulinemia. Clin Lymphoma Myeloma. 2009;9(1):97–9.
6. Nanah A, Al Hadidi S. Bing-Neel syndrome: update on the diagnosis and treatment. Clin Lymphoma Myeloma Leuk. 2022;22(3):e213–9.
7. Lu R, Richards T. A focus on Waldenström Macroglobulinemia and AL Amyloidosis. J Adv Pract Oncol. 2022;13(Suppl 4):45–56.
8. Dimopoulos MA, Panayiotidis P, Moulopoulos LA, Sfikakis P, Dalakas M. Waldenstrom's macroglobulinemia: clinical features, complications, and management. J Clin Oncol. 2000;18(1):214.
9. Shaheen SP, Talwalkar SS, Lin P, Medeiros LJ. Waldenström Macroglobulinemia: a review of the entity and its differential diagnosis. Adv Anat Pathol. 2012;19(1):11.
10. Zanwar S, Le-Rademacher J, Durot E, D'Sa S, Abeykoon JP, Mondello P, Kumar S, Sarosiek S, Paludo J, Chhabra S, Cook JM. Simplified risk stratification model for patients with Waldenström macroglobulinemia. J Clin Oncol. 2024;42(21):2527–36.
11. Vos JMI, Minnema MC, Wijermans PW, Croockewit S, Chamuleau MED, Pals ST, et al. Guideline for diagnosis and treatment of Waldenström's macroglobulinaemia. Neth J Med. 2013;71(2):54–62.

12. Zarkovic M, Kwaan HC. Correction of Hyperviscosity by Apheresis. Semin Thromb Hemost. 2003;29:535–42.
13. Kapoor P, Ansell SM, Fonseca R, Chanan-Khan A, Kyle RA, Kumar SK, Mikhael JR, Witzig TE, Mauermann M, Dispenzieri A, Ailawadhi S. Diagnosis and management of Waldenström macroglobulinemia: mayo stratification of macroglobulinemia and risk-adapted therapy (mSMART) guidelines 2016. JAMA Oncol. 2017;3(9):1257–65.
14. Treon SP, Ioakimidis L, Soumerai JD, Patterson CJ, Sheehy P, Nelson M, Willen M, Matous J, Mattern J, Diener JG, Keogh GP. Primary therapy of Waldenström macroglobulinemia with bortezomib, dexamethasone, and rituximab: WMCTG clinical trial 05-180. J Clin Oncol. 2009;27(23):3830–5.

38 Elderly Patient with Pruritus, Splenomegaly, and Constitutional Symptoms: Itchy Ignatius

Grade Moderate.

Abstract An elderly patient with an initial presentation of weakness, loss of weight, and pruritus is later admitted to a hospital with clinical features suggestive of mesenteric ischemia.

Story Ignatius has been your patient since you graduated from medical school, and you are quite attached to him. You both have a shared interest in the butterflies of Asia and spend many happy minutes discussing this in your consultation room.

Ignatius shows up one fine Friday morning for his routine monthly checkup. But he seems to be in low spirits and loath to discuss your shared hobby.

"What's up, Mr Ignatius? You don't seem to be your usual self."

"Not feeling that great honestly," Ignatius says scratching his forearm frantically.

"Is it an allergy that is troubling you?"

"I'm not sure doctor, but my whole body itches, and I feel so tired all the time."

You check his weight and are worried to see that it is 3 kg below his baseline.

"How is your appetite?"

"My appetite is ok, but I feel full after only a few morsels."

"Ok, please lie down on the examination couch, let's have a look at you."

You note that Mr Ignatius is pale. The liver is palpable 4 cm below the right costal margin, and the spleen crosses the midline.

"My legs hurt a lot, doctor," says Ignatius, and when you examine the lower limbs, you note that the left tibia and knee are palpably warmer, though nontender.

These findings concern you, and you suggest Mr Ignatius gets admitted to the hospital for a few days for a thorough evaluation.

Mr Ignatius refuses however and gets quite upset when you insist.

S. Bhat, *Clinical Conundrums to Practice Diagnostic Reasoning*,
https://doi.org/10.1007/978-981-95-0636-1_38

"My wife and I have made plans to visit our granddaughter in Paris. I absolutely won't waste any time getting admitted or getting any more blood tests," he says walking off in a huff.

You worry about Mr Ignatius for a couple of days, but the wards are full, your clinic is busy, and you hardly have time to breathe, so Ignatius' problems take a backseat in your brain.

About a month later, you are in the emergency department when you see Ignatius being wheeled in, concerned son in tow.

"What happened?" you ask as Ignatius clutches his tummy and rolls around the bed in a futile attempt to find a comfortable position.

"He's not been keeping well for almost a month, doctor, ever since he returned from his Paris trip. He has been having fever and bodyache. I've been begging him to meet a doctor, but you know how stubborn he can be. This evening my parents were at our house for dinner, and we were just relaxing after a hearty meal when he suddenly had this severe pain in the tummy, especially around the navel. He had to pass motions after that, and he says his stools were black in color."

"That must have been frightening for you," you say sympathetically.

You note that BP is 130/60 mm Hg. Pallor is present. You are a little surprised, considering the amount of pain that Ignatius is in, that his abdomen is only mildly tender.

You review the lab results which are remarkable for neutrophilic leukocytosis, increased lactate, and acidosis.

You page the GI surgeon who orders an urgent CT abdomen—this is indicative of acute mesenteric vein thrombosis.

Question Can you correlate Ignatius' initial presentation of anemia, hepatosplenomegaly, and bony pain with his second admission to hospital?

Analysis

The fact that Ignatius has presented with mesenteric vein thrombosis means that he either has a condition causing hypercoagulability, or thrombocythemia, or both. Keeping this in mind, let us analyze the first presentation. The massive splenomegaly (spleen crossing the midline) is not seen in many conditions. The diseases that cause massive splenomegaly include [1]:

(a) Myelofibrosis
(b) Chronic myeloid leukemia
(c) Essential thrombocythemia
(d) Hairy cell leukemia
(e) Visceral leishmaniasis
(f) Malaria

In this context, the pruritus and the overwhelming fatigue, along with the evidence of extramedullary hemopoiesis in the form of bone pain and warmth over the knee and tibia, are suggestive of myelofibrosis. In primary myelofibrosis, thrombocythemia may coexist with anemia and is responsible for both acute arterial and venous thrombi.

Myelofibrosis is a chronic myeloproliferative disorder due to clonal proliferation of cell lines and is characterized by splenomegaly and various constitutional symptoms [2].

There is a potential for leukemic transformation [3].

It is a disease of the elderly with most patients being older than 60 years [4].

JAK2 mutation, calreticulin gene mutation, and MPL mutation may be seen [5].

Myelofibrosis occurs due to a mutation of pluripotent hematopoietic progenitor cell. The bone marrow fibrosis is secondary to cytokines secreted by the megakaryocytes, T cells, and B cells (Fig. 38.1).

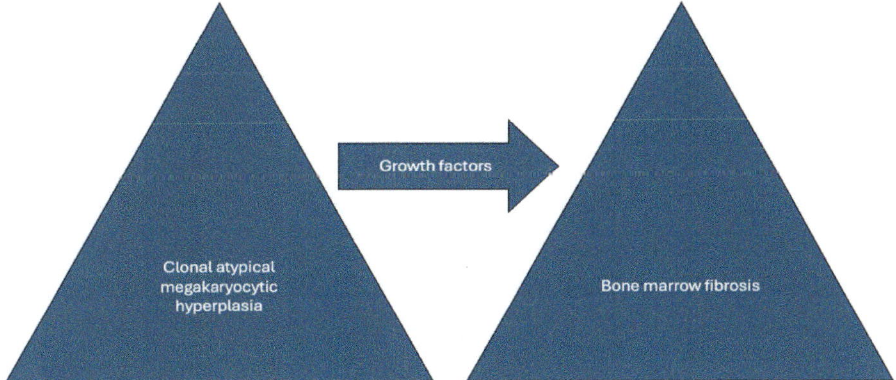

Fig. 38.1 Hyperplasia progressing to marrow fibrosis

Clinical Features

Disabling fatigue and pruritus [5] are the most common symptoms.

Other Complaints

A. Due to massive splenomegaly: Dragging pain abdomen and early satiety [6].
B. Due to hypermetabolism: Fever, night sweats, and weight loss [7].
C. Due to extramedullary hemopoiesis [1]: Warmth at knee and tibia.
D. Due to thrombocythemia [7] and hypercoagulability: Portal vein thrombosis and mesenteric thrombosis [9].

Labs Reveal [8] the Following

(a) Anemia, thrombocytopenia or thrombocytosis, leucoerythroblastic blood picture.
(b) Bone marrow aspirate often yields a dry tap, while bone marrow biopsy reveals fibrosis [11].
(c) *JAK2*, CALR, and *MPL* mutations may be seen, however, in 5% of patients; "triple-negative" disease (i.e., no *JAK2*, *CALR*, or *MPL* mutation) is also known.

Diagnosis [10]

All three major criteria and at least one minor criterion are required to make diagnosis.

Major Criteria

1. Megakaryocytic proliferation and atypia with fibrosis
2. WHO criteria for other myeloproliferative disorders, including polycythemia *not* met
3. *JAK2*, *CALR*, or *MPL* mutation

Minor Criteria

- Anemia not attributable to a comorbid condition
- Leukocytosis $\geq 11 \times 10^9$/L (>11,000/microL)
- Palpable splenomegaly
- LDH above the upper limit of normal
- Leukoerythroblastosis

Treatment

The first step is risk stratification. For high-risk patients, the definitive treatment is allogenic stem cell transplant, since most drugs do not improve survival rates. The JAK inhibitors fedratinib, pacritinib, and momelotinib have shown promising results [12].

Low-risk asymptomatic patients are observed and monitored.

Symptomatic patients may be treated as follows:

1. Anemia: Transfusion
2. Anemia with splenomegaly: Hydroxyurea [13]
3. Anemia with splenomegaly without thrombocytopenia: Ruxolitinib [14]
4. Anemia with splenomegaly with thrombocytopenia: Pacritinib [15]

Key Takeaway
Consider mesenteric ischemia in any patient presenting with abdominal pain disproportionate to physical findings, along with lab reports of leukocytosis and metabolic acidosis.

References

1. O'Reilly RA. Splenomegaly in 2,505 patients in a large university medical center from 1913 to 1995. 1913 to 1962: 2,056 patients. West J Med. 1998;169(2):78.
2. Cervantes F, Dupriez B, Pereira A, Passamonti F, Reilly JT, Morra E, Vannucchi AM, Mesa RA, Demory JL, Barosi G, Rumi E. New prognostic scoring system for primary myelofibrosis based on a study of the International Working Group for Myelofibrosis Research and Treatment. Blood J Am Soc Hematol. 2009;113(13):2895–901.
3. Vallapureddy RR, Mudireddy M, Penna D, Lasho TL, Finke CM, Hanson CA, Ketterling RP, Begna KH, Gangat N, Pardanani A, Tefferi A. Leukemic transformation among 1306 patients with primary myelofibrosis: risk factors and development of a predictive model. Blood Cancer J. 2019;9(2):12.
4. Mesa RA, Silverstein MN, Jacobsen SJ, Wollan PC, Tefferi A. Population-based incidence and survival figures in essential thrombocythemia and agnogenic myeloid metaplasia: an Olmsted County Study, 1976–1995. Am J Hematol. 1999;61(1):10–5.
5. Rumi E, Trotti C, Vanni D, Casetti IC, Pietra D, Sant'Antonio E. The genetic basis of primary myelofibrosis and its clinical relevance. Int J Mol Sci. 2020;21(23):8885.
6. Vaa BE, Wolanskyj AP, Roeker L, Pardanani A, Lasho TL, Finke CM, Tefferi A. Pruritus in primary myelofibrosis: clinical and laboratory correlates. Am J Hematol. 2012;87(2):136–8.
7. Oon SF, Singh D, Tan TH, Lee A, Noe G, Burbury K, Paiva J. Primary myelofibrosis: spectrum of imaging features and disease-related complications. Insights Imaging. 2019;10:1–4.
8. Gupta S, Krishnan AS, Singh J, Gupta A, Gupta M. Clinicopathological characteristics and management of extramedullary hematopoiesis: a review. Pediatric Hematol Oncol J. 2022;7(4):182–6.
9. Barbui T, Carobbio A, Cervantes F, Vannucchi AM, Guglielmelli P, Antonioli E, Alvarez-Larrán A, Rambaldi A, Finazzi G, Barosi G. Thrombosis in primary myelofibrosis: incidence and risk factors. Blood J Am Soc Hematol. 2010;115(4):778–82.
10. Prakash S, Orazi A. How I diagnose primary myelofibrosis. Am J Clin Pathol. 2022;157(4):518–30.

11. Abou Zahr A, Salama ME, Carreau N, Tremblay D, Verstovsek S, Mesa R, Hoffman R, Mascarenhas J. Bone marrow fibrosis in myelofibrosis: pathogenesis, prognosis and targeted strategies. Haematologica. 2016;101(6):660.
12. Nair PC, Piehler J, Tvorogov D, Ross DM, Lopez AF, Gotlib J, Thomas D. Next-generation JAK2 inhibitors for the treatment of myeloproliferative neoplasms: lessons from structure-based drug discovery approaches. Blood Cancer Discov. 2023;4(5):352–64.
13. Verstovsek S. How I manage anemia related to myelofibrosis and its treatment regimens. Ann Hematol. 2023;102(4):689–98.
14. Devos T, Selleslag D, Granacher N, Havelange V, Benghiat FS. Updated recommendations on the use of ruxolitinib for the treatment of myelofibrosis. Hematology. 2022;27(1):23–31.
15. Mascarenhas J. Pacritinib for the treatment of patients with myelofibrosis and thrombocytopenia. Expert Rev Hematol. 2022;15(8):671–84.

Low Mood and Multiple Disparate Somatic Complaints: Morose Monroe

39

Grade Easy.

Abstract A previously healthy male noted to have cognitive deterioration, depressive symptoms, and loss of weight. He gets admitted to a hospital with severe abdominal pain.

Story Monroe's boss, Basappa has reached the end of his tether. In his early days of employment as the accountant in a mid-sized cargo transport agency, Monroe was the ideal employee—punctual, competent, and cheerful. For the last 4 months, however, Monroe's behavior and efficiency have deteriorated to the point that even the parcel delivery man has noticed.

These days, Monroe walks into the office at least an hour late, with no smile for the many people who wish him "good morning." He falls into his chair looking as tired as if he is at the end of his working day, not the beginning. The only time he looks active is when he runs to the men's room, and he seems to be doing this almost hourly. He hardly eats the catered lunch that his secretary brings him at noon every day, and in his response to her concerned queries, he mumbles "I'm not hungry." His devoted secretary double-checks his work before she sends it to Basappa's office and is disturbed to see the number of mistakes in meticulous Monroe's work.

Things come to a head when the secretary has taken a day off to attend her best friend's wedding. Monroe's calculations, riddled with errors, are submitted to Basappa's office. Basappa is thunderously angry at the slipshod work, and he summons Monroe to his office. "I'm sorry, Monroe, this cannot go on any longer. I can't afford to have subpar workers in my office. Please clear your desk today, a month's pay will be credited to your bank account in lieu of notice."

Monroe barely reacts. He shuffles back to his chamber and begins clearing his desk. Suddenly, however, he screams and falls to the floor, writhing in pain and clutching his tummy. Basappa is very worried. Will he be blamed for Monroe's

S. Bhat, *Clinical Conundrums to Practice Diagnostic Reasoning*,
https://doi.org/10.1007/978-981-95-0636-1_39

illness? He panics and yells at his underlings to call for help and stands at the gate wringing his hands until an ambulance arrives.

You happen to be the doctor in the ER when Monroe is wheeled in. You can barely elicit a coherent history from Basappa, but you do note the salient points and proceed with your examination.

Your findings are as follows:

HR: 60/min; BP: 150/100 mm Hg.

The tongue is dry.

Monroe is conscious, but drowsy. He obeys simple verbal commands after a small but significant delay. Deep tendon reflexes appear diminished, but there are no lateralizing signs. There is no papilloedema.

The abdomen is soft. The right flank is tender to palpation.

Question What caused Monroe's symptoms? Is it mere stress at work, brought to a head by the tongue lashing he received from his boss? Or might there be an organic cause for his 4 months of altered behavior?

Analysis

From the story, one can glean some information about Monroe's health issues: he has depression, fatigue, polyuria, and anorexia. Examination reveals dehydration, bradycardia, and diminished tendon reflexes. Taken as a whole, along with the severe abdominal pain, this appears to be a case of hypercalcemia and renal colic. Reassuringly, for Basappa, his role in Monroe's presentation was merely coincidental.

Hypercalcemia is a true elevation in the calcium in the blood greater than 10.4 mg%. More than 90% of cases of hypercalcemia are due to primary hyperparathyroidism or malignancy-associated hypercalcemia. Hypercalcemia may be classified according to severity [1]:

Mild: 12 mg%.
Moderate: 12–14 mg%.
Severe: > 14 mg%.

Calcium in the blood exists in free and bound states. 45% is bound to albumin, 45% is ionized, and 10% is bound to anions such as phosphate and citrate. It is a crucial component of many systems—neural transmission, enzyme activity, intracellular signaling, and myocardial function.

Etiopathogenesis

Hypercalcemia may either be parathormone-dependent or independent [2] (Fig. 39.1).

Additional Causes

1. Immobilization.
2. Vitamin A toxicity.
3. Hyperthyroidism.
4. Granulomatous disorders like sarcoidosis,tuberculosis, and silicosis.

Clinical Features

The clinical manifestations of hypercalcemia develop when serum calcium is >12 mg% and depends not only on the degree of hypercalcemia but also on the rapidity with which it develops. The symptoms of hypercalcemia have been vividly described as "groans, bones, stones, moans, thrones (constipation and polyuria), and psychic overtones. Serum calcium more than 15 mg% is a medical emergency.

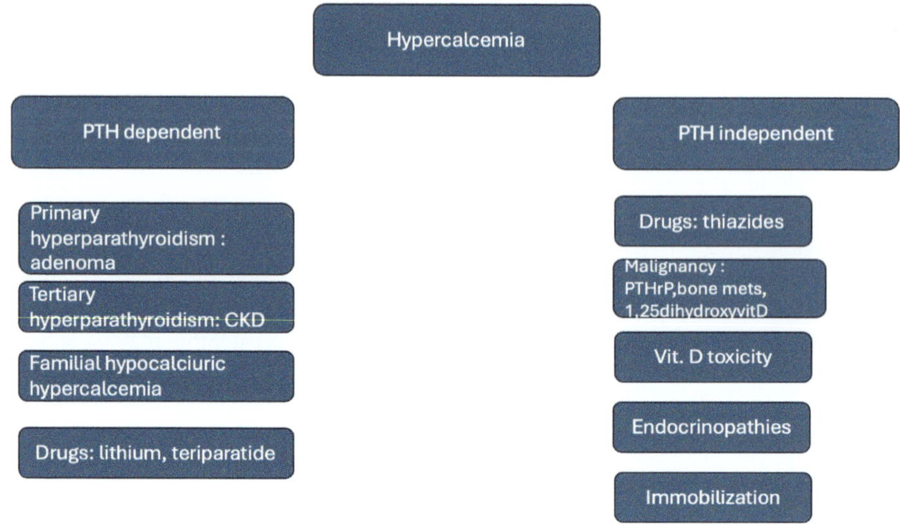

Fig. 39.1 Causes of hypercalcemia

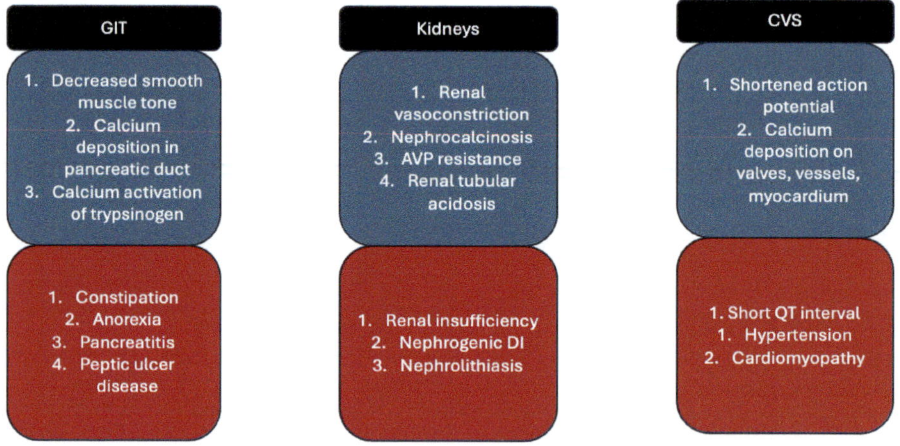

Fig. 39.2 Pathogenesis of various clinical features of hypercalcemia

1. Neuropsychiatric manifestations: High calcium causes "glutaminergic excitotoxicity." It may also inhibit neuromuscular transmission and cause muscle weakness [3].
2. Bone—osteoporosis, osteomalacia, and pathological fractures.

Other systemic manifestations and their pathogenesis are described in Fig. 39.2 [4, 5, 6].

Diagnosis

PTH, 24-h urine calcium, ECG, cancer screening if hypercalcemia of malignancy is suspected, USG kidney, thyroid, and parathyroid.

Approach (Fig. 39.3)

Treatment [7, 8]

1. IV hydration.
2. Calcitonin: 4 units/kg every 12 h [9].
3. Bisphosphonates: like zoledronic acid [10].
4. Denosumab [11].
5. Glucocorticoids [12].
6. Calcimimetics [13].
7. Dialysis [14].
8. Parathyroidectomy [15].
9. Cinacalcet [16].
10. Treatment of underlying condition.

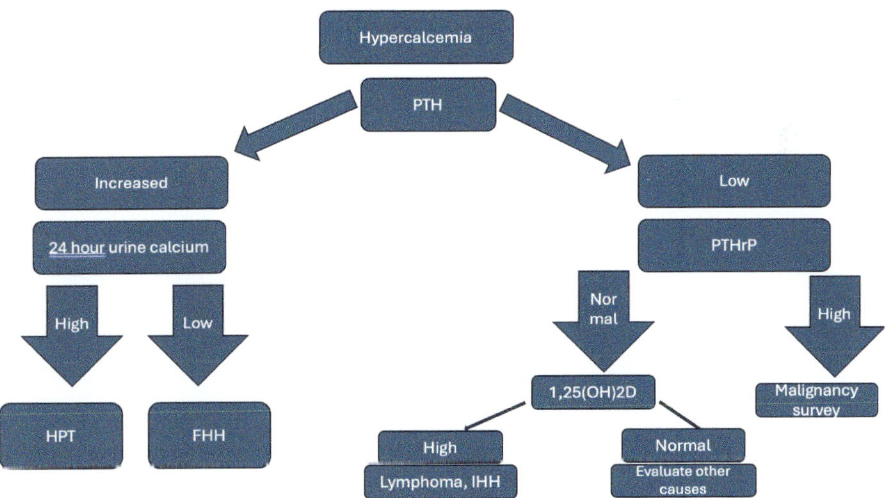

Fig. 39.3 Approach to hypercalcemia
HPT hyperparathyroidism, *FHH* Familial hypocalciuric hypercalcemia

References

1. Walker MD, Shane E. Hypercalcemia: a review. JAMA. 2022;328(16):1624–36.
2. Carroll MF, Schade DS. A practical approach to hypercalcemia. Am Fam Physician. 2003;67(9):1959–66.
3. Chou FF, Sheen-Chen SM, Leong CP. Neuromuscular recovery after parathyroidectomy in primary hyperparathyroidism. Surgery. 1995;117(1):18–25.
4. Levi M, Ellis MA, Berl T. Control of renal hemodynamics and glomerular filtration rate in chronic hypercalcemia: role of prostaglandins, renin-angiotensin system, and calcium. J Clin Invest. 1983;71(6):1624–32.
5. Ahmed R, Hashiba K. Reliability of QT intervals as indicators of clinical hypercalcemia. Clin Cardiol. 1988;11(6):395–400.
6. Bilezikian JP. Primary hyperparathyroidism. In Hypercalcemia: clinical diagnosis and management. Cham: Springer International Publishing; 2022. p. 89–110.
7. Renaghan AD. Rosner MH. Hypercalcemia: etiology and management.
8. Ralston S. Medical management of hypercalcaemia. Br J Clin Pharmacol. 1992;34(1):11–20.
9. Almuradova E, Cicin I. Cancer-related hypercalcemia and potential treatments. Front Endocrinol [Internet]. 2023 Mar 22 [cited 2025 Mar 24];14. Available from: https://www.frontiersin.org/journals/endocrinology/articles/10.3389/fendo.2023.1039490/full
10. Khan AA, Gurnani PK, Peksa GD, Whittier WL, DeMott JM. Bisphosphonate versus bisphosphonate and calcitonin for the treatment of moderate to severe hypercalcemia of malignancy. Ann Pharmacother. 2021;55(3):277–85.
11. Thosani S, Hu MI. Denosumab: a new agent in the management of hypercalcemia of malignancy. Future Oncol. 2015;11(21):2865–71.
12. El-Hajj Fuleihan G, Clines GA, Hu MI, Marcocci C, Murad MH, Piggott T, et al. Treatment of hypercalcemia of malignancy in adults: an endocrine society clinical practice guideline. J Clin Endocrinol Metab. 2023;108(3):507–28.
13. Hou YC, Zheng CM, Chiu HW, Liu WC, Lu KC, Lu CL. Role of calcimimetics in treating bone and mineral disorders related to chronic kidney disease. Pharmaceuticals. 2022;15(8):952.
14. Basok AB, Rogachev B, Haviv YS, Vorobiov M. Treatment of extreme hypercalcaemia: the role of haemodialysis. Case Reports. 2018;2018:bcr-2017.
15. Ryder CY, Jarocki A, McNeely MM, Currey E, Miller BS, Cohen MS, et al. Early biochemical response to parathyroidectomy for primary hyperparathyroidism and its predictive value for recurrent hypercalcemia and recurrent primary hyperparathyroidism. Surgery. 2021;169(1):120–5.
16. Chandran M, Bilezikian JP, Lau J, Rajeev R, Yang SP, Samuel M, Parameswaran R. The efficacy and safety of cinacalcet in primary hyperparathyroidism: a systematic review and meta-analysis of randomized controlled trials and cohort studies. Rev Endocr Metab Disord. 2022;23(3):485–501.

An Adult Male with Diverse Hematological, Skeletal, and Skin Anomalies: Tippu with Thrombocytopenia

40

Grade Moderate.

Abstract An adult male referred for evaluation of pancytopenia is found to have various congenital anomalies.

Story Mr. Tippu is referred to you for evaluation of his low platelet count. You glance at the lab reports before the patient arrives and note that the platelet count is 30,000/mL, Hb is 10 g%, and the absolute neutrophil count is 1000. The referring doctor has included details of the basic evaluation—there is no history of ethanol abuse, HIV is negative, ANA is negative, and Vitamin B12 is normal.

As Mr. Tippu walks in, you are surprised to see how short he is. You find that he has hyperpigmented patches on his neck and trunk. Some patches of hyperpigmentation, on the back in particular, remind you of café au lait spots, but you are not quite sure how this would fit in with the thrombocytopenia. His right thumb is much smaller than the other fingers and looks like it will fall off the hand any moment.

You ask Mr. Tippu about health issues among his family members, but he can hardly hear what you are saying.

He apologizes—"Sorry doctor, my hearing is not that good."

You proceed with a detailed physical examination—you detect a number of anomalies: apart from the hypoplastic right thumb, you observe a divergent squint in the right eye. The BP is 180/100 mm Hg in the right brachial artery and 150/90 mm Hg in the right femoral artery.

Question Can all these physical findings and the thrombocytopenia be explained by a single diagnosis?

S. Bhat, *Clinical Conundrums to Practice Diagnostic Reasoning*,
https://doi.org/10.1007/978-981-95-0636-1_40

Analysis

The salient features here are

1. Pancytopenia with no obvious cause—the basic evaluation for pancytopenia is noncontributory; hence, the possibility of bone marrow involvement causing the pancytopenia increases.
2. Short stature, thumb aplasia, divergent squint, and perhaps coarctation of aorta (leg BP is significantly lower)—these point toward congenital anomalies.

   If both pancytopenia and the congenital anomalies have the same cause (which is plausible), then the pancytopenia is congenital too; hence, the bone marrow failure may be congenital as well. The most common cause of inherited bone marrow failure syndrome (IBMFS) is Fanconi's anemia.

Fanconi's anemia (FA) is a rare genetic disorder characterized by progressive bone marrow failure, congenital abnormalities, and predisposition to malignancies [1]. On the one hand, FA is characterized by cytopenia and on the other by untrammelled cell proliferation, i.e., malignancy. Mutation in the genes responsible for DNA repair results in ineffective DNA repair, thus predisposing to cancer. Fanconi's anemia follows an autosomal recessive inheritance pattern in most cases, though X-linked and autosomal dominant inheritance exist as well [2].

Pathogenesis

DNA repair suppresses tumorigenesis, and the absence of an effective DNA repair system leads to genetic instability and an increased risk of cancer [3]. The pathogenesis of FA centers on defective DNA repair in the Fanconi anemia/BRCA pathway [4]. This pathway is responsible for the following:

(a) Recognition and repair of DNA interstrand crosslinks (ICLs) which are clastogenic (chromosome breaking) [5].
(b) Protection of replication forks.
(c) Maintenance of chromosomal stability.

When DNA damage occurs and ICLs are formed, the FA core complex is activated. This complex monoubiquitinates the FANCD2–FANCI protein complex, [6] which then coordinates DNA repair. In FA patients, this pathway is disrupted (Fig. 40.1) leading to:

(a) Accumulation of DNA damage.
(b) Increased chromosomal breakage.
(c) Enhanced cellular sensitivity to DNA cross-linking agents.
(d) Progressive loss of hematopoietic stem cells.
(e) Genomic instability [7] promoting cancer development.

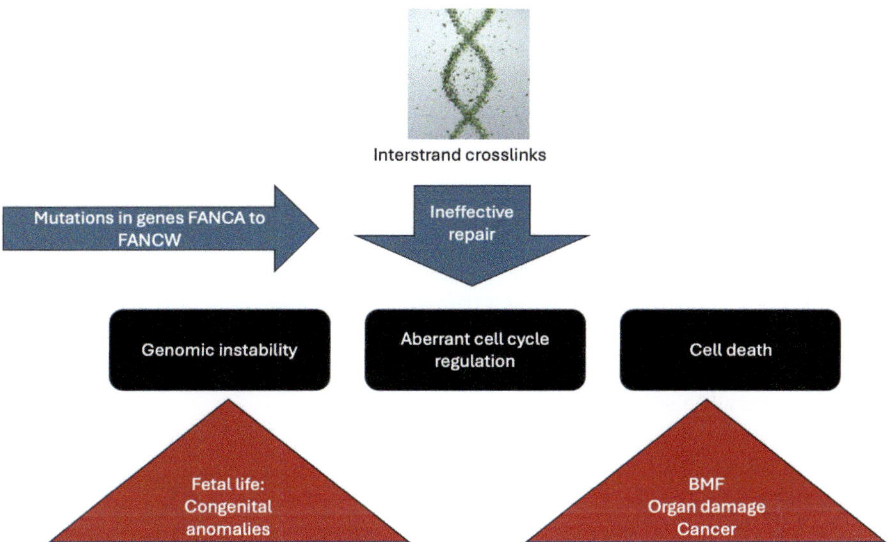

Fig. 40.1 Pathogenesis of Fanconi's anemia

Clinical Features

The clinical presentation is highly variable but typically includes:

Hematological [8]

(a) Progressive bone marrow failure (usually presenting between ages 5 and 10).
(b) Pancytopenia—especially neutropenia and thrombocytopenia,
(c) Macrocytosis.
(d) Elevated HbF.

Congenital Abnormalities [9]

(a) Short stature.
(b) Skin hyperpigmentation and café-au-lait spots.
(c) Thumb and radial ray abnormalities.
(d) Microcephaly.
(e) Characteristic facies (triangular face, small eyes).
(f) Renal anomalies.
(g) Hypogonadism.
(h) Predisposition to cancer.

(i) Acute myeloid leukemia (AML).
(j) Myelodysplastic syndrome (MDS).
(k) Solid tumors (particularly head and neck squamous cell carcinoma).

Diagnosis

1. Chromosomal breakage test (gold standard):
   Exposure of peripheral blood lymphocytes to DNA cross-linking agents (mitomycin C or di-epoxybutane) [10]. FA cells show increased chromosomal breakage.
2. Molecular genetic testing:
   Next-generation sequencing panel for FA genes.

Treatment

Hematopoietic stem cell transplantation (HSCT) is the only definitive cure [11]

Key Takeaway
Though Fanconi's anemia is a rare condition, diagnosis is especially important, as the mutations present in Fanconi's anemia affect cancer progression and response to treatment. Once Fanconi's anemia is diagnosed, regular screening for cancer is required. If cancer is detected, doses of chemotherapy must be modified.

References

1. Soulier J. Fanconi anemia. Hematology 2010, the American Society of Hematology Education Program Book. 2011; 10(1):492–7.
2. Fiesco-Roa MO, Giri N, McReynolds LJ, Best AF, Alter BP. Genotype-phenotype associations in Fanconi anemia: a literature review. Blood Rev. 2019;37:100589.
3. Harada N, Asada S, Jiang L, Nguyen H, Moreau L, Marina RJ, Adelman K, Iyer DR, D'Andrea AD. The splicing factor CCAR1 regulates the Fanconi anemia/BRCA pathway. Mol Cell. 2024;84(14):2618–33.
4. Kim H, D'Andrea AD. Regulation of DNA cross-link repair by the Fanconi anemia/BRCA pathway. Genes Dev. 2012;26(13):1393–408.
5. Su X, Huang J. The Fanconi anemia pathway and DNA interstrand cross-link repair. Protein Cell. 2011 Sep;2:704–11.
6. D'Andrea AD, Grompe M. The Fanconi anaemia/BRCA pathway. Nat Rev Cancer. 2003;3(1):23–34.
7. Niraj J, Färkkilä A, D'Andrea AD. The Fanconi anemia pathway in cancer. Ann Rev Cancer Biol. 2019;3(1):457–78.

8. Butturini A, Gale RP, Verlander PC, Adler-Brecher B, Gillio AP, Auerbach AD. Hematologic abnormalities in Fanconi anemia: an international Fanconi anemia registry study [see comments]. Blood. 1994;84(5):1650–5.
9. Glanz A, Fraser FC. Spectrum of anomalies in Fanconi anaemia. J Med Genet. 1982;19(6):412–6.
10. Auerbach AD. Diagnosis of Fanconi anemia by Diepoxybutane analysis. Curr Protoc Hum Genet. 2003;37(1):8.7.1–8.7.15.
11. de Latour RP, Porcher R, Dalle JH, Aljurf M, Korthof ET, Svahn J, Willemze R, Barrenetxea C, Mialou V, Soulier J, Cappelli E. Long-term outcome after matched allogeneic hematopoietic stem cell transplantation for Fanconi anemia on behalf of the FA Committee of the Severe Aplastic Anemia Working Party (SAA WP) and the pediatric working Party of the European Group for blood and marrow transplantation (EBMT). Blood. 2011;118(21):325.

Life-Threatening Disease Acquired in the Wilderness: The Sick Spelunker

41

Grade Difficult.

Abstract A young, fit hiker, and spelunker presenting with insomnia, tingling and numbness in the left upper limb, and weakness.

Story KK is a super-fit accountant with not a single unhealthy habit to his name. He works in a government office, but his real passion is exploring—specifically, exploring caves. He toils hard from Monday to Friday and sets off once every 2 months to South Dakota to make his way to the more remote, less-explored sections of the Wind Cave (Fig. 41.1). He is also an adept violinist and soothes with music, the occasional misery of living alone.

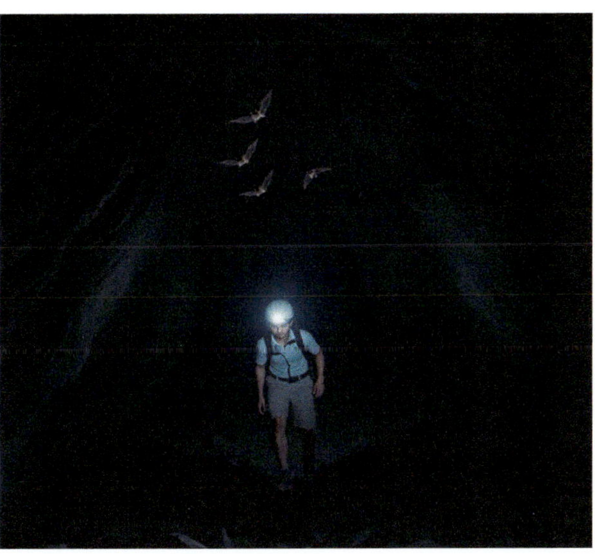

Fig. 41.1 Spelunking (created with Claude AI)

S. Bhat, *Clinical Conundrums to Practice Diagnostic Reasoning*,
https://doi.org/10.1007/978-981-95-0636-1_41

Perhaps it is the hubris of youth that makes him ignore the occasional minor niggles with his health that he has been noticing lately.

For the last week or so, he has been unable to sleep. Perhaps that is why he feels so tired and irritable all the time? Less easy to explain is the weird sensation he has on his left arm—it feels both tingly and numb and a little floppy and weak too.

He describes these problems to his colleague over lunch, who by dint of constant persuasion for 5 days ensures that KK visits a physician.

As luck would have it, you are the physician KK meets.

"Good morning, doctor."

"Good morning, KK. How may I help you today?"

"I'm afraid I'm making a big fuss about what is probably nothing, doctor."

"It's always better to be cautious. If we find that nothing is wrong with your health, it is reassuring for both of us!"

"Very true. I've been feeling a little below par for the last 10 days—actually I'm not really sure when the problem started."

"What exactly is troubling you?"

"I guess the main thing is this tingling and numbness in my left arm."

"I see. Is there any weakness in that arm? In the sense you feel you can't hold or lift things?"

"A little, I think, when compared to my right arm."

"Any weakness or tingling in the legs? Or problems with your bowels or bladder?"

"No, doctor."

"Do you have diabetes? Or hypertension?"

"No, I don't. I have been tested and found normal about 6 months ago."

"Ok. Have you had any problem with neck pain, or shooting pain down your arms?"

"Not at all."

"Is there any problem apart from that?"

"I guess I'm a little tired and cranky—at least that's what my work friends say."

You're quite convinced, as you complete the history, that there are no major health issues with KK. You reassure him, and as he smiles in relief, you note a subtle facial asymmetry, with deviation of the angle of the mouth to the right.

This prompts you to proceed with a detailed neurological examination. You note hypotonia in all four limbs, with occasional fasciculations. When you percuss the muscle to confirm fasciculations, you see a curious bump at the site of strike. Deep tendon reflexes are absent, even with reinforcement.

These findings are sufficiently worrisome, and you admit KK for further evaluation.

Question

1. What is the likely diagnosis?
2. How would you confirm it?

Analysis

This is a slightly tricky presentation, but the diagnosis may be deduced with the clues provided.

1. Patient in USA who is a spelunker.
2. Initial symptoms localized to one limb.
3. Flaccid quadriparesis with areflexia points to Guillain Barre syndrome, but the mounding on percussion (percussion myxedema) is a pointer to rabies, in this case, paralytic rabies.

In countries like the US where canine rabies has been eliminated due to a strong vaccination program, bat rabies may be seen occasionally. The presentation of bat rabies is atypical, and difficult to recognize, unlike encephalitic rabies where the clinical picture of hydrophobia, aerophobia, and agitation is fairly well known. It is important to remember that the patient may not actually volunteer a history of bat bite.

Confirmation of diagnosis: PCR on saliva and skin serum CSF.
CSF analysis: If antibodies against rabies virus are present in CSF, it confirms infection.

Rabies is a zoonotic disease caused by a lyssavirus. It is one of the rare infectious diseases that once symptomatic is almost invariably fatal [1].

It may manifest as either the paralytic or encephalitic form. In Asia, the rabies virus is enzootic and mainly seen in dogs, foxes, and mongooses [2]. However, in the Americas, the virus is maintained in bat species [3].

Etiopathogenesis

The virus reaches the peripheral nerve or motor end plate from the site of inoculation; it travels by retrograde axonal transport until it reaches the body of the neuron [4]. Here, it multiplies, gets transported across the synaptic cleft, and travels from neuron to neuron till it reaches the brain (Fig. 41.2). From the brain, it moves centrifugally down to the dorsal ganglion as well as the salivary gland [5].

Clinical Features [6, 7]

The usual incubation period is 1–3 months, though periods as long as 10 years have been described.

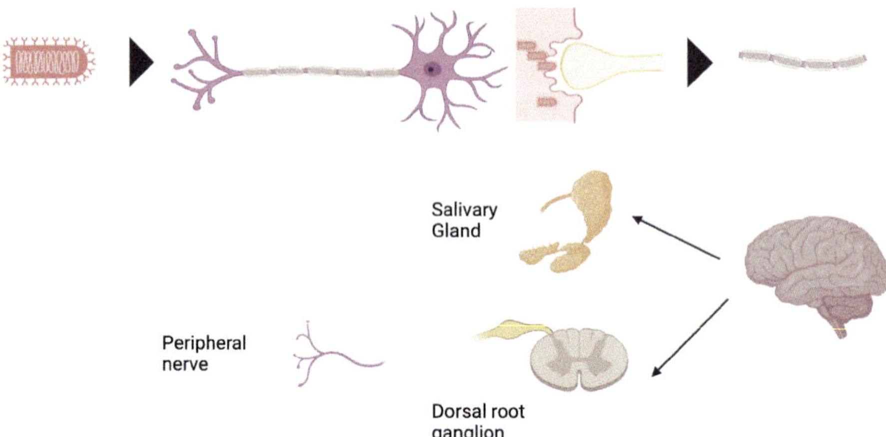

Fig. 41.2 Entry and centripetal spread of rabies virus. (Created in BioRender. Bhat, S. (2025)

In the prodromal phase, there are nonspecific symptoms of fatigue, fever, headache, insomnia, and irritability. Tingling, itching, burning, numbness at the bite site, and weakness of the affected limb may be early diagnostic pointers.

Neurologic phase—May be either encephalitic or paralytic rabies.

Encephalitic rabies:

(a) Hyperexcitability alternating with normal sensorium.
(b) Hydrophobia and aerophobia.
(c) Autonomic dysfunction in the form of hypersalivation, lacrimation, sweating, and pupil dilatation.
(d) Hyperpyrexia.
(e) Dysarthria, dysphagia, and diplopia.
(f) Hypertonia and brisk tendon reflexes with extensor plantar responses.
(g) Neck rigidity may be present.

Paralytic rabies: The symptoms are not very specific for rabies

(a) Limb weakness, fasciculations, flaccid weakness, and areflexia.
(b) Facial weakness, may point toward GBS.
(c) Bowel and bladder incontinence.

Later, the patient develops dense paraplegia with the paralysis of deglutition and respiration.

Rabies acquired from bats has a more atypical presentation [8]: Findings include cranial nerve, sensory, and motor deficits, without the characteristic hydrophobia and aerophobia. Tremor and myoclonus may be present as well.

Diagnosis Rabies is mainly diagnosed based on history and observation. Supportive investigations include

(a) Saliva RT-PCR for virus [9]
(b) Skin biopsy from the neck RT-PCR.

Differential Diagnoses

(a) Paralytic rabies must be differentiated from Guillain Barre syndrome and Japanese encephalitis.
(b) Differentials for furious rabies include delirium tremens and tetanus.

Treatment [10]

(a) Supportive.

(b) Milwaukee protocol: Antivirals and therapeutic coma have low rates of success [10].

Prevention

Post-exposure prophylaxis [11, 12]: Cell culture vaccine administered at 0, 3, 7, and 28 days.

To Note In canine rabies, the virus can multiply in the motor end plate, hence deep bites are more likely to cause the infection. However, in bat rabies, rabies-like viruses can be transmitted even after a scratch since these viruses multiply in the epidermis.

References

1. Jackson AC. Rabies pathogenesis. J Neurovirol. 2002;8(4):267–9.
2. Leung AK, Davies HD, Hon KL. Rabies: epidemiology, pathogenesis, and prophylaxis. Adv Ther. 2007;24:1340–7.
3. Fooks AR, Banyard AC, Horton DL, Johnson N, McElhinney LM, Jackson AC. Current status of rabies and prospects for elimination. Lancet. 2014;384(9951):1389–99.
4. Farihah IH, NR AD, Arsiazi BA, Nabila C, Anggrayani P. Neuropathogenesis of human rabies. KESANS. 2022;1(4):376–86.
5. Gluska S, Zahavi EE, Chein M, Gradus T, Bauer A, Finke S, Perlson E. Rabies virus hijacks and accelerates the p75NTR retrograde axonal transport machinery. PLoS Pathog. 2014;10(8):e1004348.

6. Warrell MJ, Warrell DA. Rabies and other lyssavirus diseases. Lancet. 2004;363(9413):959–69.
7. Warrell MJ, Warrell DA. Rabies: the clinical features, management and prevention of the classic zoonosis. Clin Med. 2015;15(1):78–81.
8. Kuzmin IV, Bozick B, Guagliardo SA, Kunkel R, Shak JR, Tong S, Rupprecht CE. Bats, emerging infectious diseases, and the rabies paradigm revisited. Emerg Health Threat J. 2011;4(1):7159.
9. Candia-Puma MA, Pola-Romero L, Barazorda-Ccahuana HL, Goyzueta-Mamani LD, Sobreira Galdino A, Machado-de-Ávila RA, Cordeiro Giunchetti R, Ferraz Coelho EA, Chávez-Fumagalli MA. Rabies test accuracy: comprehensive systematic review and meta-analysis for human and canine diagnostics. medRxiv. 2024;5:2024–11.
10. Lacy M, Phasuk N, Scholand SJ. Human rabies treatment—from palliation to promise. Viruses. 2024;16(1):160.
11. Ledesma LA, Lemos ER, Horta MA. Comparing clinical protocols for the treatment of human rabies: the Milwaukee protocol and the Brazilian protocol (Recife). Rev Soc Bras Med Trop. 2020;53:e20200352.
12. Chen SJ, Rai CI, Wang SC, Chen YC. Infection and prevention of rabies viruses. Microorganisms. 2025;13(2):380.

42 Collapse While Standing at a Live Performance: The Deadly Laugh

Grade Easy.

Abstract A young woman with no previous comorbidities collapses at a comedy performance. However, there is no post-episode amnesia or drowsiness.

Story You hear their voices through your cabin walls—loud and opinionated. You mentally gird your loins for what you feel will be a slightly unpleasant consultation. You have seen your fair share of know-it-alls and you know it is always tricky to convince them about investigations and treatment. The couple walks in—he is in a blinding green shirt, and she wears so much jewelry that she jangles as she walks.

"I'm Shankar," says the man "and this is my wife Rashmi."

"Hello, doctor."

"Good afternoon. How may I help you today?"

"Well, we were at a stand-up comedy by KK—I'm sure you've heard of him" Shankar begins. "Front row of course."

"Of course," you echo. You personally do not consider KK's performances to be funny at all, but tastes vary, of course.

"What happened there?"

"Well, it was a particularly good show, all of us in the audience were standing up and clapping —it was so good —and Rashmi couldn't stop laughing."

"And then?"

"And then ....well she collapsed."

"Collapsed?! Meaning?!" you ask concerned and interested.

"She just fell to the ground."

"For how long was she unconscious?"

"Oh, I don't think she was unconscious! Her eyes were open."

"Did she bite her tongue or pass urine involuntarily when she was unconscious?"

S. Bhat, *Clinical Conundrums to Practice Diagnostic Reasoning*,
https://doi.org/10.1007/978-981-95-0636-1_42

"No, no of course not!" Rashmi interjects. "I was aware of what was going on around me. I wasn't unconscious, doctor. I just felt for a moment or two that there was no strength in my legs."

"Have you had any health issues prior to this?"

"No, doctor."

"Oh, she did have a bad cold and fever and body ache 4 months ago. Our family doctor said it was a mild form of flu," says Shankar.

"I don't think I have completely recovered from that flu, doctor. I feel quite tired and sleepy all the time."

"That's true!" chimes in her husband. "The drive from home to hospital took only 10 minutes, but she started snoring even in that brief time" he guffaws and earns a severe frown from his wife.

"It's not funny. I can't sleep well at night because you snore so loudly. That's why I grab a moment of shuteye whenever I can."

"Ha! Snoring! Snoring is better than those weird things you say when you sleep."

"What? What do I say?"

"Sorry love, I didn't mean that."

"No, tell me. What do I say when I'm asleep?"

Shankar shakes his head ruefully. "I really shouldn't have said that. The thing is doctor, she lost her grandfather a couple of months ago, and I think she dreams about him. She talks to him in her dreams."

Rashmi covers her face with her hands and weeps silently. "It's true—I have very vivid dreams almost every night —that he's talking to me, giving me advice about many things," she confesses.

Shankar takes some time to console her. You are feeling desperately sorry for Rashmi now.

"Is there any stressor I should know about?"

"No, doctor, apart from this bereavement."

"May I ask, are you taking any medicine to help you sleep?" "No, but I use a pillow spray."

You perform a fairly detailed physical examination, but this is essentially normal apart from a BMI of 31. There are no focal neurological deficits, and the fundus is normal.

Holter monitoring, EEG, MRI, and thyroid function are all normal.

Questions

What investigations do you ask for?

What line of treatment is preferred for the most likely diagnosis with the above description?

Analysis

The fall, not associated with loss of consciousness, is "cataplexy", which is fairly characteristic of narcolepsy. Cataplexy can be precipitated by laughter, excitement or anger. The auditory hallucinations as she is falling asleep and the daytime sleepiness corroborate the diagnosis of narcolepsy.

Diagnosis

Narcolepsy is defined as chronic daytime sleepiness with or without cataplexy, sleep disruption, sleep paralysis, and hypnogogic hallucinations [1].

Narcolepsy is classified as follows [2]:

NT1—the classical form—due to orexin deficiency.
NT2—cataplexy is absent, and orexin levels are normal.

Narcolepsy affects males and females equally and is most common between the ages of 20 and 40.

Etiopathogenesis

Narcolepsy is genetically determined, and DQB1*0602 haplotype is present in more than 95% of patients [3]. Infections, particularly flu and streptococcus, appear to precipitate narcolepsy in those genetically predisposed [4]. Autoimmunity has also been proposed as a mechanism by which orexin-producing neurons are destroyed in the genetically predisposed [5].

Orexin plays a key role in maintaining wakefulness and preventing transition into sleep (Fig. 42.1). Low orexin levels result not only into an inappropriate transition into sleep but also demonstration of REM-related phenomena—cataplexy, hypnogogic hallucinations, and sleep paralysis (Fig. 42.2).

Clinical Features

Patients with narcolepsy are more likely to be obese, have neuropsychiatric disorders, and fragmented sleep.

(a) Daytime sleepiness: Apart from excessive daytime sleepiness where the sensation of well-being and rest is restored by short naps, patients with narcolepsy suffer from "sleep attacks." Sleep attacks are described as sudden severe drowsiness, resulting in the patient falling asleep with no warning [7].

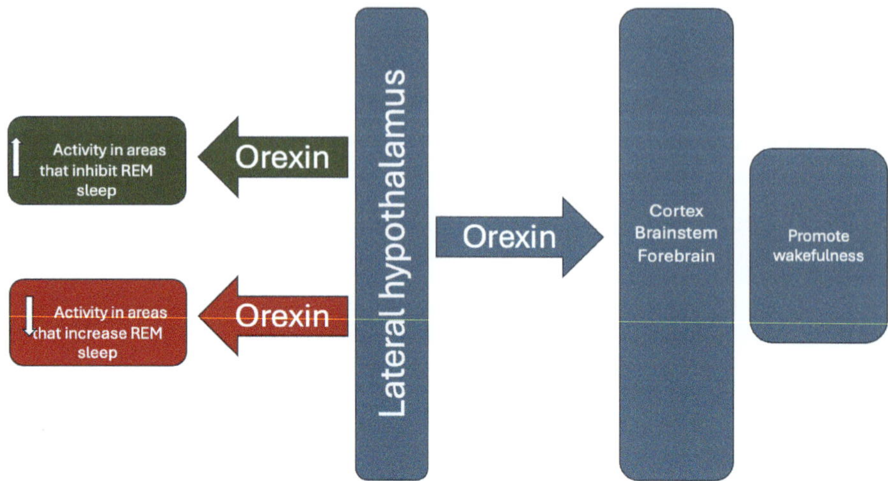

Fig. 42.1 The role of Orexin in maintaining wakefulness [6]

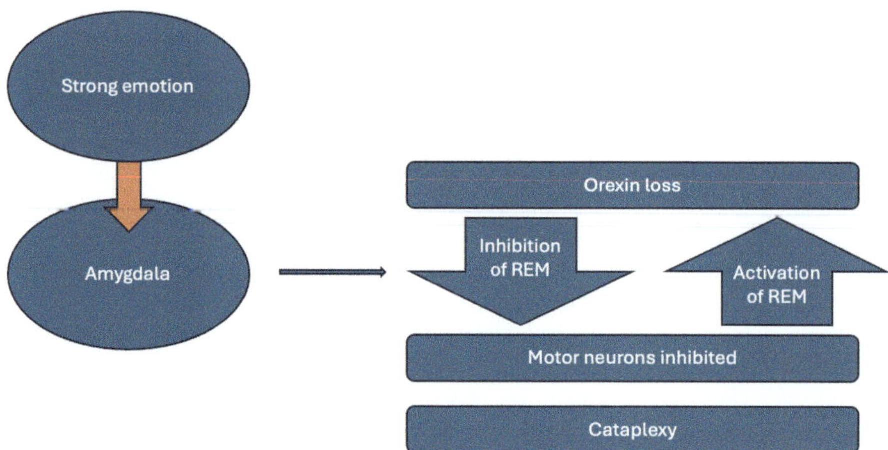

Fig. 42.2 Mechanism of cataplexy in narcolepsy

(b) Cataplexy: It is one of the more frightening symptoms of narcolepsy. Cataplexy is precipitated by strong positive emotions (laughter, in this case). There is sudden loss of muscle tone—in the face, jaw, and lower limbs which may be severe enough to cause a fall. However, consciousness is preserved during the attack of cataplexy [8].
(c) Hypnagogic hallucinations: Vivid, sometimes frightening auditory or visual, hallucinations at the onset of sleep or wakefulness [9].
(d) Sleep paralysis: Inability to move while falling asleep accompanied by a feeling of suffocation [10].

Investigations [11]

1. Polysomnography.
2. Multiple sleep latency test.
3. CSF orexin.

Treatment

(a) Daytime naps.
(b) Sleep hygiene practices.
(c) Treat comorbidities like hypertension and obstructive sleep apnea.
(d) Modafinil [12]
(e) Oxybates [13] or methylphenidate for those with disabling sleepiness.

References

1. Barateau L, Pizza F, Plazzi G, Dauvilliers Y. 50th anniversary of the ESRS in 2022-JSR special issue. J Sleep Res. 2022;31(4)
2. Bassetti CL, Adamantidis A, Burdakov D, Han F, Gay S, Kallweit U, Khatami R, Koning F, Kornum BR, Lammers GJ, Liblau RS. Narcolepsy—clinical spectrum, aetiopathophysiology, diagnosis and treatment. Nat Rev Neurol. 2019;15(9):519–39.
3. European Narcolepsy Network (EU-NN). DQB1 locus alone explains most of the risk and protection in narcolepsy with cataplexy in Europe. Sleep. 2014;37(1):19–25.
4. Aran A, Lin L, Nevsimalova S, Plazzi G, Hong SC, Weiner K, Zeitzer J, Mignot E. Elevated anti-streptococcal antibodies in patients with recent narcolepsy onset. Sleep. 2009;32(8):979–83.
5. Hallmayer J, Faraco J, Lin L, Hesselson S, Winkelmann J, Kawashima M, Mayer G, Plazzi G, Nevsimalova S, Bourgin P, Hong SC. Narcolepsy is strongly associated with the T-cell receptor alpha locus. Nat Genet. 2009;41(6):708–11.
6. Yamanaka A, Tsujino N, Funahashi H, Honda K, Guan JL, Wang QP, Tominaga M, Goto K, Shioda S, Sakurai T. Orexins activate histaminergic neurons via the orexin 2 receptor. Biochem Biophys Res Commun. 2002;290(4):1237–45.
7. Morrison I, Riha RL. Excessive daytime sleepiness and narcolepsy—an approach to investigation and management. Eur J Intern Med. 2012;23(2):110–7.
8. Sardar H, Goldstein-Piekarski AN, Giardino WJ. Amygdala neurocircuitry at the interface between emotional regulation and narcolepsy with cataplexy. Front Neurosci [Internet]. 2023 Apr 21 [cited 2025 Mar 31];17. Available from: https://www.frontiersin.org/journals/neuroscience/articles/10.3389/fnins.2023.1152594/full
9. Foffani G. To be or not to be hallucinating: implications of hypnagogic/hypnopompic experiences and lucid dreaming for brain disorders. PNAS Nexus. 2024;3(1):pgad442.
10. Terzaghi M, Ratti PL, Manni F, Manni R. Sleep paralysis in narcolepsy: more than just a motor dissociative phenomenon? Neurol Sci. 2012;33(1):169–72.
11. Morgenthaler TI, Kapur VK, Brown TM, Swick TJ, Alessi C, Aurora RN, Boehlecke B, Chesson AL Jr, Friedman L, Maganti R, Owens J. Practice parameters for the treatment of narcolepsy and other hypersomnias of central origin. Sleep. 2007;30(12):1705–11.
12. Scammell TE, Estabrooke IV, McCarthy MT, Chemelli RM, Yanagisawa M, Miller MS, Saper CB. Hypothalamic arousal regions are activated during modafinil-induced wakefulness. J Neurosci. 2000;20(22):8620–8.
13. Vienne J, Bettler B, Franken P, Tafti M. Differential effects of GABAB receptor subtypes, γ-hydroxybutyric acid, and baclofen on EEG activity and sleep regulation. J Neurosci. 2010;30(42):14194–204.

43 Acneiform Eruptions and Oral Ulcers in a Young Adult Male: Acne Angst

Grade Easy

Abstract Young adult male with the initial complaint of severe acne and mouth ulcers admitted to hospital with hemoptysis.

Story Last April, worried about burnout and desperate for a holiday, you had a wonderful solo holiday in Istanbul, Cappadocia, and Pamukkale. While in Cappadocia, your guide was an utterly gorgeous Turkish man named Altan. You have fond memories of him accompanying you on the hot air balloon ride, the Kaymakli underground city, and the village of Goreme. You are surprised to receive an email from him.

"Hey, doc. I hope you are well…I need your help. My cousin Eren is travelling with his pals through your beautiful country and he's in your city tomorrow. He's having some issues with his health. Would you mind having a look?

"Of course, no problem," you mail back and write Eren's name in your appointment chart for the next day.

Eren, tall and richly pimpled, walks into your office the next morning.

"Good morning, Eren. Your cousin mailed that you are not keeping well. Can you tell me what exactly the problem is?"

Eren sadly indicates his face.

"Ah, I see. Well, you'll be happy to know that there are various therapies available for acne, even when it's as severe as yours. Is there anything else troubling you?"

"I used to get sores in my mouth quite often, but that kind of settled once I started smoking."

"Started or stopped smoking?!"

"Started doctor. Things became better when I smoked."

"I see," you say doubtfully.

S. Bhat, *Clinical Conundrums to Practice Diagnostic Reasoning*,
https://doi.org/10.1007/978-981-95-0636-1_43

Eren whispers something.

"Sorry, I didn't quite get that?"

"Sometimes, I get sores there too," he says waving shyly at his crotch area.

"OK."

You proceed to perform a detailed examination. You note that both eyes are red and that the right knee and ankle are both swollen and tender to palpation.

You order some investigations, ask for a dermatology consult, and tell Eren to meet you in a week with the test reports.

Unfortunately, Eren is admitted the very next day with the complaint of coughing out blood.

Questions What do you think is happening to Eren. Are the first and second presentations related?

Analysis

The following clues may be discerned by an astute reader:

(a) The fact that Eren is from Turkey.
(b) The combination of oral ulcers, acneiform eruptions, and genital ulcers.
(c) The red eye.
(d) The oligoarticular arthritis.

In combination, these are clear clues to Behcet's disease. The admission to hospital with hemoptysis may be secondary to pulmonary artery aneurysm.

Behçet's syndrome (BS), also known as Behçet's disease, is a chronic, inflammatory vasculitis characterized by recurrent mucocutaneous ulcers and various systemic manifestations [1].

Epidemiology

The highest prevalence of Behçet's disease is along the so-called "Ancient Silk Road" which extends from Eastern Asia to the Mediterranean. It is especially common in Turkey, affecting young adult males [2].

Etiology

The exact cause of BS remains unknown, but it is believed to involve a combination of genetic and environmental factors.

Genetic Factors There is a strong association with the HLA-B51 gene [3]. However, this association is not consistent across all populations, and its role in determining disease severity is debated. Other genes outside the major histocompatibility complex (MHC) may also contribute to the pathogenesis of BS.

Environmental Factors Various environmental triggers such as infections, trauma, and stress have been implicated in the disease process. There is also evidence suggesting a role for the microbiome [4].

Pathogenesis The pathogenesis of Behçet's syndrome involves a complex interplay of immune system dysfunction and vascular inflammation.

(a) Vasculitis: Many of the clinical manifestations are thought to result from vasculitis, affecting blood vessels of all sizes, both arterial and venous. The classic lesion is a necrotizing, leukocytoclastic, obliterative perivasculitis and venous thrombosis, with infiltration of neutrophils and CD4+ T lymphocytes [5].

(b) Immune system: The disease is associated with increased levels of antibodies to mycobacterial heat shock protein epitopes. T cells and antibodies may recognize these epitopes. There is an imbalance in cytokine production, with a Th1-dominant response observed in some patients, while Th2 association is also observed [6]. Other factors such as oxidative stress and increased levels of homocysteine may contribute to the pathogenesis of BS.
(c) Innate immunity: The innate immune system also appears to be involved, with an increased expression of toll-like receptor 6 on granulocytes and monocytes in BS patients.

Clinical Features

BS is a multisystem disorder with a wide range of clinical manifestations, which can vary in severity and presentation:

(a) Mucocutaneous lesions: Recurrent painful oral aphthous ulcers are a hallmark of the disease. The ulcers heal spontaneously over weeks but have a tendency to recur. Interestingly, these oral ulcers are less common in smokers [7].
(b) Painful genital ulcers, especially scrotal ulcers with scarring are fairly specific for Behcet's syndrome [8]. Skin lesions can include erythema nodosum, papulopustular lesions, and acneiform eruptions. Histology of the erythema nodosum reveals a septal panniculitis with medium-sized vasculitis [9]. Pathergy and dermographism may be demonstrated.
(c) Ocular involvement is in the form of posterior uveitis, pan uveitis, hypopyon, and retinal vasculitis [10].
(d) Neurological manifestations [11] may be either parenchymal lesions (presenting as headache, dysarthria, ataxia, and hemiparesis) or disease secondary to vasculitis, e.g., cerebral venous thrombosis.
(e) Pulmonary artery aneurysms may present as cough, hemoptysis, dyspnea, fever, and pleuritic chest pain [12]. These symptoms may also be secondary to eosinophilic pneumonias.
(f) Gastrointestinal manifestation of Behcet's may mimic inflammatory bowel disease with symptoms of abdominal pain, diarrhea, gastrointestinal ulcers, and bleeding [13]. Volcano-shaped ulcers in the ileocecal area are not often seen in conditions other than Behcet's.
(g) Musculoskeletal system: Asymmetric nondeforming large joint arthritis which causes severe pain and functional limitation [14].

Diagnostic Criteria In addition to the involvement of eye, skin, and oral and genital ulcers, a positive pathergy test is one of the diagnostic criteria of Behcet's.

Pathergy Test A positive pathergy test is due to skin hyperreactivity to minor trauma. It is performed by inserting a 20 gauge needle obliquely into the skin. A positive test is indicated by the development of a papule at least 2 mm in size within 2 days [15].

Femoral vein thickness measurement (thickness is increased) can be a useful diagnostic tool, with a cutoff value of 0.5 mm showing good sensitivity and specificity.

Disease activity: The simplified Behcet's disease current activity form (BDCAF) [16] is a tool used to evaluate the disease activity. It considers symptoms such as headaches, oral and genital ulcers, skin lesions, joint involvement, gastrointestinal, eye and nervous system symptoms, and major vessel involvement.

Treatment [17]

1. Topical corticosteroids/colchicine or apremilast for oral and/or genital ulcers.
2. Arthritis is initially treated with colchicine and NSAIDs. For refractory arthritis, treatment may be escalated to azathioprine, interferon-alpha, and methotrexate.
3. The other systemic manifestations of Bechet's are managed by gradually escalating immunosuppression with mycophenolate methotrexate and cyclophosphamide.

Note: Approach to Oral Ulcers

Recurrent aphthous stomatitis is a frequent presenting complaint in outpatient clinics. Generally harmless, they can occasionally portend more serious conditions. Aphthous ulcers by definition are oval/round, encircled by an erythematous rim, and are *less than 5 mm in size.*

Classification

(a) Minor.
(b) Major.
(c) Severe.

The following have been implicated in the causation of aphthous ulcers

(a) Genetic susceptibility.
(b) Gut microbiota alteration.
(c) Smoking.
(d) Stress.
(e) Certain medications like methotrexate and nicorandil.
(f) Vitamin and mineral deficiency.

Oral ulcers are seen in the following conditions:

1. Herpes simplex virus infection.
2. Oral erosive lichen planus.
3. Autoimmune bullous disease.
4. Drug-induced mucosal ulcers.
5. Behçet syndrome.
6. Systemic lupus erythematosus.
7. MAGIC syndrome.
8. Celiac disease.
9. Inflammatory bowel disease.
10. HIV infection.

Aphthous ulcers are most often present on the buccal and oral mucosae and begin as painful pinpoint lesions which increase in size over the next 3–4 days and regress within 10 days.

Major recurrent aphthous ulcers are larger than 1 cm in size, deep, and may heal with scarring. Systemic symptoms are absent.

In a patient presenting with RAS, the following points in history must be looked into:

1. Temporal profile.
2. Symptoms of pruritus and pathergy.
3. H/o rash and other mucocutaneous lesions—especially in the anogenital area.
4. Other symptoms suggestive of mucosal involvement—dysphagia, hoarseness, stridor, ocular irritation, dysuria, dyspareunia, and hematuria.
5. Symptoms of other system involvement—respiratory, neurological, and gastrointestinal.
6. Relevant prescription history—immunosuppressants, methotrexate, and beta-blockers.

Examination

1. Local examination.
2. Anogenital area and scalp nails.

Treatment

A. Topical corticosteroids.
B. Topical anesthetic for pain relief.
C. Topical hyaluronate.

References

1. Dalvi SR, Yildirim R, Yazici Y. Behcet's syndrome. Drugs. 2012;72:2223–41.
2. Khairallah M, Accorinti M, Muccioli C, Kahloun R, Kempen JH. Epidemiology of Behçet disease. Ocul Immunol Inflamm. 2012;20(5):324–35.
3. Mendoza-Pinto C, García-Carrasco M, Jiménez-Hernández M, Hernández CJ, Riebeling-Navarro C, Zavala AN, Recabarren MV, Espinosa G, Quezada JJ, Cervera R. Etiopathogenesis of Behcet's disease. Autoimmun Rev. 2010;9(4):241–5.
4. Ma X, Wang X, Zheng G, Tan G, Zhou F, Wei W, Tian D, Yu H. Critical role of gut microbiota and epigenetic factors in the pathogenesis of behçet's disease. Front Cell Dev Biol. 2021;9:719235.
5. Handa R, Handa R. Behcet's Syndrome. Clin Rheumatol. 2021:185–9.
6. Tong B, Liu X, Xiao J, Su G. Immunopathogenesis of Behcet's disease. Front Immunol. 2019;10:665.
7. Nakamura K, Tsunemi Y, Kaneko F, Alpsoy E. Mucocutaneous manifestations of Behçet's disease. Front Med. 2021;7:613432.
8. Disease ISGfBs. Criteria for diagnosis of Behcet's disease. International Study Group for Behcet's Disease. Lancet. 1990;335(8697):1078–80.
9. Demirkesen C, Tüzüner N, Mat C, Senocak M, Büyükbabani N, Tüzün Y, Yazici H. Clinicopathologic evaluation of nodular cutaneous lesions of Behçet syndrome. Am J Clin Pathol. 2001;116(3):341–6.
10. Zamir E, et al. Conjunctival ulcers in Behçet's disease. Ophthalmology. 2003;110(6):1137–41. https://doi.org/10.1016/S0161-6420(03)00265-3.
11. Uluduz D, Kürtüncü M, Yapıcı Z, Seyahi E, Kasapçopur Ö, Özdoğan H, Saip S, Akman-Demir G, Siva A. Clinical characteristics of pediatric-onset neuro-Behçet disease. Neurology. 2011;77(21):1900–5.
12. Giannessi C, Smorchkova O, Cozzi D, Zantonelli G, Bertelli E, Moroni C, Cavigli E, Miele V. Behçet's disease: a radiological review of vascular and parenchymal pulmonary involvement. Diagnostics. 2022;12(11):2868.
13. Nguyen A, Upadhyay S, Javaid MA, Qureshi AM, Haseeb S, Javed N, Cormier C, Farooq A, Sheikh AB. Behcet's disease: an in-depth review about pathogenesis, gastrointestinal manifestations, and management. Inflamm Intes Dis. 2021;6(4):175–85.
14. Kötter I, Lötscher F. Behçet's syndrome apart from the triple symptom complex: vascular, neurologic, gastrointestinal, and musculoskeletal manifestations. A mini review. Front Med. 2021;8:639758.
15. Davatchi F. Diagnosis/classification criteria for Behcet's disease. Pathol Res Int. 2012;2012(1):607921.
16. Neves FD, Caldas CA, Medeiros DM, Moraes JC, Gonçalves CR. Adaptação transcultural da versão simplificada (s) do Behçet's Disease Current Activity Form (BDCAF) e comparação do desempenho das versões brasileiras dos dois instrumentos de avaliação da atividade da Doença de Behçet: BR-BDCAF e BR-BDCAF (s). Rev Bras Reumatol. 2009;49:20–31.
17. Yazici H, Seyahi E, Hatemi G, Yazici Y. Behçet syndrome: a contemporary view. Nat Rev Rheumatol. 2018;14(2):107–19.

Elderly Male with Difficulty in Swallowing, Unsteadiness of Gait, and Slurred Speech: The Sad Reunion

44

Grade Difficult.

Abstract An elderly patient with gait instability, frequent falls, slurred speech, and dysphagia.

Story You are visiting the town where you went to medical school. You head toward the bar with live music where you spent many happy evenings as a student. As you sip on your Jack and Coke, you scan the room slowly, looking for familiar faces.

You say to yourself "Oh my God! I can't believe it!" It's your favorite teacher—the one who inspired you to take general surgery as your speciality.

"Professor!" you call as you walk toward him. "Professor George!"

Doctor George leaps out of his chair so fast that you are worried he will fall down.

He shakes your hand with a stiff, strong grip and gazes at you with a weirdly fixed look. He says "Dinesh, how are you? it's so nice to see you. Come, sit at my table. The next one is on me." You walk back toward the bar, and you are dismayed to see that George is swaying more than a little bit. You are not surprised, though, as he was never able to hold his alcohol, even as a younger man.

"So, how have you been, Professor? Are you still inspiring your students every day? The techniques that you taught me are what gets me through surgery after surgery." George does not reply for some minutes—he gazes dully around the bar.

"That's nice to know Dinesh, Dinesh, Dinesh." George says—his words seem a little slurred. You wonder why he is looking so astonished as you speak to him.

You pass him a plate of mixed nuts, but he says "Sorry, I stick to soft cheese now. These nuts don't go down easy." He then spits repeatedly on the floor which you find surprising, because he didn't eat the nuts at all, so why is he spitting?

"Is everything ok, professor? Is something wrong with your health?"

S. Bhat, *Clinical Conundrums to Practice Diagnostic Reasoning*, https://doi.org/10.1007/978-981-95-0636-1_44

"Nothing, nothing at all," he says expansively. "It's just that I find it difficult to sleep—maybe that's what's hampering my functioning." He springs out of his chair again. "I have to head home—my wife is waiting for me."

"May I drive you home, sir?"

"Why?" he asks offended.

"Just to give you company," you say diffidently.

"No —*I* think that *you* think I'm drunk. Believe me, Dinesh I have not had more than half a mug of beer. Hold on a sec, let me get the bill." He grabs the bill from a waiter, almost falling backward in the process. You support him just in time, and tell him

"Relax prof., take it easy."

"I'm ok. Let me just sign the bill." He writes his name painstakingly—a tiny signature that is difficult to read.

As George walks toward the door, you observe that his gait is a little strange. He stands very straight and tall, like a soldier, and his arms are held away from his body.

You sit back down to finish your drink and ruminate on what you have just seen. It is easy to assume that the slurred speech, the unsteady walk, and the slightly strange behavior are due to alcohol, but maybe—just maybe—something else is going on. You decide to return to town with your friend, Dr. Vimla—a renowned neurologist—so you can figure out what exactly is happening with Professor George. You call his wife to find out if he has reached home safe. Mrs. George answers the call and after the mandatory chit chat, you say "I've noticed professor doesn't seem to be in his usual state of health. What happened?"

"It's very worrying," Mrs. George says. "It started maybe 6 months ago. He fell once or twice at home, even in the hospital. We took him to a neurologist who said it looked like Parkinson's and started him on carbidopa, but there has been hardly any improvement."

Questions Can you think of a diagnosis for Professor George's condition?

Analysis

The history of instability, at this age, with the tendency to fall, points toward a diagnosis of Parkinson's disease (PD). However, George's walk has been described as very straight and tall like a soldier, unlike the classic stooped posture of PD. Another strong clue to the diagnosis is the "Rocket Sign" [1] where the patient leaps out of the chair—this impulsivity is secondary to frontal lobe involvement. Also, the immobile face with the look of surprise (Procerus sign) [2] is a feature of Progressive Supranuclear Palsy, as is the palilalia [3] (repetition of one word).

Progressive supranuclear palsy (PSP) is a rare, age-related neurodegenerative disorder that belongs to a group of atypical parkinsonian disorders. It is characterized by progressive postural instability, vertical supranuclear gaze palsy, akinesia, rigidity, and cognitive and behavioral changes [4]. PSP's clinical spectrum is broader than that initially described.

The classic syndrome of PSP is widely recognized as a combination of down gaze palsy with progressive rigidity and imbalance leading to falls (typically backward). The typical phenotype is termed Richardson's syndrome. However, other phenotypes have been described. These include PSP-parkinsonism (PSP-P), which resembles Parkinson's disease, pure akinesia with gait freezing, and PSP with predominant cerebellar ataxia [5]. Some patients may present with the behavioral variant frontotemporal dementia, nonfluent aphasia, or corticobasal syndrome.

PSP is a sporadic disorder with a mean age of onset in the late 60 s to early 70 s. It is one of the most common atypical parkinsonian degenerative disorders, though still rare. The prevalence ranges from 1.39 to 6.4 per 100,000 individuals [6].

Etiopathogenesis

PSP is characterized by the aggregation of tau protein in the brain. It is considered a non-Mendelian disorder, although genetic factors may play a role [7]. Some studies suggest an association with an extended 5′-tau susceptibility haplotype.

The pathogenesis of PSP involves neurofibrillary tangles and neuropil threads composed of abnormal tau protein [8]. These pathological changes are prominent in the basal ganglia, brainstem, and cerebellum. Alterations of GABAergic neurons in the basal ganglia have been reported. Mitochondrial dysfunction and oxidative stress may also contribute [9].

Clinical Features [10]

The clinical presentation of PSP is variable. Common features include:

(a) Motor: Bradykinesia, rigidity, and postural instability with frequent falls, often early in the disease course. Axial rigidity with nuchal dystonia is typical. The gait is referred to as "drunken sailor gait."

(b) Oculomotor: Vertical supranuclear gaze palsy, particularly downgaze palsy, is a characteristic feature, although it may develop later in the disease. Gaze-evoked nystagmus may be present. Apraxia of lid opening can occur.
(c) Cognitive and behavioral: Frontal lobe dysfunction, including executive dysfunction, apathy, and behavioral changes. Neuropsychiatric symptoms such as depression, anxiety, and obsessive–compulsive behaviors may be observed. Impulsivity is common.
(d) Speech and swallowing: Dysarthria and dysphagia are common and can lead to aspiration pneumonia. Swallowing evaluations are important to assess the aspiration risk.

Other clinical features of PSP are [11]: Sleep abnormalities, including REM sleep behavior disorder, may occur (though less frequently in comparison to synucleinopathies). Urinary incontinence is also reported. Autonomic dysfunction can be present.

Investigations

(a) MRI [12]: Brain MRI may show midbrain atrophy, often described as the "hummingbird" or "penguin" sign (Fig. 44.1).

Measurement of the midbrain diameter and the midbrain-to-pons ratio can aid in differentiating PSP from Parkinson's disease. Atrophy of the superior cerebellar peduncle may also be evident.

(b) PET: Positron emission tomography (PET) may reveal hypometabolism in the midbrain and other brain regions.

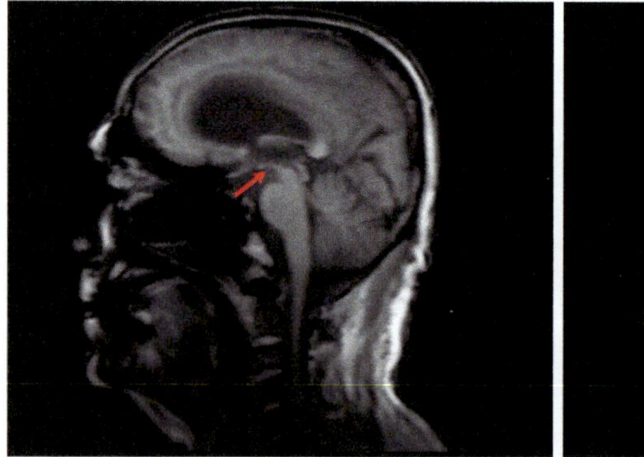

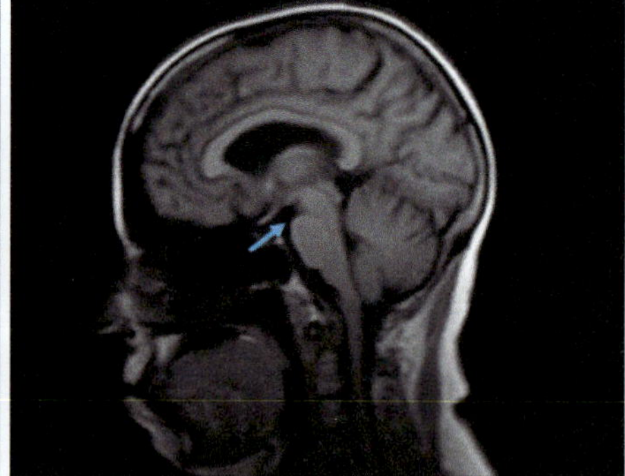

T1W MRI Saggital section , showing the marked atrophy of the midbrain (indicated by red arrow and normal midbrain indicated by blue arrow for comparison)

Fig. 44.1 Marked atrophy of midbrain (Panel 1, red arrow) compared to normal midbrain shown for comparison (Panel 2, blue arrow)
Image contributed by Dr. Vimala Colaco, neurologist, FMMC

(c) (Dat)SPECT: SPECT can be used to assess dopaminergic function.
(d) CSF biomarkers: Cerebrospinal fluid (CSF) biomarkers may assist in differential diagnosis.
(e) Skin biopsies: Tau protein quantification in skin biopsies has shown promise in differentiating tauopathies.

Diagnosis The Movement Disorder Society (MDS) criteria [13] are used for the clinical diagnosis of PSP. These criteria incorporate clinical features and neuroimaging findings to improve diagnostic accuracy.

Differential Diagnosis PSP should be differentiated from other parkinsonian disorders, including Parkinson's disease (PD), multiple system atrophy (MSA), and corticobasal degeneration (CBD). Other considerations include vascular parkinsonism, dementia with Lewy bodies, and frontotemporal dementia.

Treatment

The management of PSP is primarily supportive, as there is no cure or proven disease-modifying treatment.

Pharmacological Therapy Levodopa may provide some benefit for motor symptoms in some patients, particularly those with the PSP-P phenotype, but the response is generally limited. Amantadine may be tried. Tricyclic antidepressants [14], such as amitriptyline, have been used for depression, but their effectiveness is not well-established. Zolpidem has been reported to improve motor function in some cases.

Nonpharmacological Therapy Physical therapy and occupational therapy can help maintain mobility and function. Speech therapy can assist with dysarthria and swallowing difficulties. Dietary modifications and feeding tubes may be necessary for dysphagia.

Investigational Therapies Several clinical trials are underway to evaluate potential disease-modifying therapies, including microtubule-stabilizing agents and immunotherapies.

References

1. Rehman HU. Progressive supranuclear palsy. Postgrad Med J. 2000;76(896):333–6.
2. Pantelyat A. Progressive supranuclear palsy and corticobasal syndrome. Continuum: lifelong learning. Neurology. 2022;28(5):1364–78.
3. Kluin KJ, Foster NL, Berent S, Gilman S. Perceptual analysis of speech disorders in progressive supranuclear palsy. Neurology. 1993;43(3_part_1):563.

4. Armstrong MJ. Progressive supranuclear palsy: an update. Curr Neurol Neurosci Rep. 2018;18:1–9.
5. Lopez G, Bayulkem K, Hallett M. Progressive supranuclear palsy (PSP): Richardson syndrome and other PSP variants. Acta Neurol Scand. 2016;134(4):242–9.
6. Swallow DM, Zheng CS, Counsell CE. Systematic review of prevalence studies of progressive supranuclear palsy and corticobasal syndrome. Mov Disord Clin Pract. 2022;9(5):604–13.
7. Wen Y, Zhou Y, Jiao B, Shen L. Genetics of progressive supranuclear palsy: a review. J Parkinsons Dis. 2021;11(1):93–105.
8. De Bruin VM, Lees AJ. Subcortical neurofibrillary degeneration presenting as Steele-Richardson-Olszewski and other related syndromes: a review of 90 pathologically verified cases. Mov Disord. 1994;9(4):381–9.
9. Jellinger KA. Pathomechanisms of cognitive impairment in progressive supranuclear palsy. J Neural Transm. 2023;130(4):481–93.
10. Litvan I, Agid Y, Jankovic J, Goetz C, Brandel JP, Lai EC, Wenning G, D'Olhaberriague L, Verny M, Chaudhuri KR, McKee A. Accuracy of clinical criteria for the diagnosis of progressive supranuclear palsy (Steele-Richardson-Olszewski syndrome). Neurology. 1996;46(4):922–30.
11. Maher ER, Lees AJ. The clinical features and natural history of the Steele-Richardson-Olszewski syndrome (progressive supranuclear palsy). Neurology. 1986;36(7):1005.
12. Kim S, Suh CH, Shim WH, Kim SJ. Diagnostic performance of the magnetic resonance parkinsonism index in differentiating progressive supranuclear palsy from Parkinson's disease: an updated systematic review and meta-analysis. Diagnostics. 2021;12(1):12.
13. Höglinger GU, Respondek G, Stamelou M, Kurz C, Josephs KA, Lang AE, Mollenhauer B, Müller U, Nilsson C, Whitwell JL, Arzberger T. Clinical diagnosis of progressive supranuclear palsy: the movement disorder society criteria. Mov Disord. 2017;32(6):853–64.
14. Newman GC. Treatment of progressive supranuclear palsy with tricyclic antidepressants. Neurology. 1985;35(8):1189.

Headache, Diplopia, and Drowsiness in a Previously Healthy Young Female: The Pernicious Pimple

45

Grade Moderate.

Abstract A young female anticipating a social event is unable to attend because she has eyelid swelling, diplopia, headache, and drowsiness.

Story Satya is very excited indeed—her dearest cousin Madhavi is getting married in a month, and Satya foresees a major role for herself in the celebrations. Keeping this in mind, she has prevailed upon her doting mother, Megha, to buy her some outfits for the function—each one is more beautiful than the next. What joy Satya feels as she gazes at the finery hanging in her wardrobe—the emerald green lehenga for the sangeet, the ruby red Kanjeevaram sari for the wedding ceremony, and the gold embroidered salwar suit for the reception.

The happiness evaporates 2 days before the ceremony when she sees an incipient pimple on the left side of her nose. "Oh no!" she moans and calls for her mum to come sort things out.

"What happened, beti?" Satya's mother bustles in.

"Ma, there's a pimple on my face!"

"It's ok, I will apply an ubtan tonight. Be patient. It will be ok by the day of the wedding."

That night, Satya gazes malevolently at her reflection, at the ugly eruption disfiguring her peachy complexion.

"Out, damned spot," she mutters, pressing on the pustule.

The next day, Megha notices that Satya looks a little out of sorts and attempts to cheer her up.

"Don't worry, it will be ok by tomorrow."

"Ok," Satya responds listlessly.

On the day of the wedding, Satya comes to the kitchen asking for a cup of tea.

S. Bhat, *Clinical Conundrums to Practice Diagnostic Reasoning*,
https://doi.org/10.1007/978-981-95-0636-1_45

"What happened my dear, it looks like you've been crying?", she says, looking at Satya's swollen eyelids and red eyes.

"No. I haven't. But I don't want to come for the wedding.""Why? You look ok, don't worry. We can conceal the boil with makeup."

"No, Ma. I'm just not in the mood. You go. My head aches."

"It will look really odd if you don't come. Madhavi will be so upset."

"I don't care. You go," says Satya miserably.

Satya's parents try to persuade her, but she is stubborn in her refusal.

Saddened, Megha and her husband leave for the wedding ceremony.

It is quite late by the time they get back, and they peep into Satya's room to see that she is asleep.

The next day when Megha wakes Satya up, she is worried to see that Satya is in tears. "What happened, dear? Why are you crying?"

"Nothing happened. I'm not crying, for heaven's sake. My eyes are burning and tearing."

"Shall we take you to the doctor?"

"For sore eyes? No, thank you. Let me rest a bit. Please stop fussing."

Megha touches her daughter's forehead and says, "You've got a temperature too."

"I'm ok, ma. Please let me rest. I will be fine by tomorrow."

The next evening, however, Satya is significantly worse. She looks dull and drowsy and tells her mum "My head aches so much I feel like it is exploding. I can't see clearly. Everything looks blurred."

Satya's parents panic and bring her immediately to the emergency room. You are on duty. You note that the patient is febrile, hemodynamically stable, and drowsy. Her eyes appear red, and her left eye is deviated medially. The rest of the neurological examination is essentially normal, apart from minimal hypoesthesia on the left side of the nose and the left cheek.

Question What do you think is going on with Satya? It is obviously something more than sadness at having missed a much anticipated event.

Analysis

The answer to this puzzle lies in the first problem that Satya complained of.

She had a pimple on the side of her nose. This is part of the area that is referred to as the "danger triangle."' The severe headache ("My head aches so much I feel like it is exploding") in combination with the lateral rectus palsy (left eye deviated medially) are pointers to cavernous sinus thrombosis. In this case, it is most probably secondary to the pustule in the dangerous area of the face.

Cavernous sinus thrombosis is a rare but serious condition that occurs most often due to infections in the danger triangle of the face.

Etiopathogenesis

The cavernous sinuses are paired dural venous sinuses located at the base of the skull, lateral to the sella turcica and the sphenoid sinuses. They receive blood from the superior and inferior ophthalmic veins and superficial cortical veins and drain into the basilar plexus via the superior and inferior petrosal sinuses. The cavernous sinuses are closely realted to the internal carotid artery, the sympathetic plexus, and cranial nerves III, IV, V (ophthalmic and maxillary branches), and VI (Fig. 45.1).

The danger triangle of the face includes the bridge of the nose and the maxilla and extends to the corner of the mouth [1]. Veins draining this area are valveless and communicate directly with the intracranial cavernous sinuses. Hence, even trivial infections of this region of the face may spread intracranially [2].

Facial cellulitis, dental infections, otitis media, mastoiditis, and furuncles on the face are commonly implicated in the causation of cavernous sinus thrombosis [3].

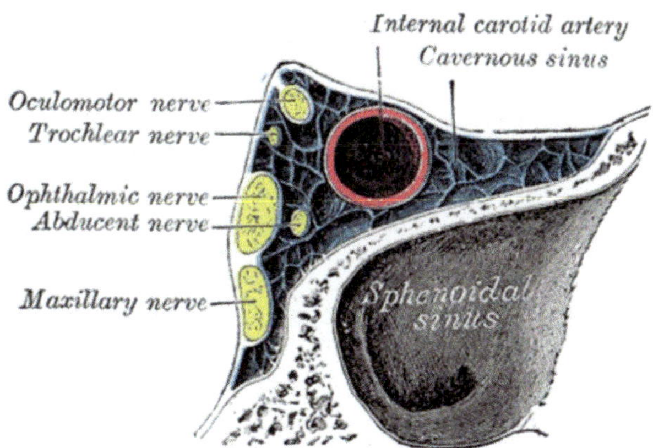

Fig. 45.1 Gray's Anatomy 20th US edition (public domain) https://archive.org/details/anatomyofhumanbo1918gray/page/658/mode/2up?q=cavernous+sinus+anatomy

Translocation of bacteria and septic embolization into the cavernous sinus from the veins draining the danger triangle cause thrombus formation in the sinus, resulting in congestion and cranial nerve compression. The lack of valves in the dural venous system allows the thrombus to propagate further.

Clinical Features [4, 5]

1. Headache: severe and retro-orbital.
2. Periorbital edema and chemosis.
3. Ptosis and proptosis.
4. Lateral rectus palsy and diplopia.
5. Mydriasis.
6. Numbness or paresthesia around the eyes, nose, and forehead results from compression of the ophthalmic and maxillary branches of the trigeminal nerve.
7. May progress to complete external ophthalmoplegia.
8. Fever confusion, seizures, or stroke.

Differential Diagnoses [6]

(a) Orbital cellulitis.
(b) Orbital abscess.
(c) Cavernous sinus neoplasm.

Investigations

(a) CT or MRI with venography [7] (Fig. 45.2).
(b) Blood cultures.

Treatment [2]

Prolonged treatment with antibiotics (a third-generation cephalosporin along with vancomycin and metronidazole if the source is likely to be anaerobic).

Key Takeaway
Always rule out cavernous sinus thrombosis in a patient who presents with severe headache and lateral rectus palsy.

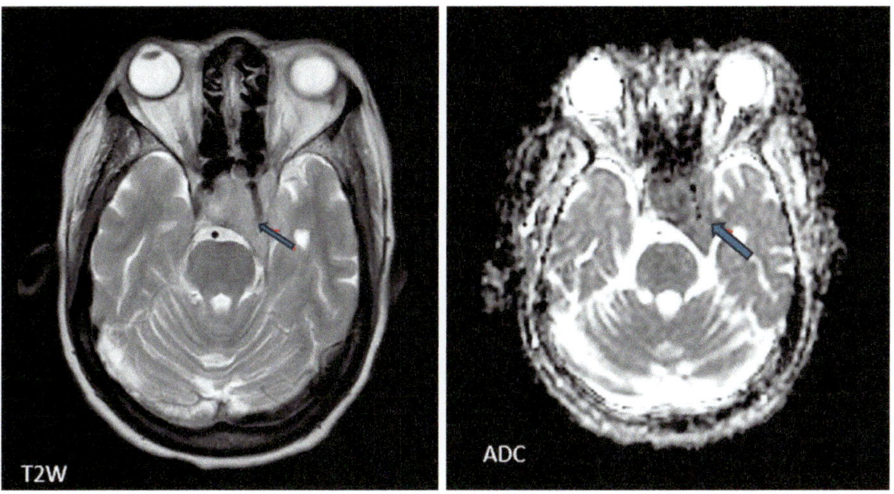

Fig. 45.2 MRI brain showing obliteration of cavernous sinus (Blue arrow). (Image contributed by Dr. Vimala Colaco, Neurologist, FMMC)

References

1. Pannu AK, Saroch A, Sharma N. Danger triangle of face and septic cavernous sinus thrombosis. J Emerg Med. 2017;53(1):137–8.
2. Ali S. Cavernous sinus thrombosis: efficiently recognizing and treating a life-threatening condition. Cureus. 13(8):e17339.
3. Khatri IA, Wasay M. Septic cerebral venous sinus thrombosis. J Neurol Sci. 2016;362:221–7.
4. Caranfa JT, Yoon MK. Septic cavernous sinus thrombosis: a review. Surv Ophthalmol. 2021;66(6):1021–30.
5. Hsu CW, Tsai WC, Lien CY, Lee JJ, Chang WN. The clinical characteristics, implicated pathogens and therapeutic outcomes of culture-proven septic cavernous sinus thrombosis. J Clin Neurosci. 2019;68:111–6.
6. Lee JH, Lee HK, Park JK, Choi CG, Suh DC. Cavernous sinus syndrome: clinical features and differential diagnosis with MR imaging. Am J Roentgenol. 2003;181(2):583–90.
7. Bhatia H, Kaur R, Bedi R. MR imaging of cavernous sinus thrombosis. Eur J Radiol Open. 2020;7:100226.

Post-coital Headache: Not Tonight, John

46

Grade Moderate.

Abstract Post-coital headache and tinnitus in a young woman.

Story Mr. Sanoof looks disgruntled and grumpy when he brings his wife, Afeefa, to your clinic. They are an odd couple—Sanoof is short and stocky and has a permanent frown, while Afeefa is very tall and slender. She looks quite stressed. You foresee a stormy consultation, mentally prepare yourself, and invite them both to sit down.

"How may I help you today?" you ask Afeefa, knowing quite well as you do so, that Sanoof will answer for his wife.

"I just got back home yesterday from a business trip to Dubai," Sanoof says.

"Oh sorry…" you say, confused. "I thought Afeefa was the patient."

"Yes, yes,doctor, she is. I'm just telling you what happened," Sanoof grumbles.

"Ok, please go ahead."

"As I was saying, I have been in Dubai for the last 2 weeks. I returned last evening."

"Ok…," you say, wondering where this was going.

"What does a man expect when he gets back home after a long trip?"

"I'm really not sure," you say glancing at your patient who has still not spoken.

"Intimate relations with his wife, of course!"

"I see …and you couldn't…." you say delicately.

"No, no. All that was fine. But after that, she started complaining of a severe headache. If she doesn't want sex all she has to do is say so, not invent imaginary ailments."

Afeefa says tearfully "I'm not inventing it, Sanoof, truly I am not."

"Tell me what happened," you ask Afeefa gently.

S. Bhat, *Clinical Conundrums to Practice Diagnostic Reasoning*,
https://doi.org/10.1007/978-981-95-0636-1_46

"It's like he said doctor. We did have intercourse, but towards the end, I developed a severe pain in my head, and it hasn't disappeared yet."

"Where exactly is the headache—is it on the whole head?"

"No just on the left," Afeefa says pointing to the left side of her face and head.

"Anything apart from that?"

"Theres a kind of whooshing sound in my ear."

"Whooshing?!" Sanoof scoffs. "That's a new one! If you don't want sex just tell me. You don't have to create these crazy stories."

"Please, Mr Sanoof give me a moment to speak to the patient."

You examine Afeefa—you check the pulse, enviously eyeing the beautiful jade rings on Afeefa's long and slender fingers as you do so.

The pulse rate is 100/minute. Your other findings are as follows:

BP: 140/90 mm Hg.
No focal neurological deficit.
The neck is supple.
Cardiovascular system normal.

You feel that there is something a little off about her face, but maybe it is because she is stressed with Sanoof's continuous barrage of criticism.

"So, Mrs Afeefa, I can't really find anything abnormal on physical examination."

"Ha!" says Sanoof "No surprise there."

"It sounds like something called a post-coital headache".

"Is that another term for 'Not tonight, John'?" Sanoof mutters.

You ignore him.

"However, to be on the safer side, since this is the first episode of a severe headache, I would like to get at least a CT scan done."

"Is it really necessary doc?" asks Sanoof. "Can't she take an aspirin and sleep it off?"

"I really think it is essential."

You prescribe some paracetamol and schedule a CT scan. A while later, the radiologist calls, telling you that the scan is normal. You call in the couple to the consulting room, inform them of their reports, prescribe pain relief, and tell them to review in 2 days if she does not feel better.

The day goes on—outpatients, ward rounds, a webinar where you moderate a panel discussion, and a hurried lunch. You are very busy, but there is a background niggle, something worrying you, and you are not sure what. As you sit down for a coffee with your colleagues, your mind goes back to the morning's consultation with Afeefa. Did you miss something? You try to reassure yourself that the CT was normal—there was something else, however. Something about the face, the fingers …

"Oh, shit" you exclaim, standing up suddenly and spilling your colleague's coffee.

"What's up with you?"

"Her face did not look symmetrical," you exclaim and rush to the clinic to call Afeefa, while your colleagues shake their heads, mystified.

Question What was wrong with Mrs. Afeefa? Was it something more than a post-coital headache?

Analysis

The following points must be taken in to account:

(a) Tall slim lady, with long slender fingers.
(b) Headache precipitated by sexual intercourse—however, this patient's headache was unilateral, whereas post-coital headache is more often bilateral.
(c) Whooshing sound in the ear: pulsatile tinnitus.
    Though the CT scan was normal, plain CT scan can miss infarcts and carotid dissection in 12% of cases of carotid artery dissection (CAD) [1].
    The facial asymmetry that you suddenly recalled was perhaps due to the eyelid drooping due to a partial Horner's syndrome.

Putting all the above together, it is likely to be a carotid artery dissection.

Arterial dissection occurs when blood penetrates the arterial wall through an intimal tear, creating a false lumen between the intimal and medial layers. It can potentially result in intramural hematoma and luminal narrowing.

Epidemiology

CAD accounts for approximately 2.5% of all strokes in the general population but is responsible for up to 25% of strokes in patients under 45 years of age [2]. The annual incidence is estimated at 2.6–3.0 per 100,000 individuals [3]. The condition affects men and women equally, with a median age of onset in the early 40 s. Seasonal variation has been observed, with higher occurrence rates during autumn and winter.

Etiology

CAD can be categorized into spontaneous and traumatic dissections. Spontaneous dissections are often associated with underlying arteriopathies [4]. Though a genetic predisposition has been suggested, this has not been proven unequivocally [5].

Spontaneous dissections may be associated with

- Fibromuscular dysplasia.
- Ehlers–Danlos syndrome type IV.
- Marfan syndrome.
- α1-antitrypsin deficiency,

Traumatic dissections may result from:

- Road traffic accidents.
- Sudden neck movements, chiropractic manipulation.

- Sports-related injuries.
- Prolonged hyperextension of the neck.

Pathogenesis

The initial event involves damage to the vessel wall with an intimal tear. Blood enters through this tear, creating a false lumen within the arterial wall (Fig. 46.1). This process can lead to:

1. Luminal stenosis or occlusion from expanding hematoma.
2. Thromboembolism from the damaged endothelial surface.
3. Aneurysmal dilation of the weakened vessel wall.

Clinical Features

The classic triad includes:

1. Unilateral headache/neck pain (present in 80% of cases)—ipsilateral periauricular, periorbital, or cervical area.
2. Partial Horner syndrome (due to compression of sympathetic fibers by the enlarged carotid artery).
3. Cerebral/retinal ischemia—TIA, cerebrovascular accident (cortical or large subcortical infarcts).

Additional manifestations include:

- Pulsatile tinnitus.
- Lower cranial nerve palsies.
- Transient ischemic attacks.
- Amaurosis fugax.

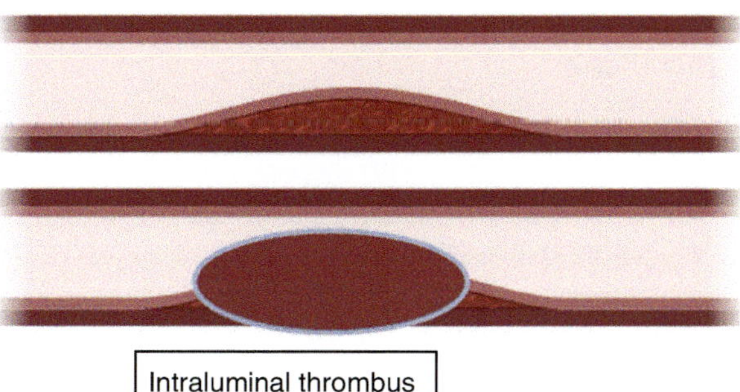

Fig. 46.1 Occlusion of lumen by intramural hematomaCreated in BioRender. Bhat, S. (2025) https://BioRender.com/g0pc20t

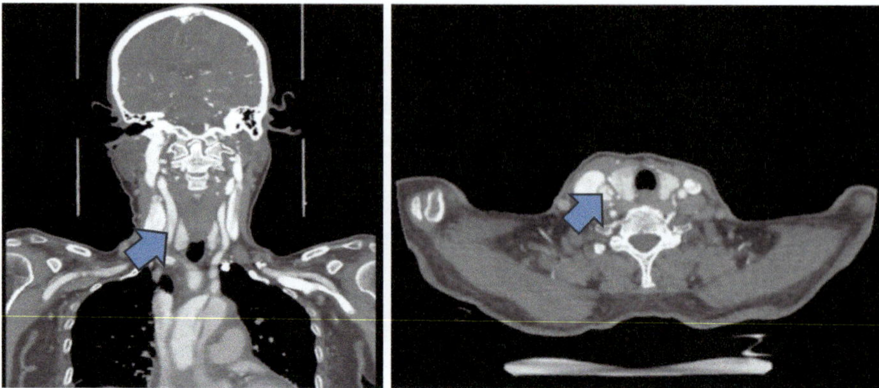

Fig. 46.2 CT angio of head and neck vessels—blue arrows indicate dissection flap. Image contributed by Dr. Vimala Colaco, neurologist, FMMC

Investigations

- CT brain: Relatively insensitive.
- CTA (computed tomographic angiography) (Fig. 46.2).
- MRA (magnetic resonance angiography).
- Conventional angiography.
- Ultrasound: Limited utility but useful for monitoring.

Suggestive Findings

- String sign on angiography.
- Intramural hematoma on fat-suppressed T1-weighted MRI.
- Double lumen sign.
- Irregular luminal stenosis.

Treatment

Acute Phase:

1. Antithrombotic therapy:
   - Anticoagulation with heparin, followed by warfarin for 3–6 months in most cases.
   - Alternatively, antiplatelet therapy with aspirin in selected cases.
   - However, neither antiplatelet nor anticoagulant therapy lowers the risk of recurrent stroke after carotid artery dissection [6].

2. Blood pressure control:
   - Target systolic BP <140 mmHg.
   - BP control must be undertaken cautiously if the carotid artery dissection is complicated by stroke.

Endovascular/Surgical Intervention [7].

Reserved for cases with:

- Progressive neurological symptoms despite medical therapy.
- Expanding aneurysms.
- Recurrent thromboembolic events.

Prognosis is generally favorable, with complete recovery in 70–85% of patients. Recurrence rates are approximately 2% annually. Long-term follow-up is essential to monitor for complications and prevent recurrence.

References

1. Shaw M, Whittaker TJ. Horner's syndrome caused by carotid dissection missed on radiological reports. Invest Ophthalmol Vis Sci. 2010;51(13):1458–8.
2. Schievink WI. Spontaneous dissection of the carotid and vertebral arteries. N Engl J Med. 2001;344(12):898–906.
3. Lee VH, Brown RD Jr, Mandrekar JN, Mokri B. Incidence and outcome of cervical artery dissection: a population-based study. Neurology. 2006;67(10):1809–12.
4. Keser Z, Chiang CC, Benson JC, Pezzini A, Lanzino G. Cervical artery dissections: etiopathogenesis and management. Vasc Health Risk Manag. 2022;18:685–700. https://doi.org/10.2147/VHRM.S362845.
5. Debette S, Markus HS. The genetics of cervical artery dissection: a systematic review. Stroke. 2009;40(6):e459–66.
6. Markus HS, Levi C, King A, Madigan J, Norris J. Antiplatelet therapy vs anticoagulation therapy in cervical artery dissection: the cervical artery dissection in stroke study (CADISS) randomized clinical trial final results. JAMA Neurol. 2019;76(6):657–64.
7. Garg K, Rockman CB, Lee V, Maldonado TS, Jacobowitz GR, Adelman MA, Mussa FF. Presentation and management of carotid artery aneurysms and pseudoaneurysms. J Vasc Surg. 2012;55(6):1618–22.

Subacute Confusion in the Previously Well: The Muddled Model

47

Grade Moderate.

Abstract An aspiring model is brought by her flatmate to your hospital. There is a history of confusion, odd behavior, and disinterest.

Story Rainbow is a 22-year-old who is just beginning to make her name in modeling. She has a few print ads for local businesses in her portfolio, as well as a television advertisement for a nationally known company that she is justifiably proud of. Ad agencies like to employ her, as she is professional as well as disciplined, and unlike many other of her contemporaries, is neither fussy nor demanding. She is slim and pretty and fits into almost any role that is assigned to her.

You are in charge of the emergency department on a quiet Saturday night. A junior resident runs in to the room excitedly and says "It's Rainbow! That model! Come quick."

Rainbow is accompanied by another young lady who introduces herself as Gloria, the model's flatmate. You assure yourself that the patient is hemodynamically stable, get a glucometer sugar done which shows 150 mg %, and then proceed to obtain a history.

"I'm very concerned about Rainbow,"Gloria says. "She's been acting weird for the last 2 weeks."

"Weird in the sense?"

"It's difficult to describe, doctor. She looks really confused—doesn't seem to be paying attention. And her face looks a little strange. There's something not quite right about her eyes, but I can't figure it out."

"What's brought this on?" you ask. "Has there been anything unusual going on in her life?"

"I'm not really sure, doctor, she just moved in as my flatmate a month ago."

S. Bhat, *Clinical Conundrums to Practice Diagnostic Reasoning*,
https://doi.org/10.1007/978-981-95-0636-1_47

While you are having this conversation, Ms. Rainbow gazes around the room, completely uninterested in what you both are talking about. She does not respond when she is spoken to and looks quite unaware of what is going on.

"Does she drink, smoke or take recreational drugs?"

"No, I'm sure about that, doctor. She is very careful about what goes into her body and is extremely health-conscious. She drinks only green tea and fruit juice."

Maybe, unintentionally, you look a little skeptical because Gloria says "I know how important it is to give an accurate history. Both my parents are doctors. I swear I am not bluffing. There is no substance abuse at all."

"Have there been any hospital admissions in the past?"

"Not as far as I know. She's been perfectly healthy till recently. In fact, she had begun to lose that skeletal skinniness. Actually, she was a little tense about the half to one kilogram weight she had gained. She told me that she used to be very overweight as a teen, and she would never go down that road again. She was doing very well until a month ago when she started acting strange and it's only gotten worse since then."

"Did anything out of the ordinary happen 30 days ago?"

"Not anything untoward. She visited her parents' home in Bangalore. She said she required elective surgery."

"What was the surgery for?"

"I really don't know, doctor. I did ask her once, but she was quite cagey about it, and I was reluctant to poke my nose into personal matters."

Ms. Rainbow lies on the examination couch, passive and unresponsive, and permits you to examine her.

Physical examination findings are as follows:

Blood pressure: 100/60 mm Hg.

The BMI is 18 kg/m^2. The patient looks pale, and there is some evidence of cheilitis and glossitis. There is koilonychia as well.

Rainbow scores 19 on her MMSE. There is no papilloedema and no signs of meningeal irritation. Power in all four limbs is normal, though she does have a slightly wide-based ataxic gait. Her speech seems fine, and there is no limb ataxia. Her systemic examination is essentially normal, though you do notice what are possibly laparoscopic scars on her abdomen.

You perform a focused neurological examination and note that there is a horizontal nystagmus and bilateral lateral rectus palsy. Pupils are equal but sluggishly reactive.

The ankle jerk is absent.

Question What is wrong with Ms. Rainbow? Do you think she is bluffing about the alcohol and drug consumption?

Analysis

The salient points are as follows:

(a) A model who is concerned about her weight gain undergoes elective surgery—perhaps it is bariatric surgery.
(b) Signs of malnutrition in the form of low BMI, cheilitis, glossitis, and koilonychia.
(c) Subacute onset, rapidly progressive neurological deficit in the form of confusion, oculomotor abnormalities, and gait ataxia.

The astute clinician, if aware of the neurological complications of bariatric surgery, will consider Wernicke's encephalopathy (WE) in this patient and promptly commence treatment for this neurological emergency.

Diagnosis of WE

It is based on Cain's criteria [1].

- Dietary deficiency.
- Oculomotor abnormalities.
- Cerebellar dysfunction.
- Either altered mental status or mild memory impairment.

WE, due to the deficiency of thiamine, is an acute neurological emergency which causes death and disability if not treated urgently.

Etiopathogenesis [2]

- Chronic heavy alcohol use.
- Anorexia nervosa.
- Hyperemesis gravidarum.
- Prolonged intravenous feeding with inadequate nutrient prescription.
- Prolonged fasting.
- Gastrointestinal disease.
- Bariatric surgery.
- Acquired immune deficiency syndrome.

Thiamine is a cofactor for enzymes involved in energy metabolism, like transketolase and pyruvate dehydrogenase [3]. Thiamine deficiency affects areas of the brain which are most metabolically active and causes excitotoxicity, generation of ROS, and disruption of the blood brain barrier [4].

Clinical Features

Symptoms The patient presents with a history of insidious onset, gradually progressive neurological deficit in the form of confusion and gait instability.

Signs The classic triad of WE includes the following:

(a) Confusion, disorientation, and inattentiveness.
(b) Oculomotor dysfunction: Nystagmus (usually horizontal, sometimes downbeat), lateral rectus palsy, and conjugate gaze palsies.
(c) Ataxia: Gait ataxia in WE is due to the combination of cerebellar involvement and polyneuropathy. Since only anterior and superior vermis are involved, limb ataxia and speech abnormalities are not present.

    It is important to remember that this clinical triad is present in only a third of patients, with most patients usually presenting with two of the three features.

Lab Abnormalities WE is mainly a clinical diagnosis; however, erythrocyte transketolase may be elevated [5].

Neuroimaging may show increased signal intensity in mammillary bodies, dorsomedial thalami, tectal plate, periaqueductal grey matter, and around the third ventricle (Fig. 47.1).

Treatment [6]

1. 500 mg thiamine iv eighth hourly for 2–3 days
2. Followed by 250 mg od for 5 days.
3. Followed by 100 mg daily orally to continue.
4. Magnesium replacement if required.

Key Takeaway

Diagnosing a case of WE with the triad of encephalopathy, oculomotor dysfunction, and ataxia in a patient with alcohol abuse is simple enough. However, the expertise of the clinician lies in diagnosing a case of WE with only one or two components of the triad in a patient with a risk factor other than ethanol abuse. WE should be considered a possible cause of all acute onset delirium with or without ataxia, regardless of the absence of history of ethanol use [7]. In any patient with acute onset delirium, thiamine must be administered parenterally on an emergent basis, even before investigations to confirm the diagnosis.

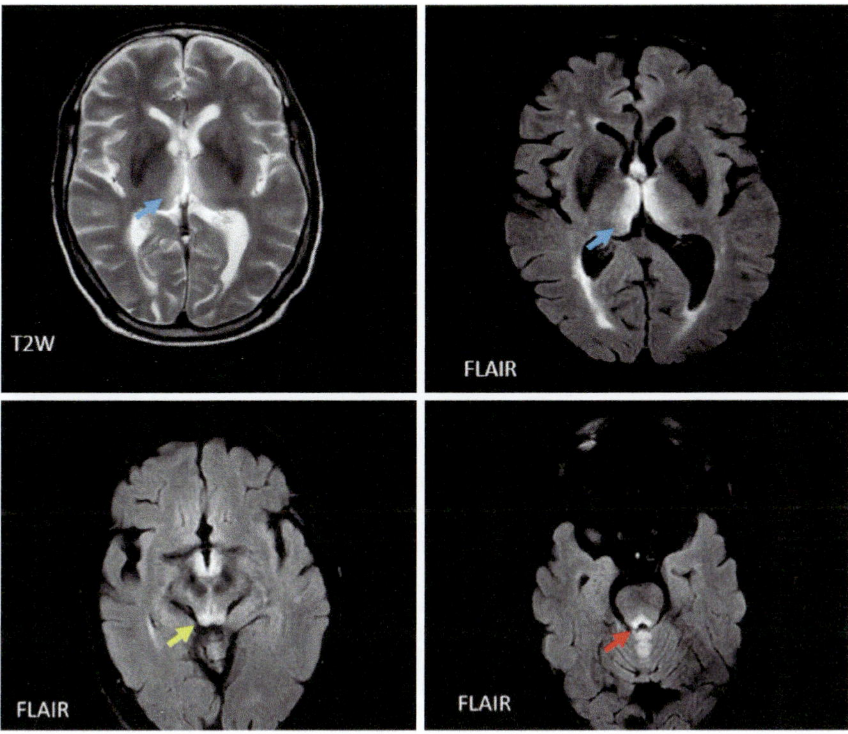

Classic MRI findings in Wenicke encephalopathy- T2 Flair hyperintensities affecting the dorsomedial thalami(blue arrow), mammillary bodies(yellow arrow), peri aqueductal grey matter(red arrow)

Fig. 47.1 MRI findings in Wernicke's Encephalopathy (Image contributed by Dr. Vimala Colaco, neurologist, FMMC)

References

1. Tanasescu R, Dumitrescu L, Dragos C, Luca D, Oprisan A, Coclitu C, Simionescu O, Cojocaru L, Stan M, Carasca A, Gitman A, Wernicke's encephalopathy. Miscellanea on encephalopathies—a seconf look. 1st ed. Rijeka: IntechOpen; 2012. p. 327–64.
2. Desjardins P, Butterworth RF. Role of mitochondrial dysfunction and oxidative stress in the pathogenesis of selective neuronal loss in Wernicke's encephalopathy. Mol Neurobiol. 2005;31:17–25.
3. Foster JB. The Wernicke-Korsakoff syndrome and related neurologic disorders due to alcoholism and malnutrition. J Neurol Neurosurg Psychiatry. 1989;52(10):1217.
4. Martin PR, Singleton CK, Hiller-Sturmhöfel S. The role of thiamine deficiency in alcoholic brain disease. Alcohol Res Health. 2003;27(2):134.

5. Leigh D, McBurney A, Mcllwain H. Erythrocyte transketolase activity in the Wernicke-Korsakoff syndrome. Br J Psychiatry 1981;139(2):153–6./.
6. Cook CC, Hallwood PM, Thomson AD. B vitamin deficiency and neuropsychiatric syndromes in alcohol misuse. Alcohol Alcohol. 1998;33(4):317–36.
7. Wernicke-Korsakoff syndrome despite no alcohol abuse: A summary of systematic reports—ScienceDirect [Internet]. [cited 2025 Jan 27]. Available from: https://www.sciencedirect.com/science/article/pii/S0022510X21001763

Acute Confusion in an Elderly Gentleman: Grandad in the Department Store

48

Grade Difficult.

Abstract An elderly gentleman is confused and flustered. He forgets where he is and what is said to him.

Story You are using your weekly holiday well—equipped with a couple of free hours and a huge credit card limit you decide yourself to treat yourself to clothing and jewelry at the city's premium department store. As you debate between a lilac blouse and a gray silk shirt, you note that the elderly gentleman shopping in the aisle appears a little confused.

"Sir, are you ok?"

"Yes, I am. Can you please tell me the way to the cashiers desk?" "Sure, I will take you there," you say kindly. As you walk to the desk, the gentleman asks again "Can you tell me the way to the cashiers desk?"

You are a little concerned now. You say "I'm Dr. Raksha, sir, it's a pleasure to meet you. I will take you to the cashier's desk."

"Nice to meet you," the man responds. "My name is Raghavan. Can you tell me the way to the cashier's desk?"

You walk together to the desk and you watch, worried, as Raghavan fumbles for his wallet. It falls to the floor. He gets flustered, bends down to pick it up, and things start falling out of his pocket. He gets up, looks around helplessly, and is almost in tears. He grabs your sleeve and says in exactly the same tone as before "Can you tell me the way to the cashier's desk? ".

S. Bhat, *Clinical Conundrums to Practice Diagnostic Reasoning*, https://doi.org/10.1007/978-981-95-0636-1_48

You discreetly murmur to the cashier "Can you cancel this order? This gentleman needs to go to hospital now." As you accompany Raghavan to your car, to drive him to hospital, you note that he has no difficulty in walking. There is no facial asymmetry, and the speech, though confused, is not slurred.

On the way to the hospital, you say, "Mr Raghavan, there's nothing to worry about. I'm just taking you to the hospital for a quick check up."

"Ok," he replies amiably.

"Can you tell me if you are on regular medication for anything? High blood sugar, high blood pressure, anything like that?"

"Yes, high blood pressure. And also medicines to prevent migraine."

You reach the hospital and take Mr. Raghavan to the neurologist.

Questions What is happening to poor Mr. Raghavan? Why is that he remembers his name and details of his previous medical history but not what is said to him even a minute prior?

Analysis

The clues here are in the demography (elderly male), the past history (hypertension and migraine), as well as the antegrade and retrograde memory dysfunction with the preservation of remote memory. In fact, Mr. Raghavan appears to have developed transient global amnesia (TGA).

Transient Global Amnesia

TGA is a syndrome of reversible, temporary anterograde and retrograde memory dysfunction [1]. It mainly affects adults between the ages of 50 and 80 years with a slight male preponderance. Hypertension, dyslipidemia, hypothyroidism, coronary artery disease, and a previous history of Transient Ischemic Attack (TIA) are more common in patients with TGA than in the normal population. Migraine is strongly associated with TGA [2]. Obstructive sleep apnea is more common in patients with TGA [3].

Etiopathogenesis [4]

Interestingly, attacks of TGA may be precipitated by either mental or physical pressure—like emotional stress, physical stress, and physical effort [5]. TGA is perhaps secondary to ischemia, affecting the medial temporal lobe and thalamus or involvement of the posterior cerebral circulation. Neurons of the CA1 region of the hypothalamus are particularly vulnerable to metabolic stress [6]. Functional neuroimaging: During episodes of TGA, apart from hypoperfusion, decreased connectivity of the hippocampi, Para hippocampi, and amygdala have been found [7, 8].

Clinical Features

It is important to remember that remote memories remain unaffected (Ribot's law). [9] The ability to form and retain memories is restored within 24 h, but the patient remains amnesic about the period of TGA.

Episodes of TGA usually last between 4 to 6 h but can range from 30 min to 24 h. The primary clinical features include:

Anterograde amnesia: Profound inability to form new memories. Inability to retain new information leads to the characteristic repetitiveness of questions and sentences.

Retrograde amnesia: Variable impairment of past memories. In particular, patients may have difficulty recalling events from the recent past.

The symptoms appear abruptly and are often preceded by a triggering event.

Preserved cognitive functions: Language, reasoning, and spatial awareness remain intact. There is no clouding of consciousness or loss of personal identity.

Mild constitutional symptoms such as headache, nausea, or dizziness can occur during the acute phase.

Investigations

Diffusion-weighted MRI may show transient punctate lesions in the CA1 field hippocampus, along with subtle focal areas of diffusion restriction (Fig. 48.1).

EEG: An electroencephalogram (EEG) to rule out post-ictal disorders or nonconvulsive status epilepticus.

SPECT.

FDG PET scan.

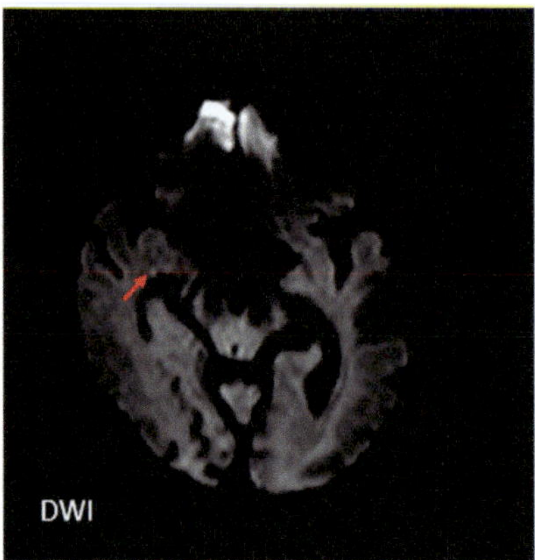

Subtle focal area of diffusion restriction in the right temporal lobe (indicated by the red arrow) This pattern is highly suggestive of transient global amnesia (TGA), given its characteristic involvement of the CA1 sector of the hippocampus.

Fig. 48.1 Diffusion restriction in right temporal lobe (Image contributed by Dr. Vimala Colaco, neurologist, FMMC)

Diagnostic Criteria

1. Attack is witnessed.
2. Dysfunction limited to repetitive queries and amnesia.
3. No other major neurologic signs or symptoms.
4. Memory loss is transient, usually lasting hours to a day.

Differential Diagnosis

(a) Transient epileptic amnesia (TEA): Characterized by recurrent, brief amnesic episodes, often upon waking.
(b) Stroke: Posterior circulation strokes or transient ischemic attacks (TIAs) can cause acute amnesia.
(c) Psychogenic amnesia: Due to psychological trauma or stress.
(d) Post-traumatic amnesia.
(e) Toxic/drug-related amnesia.
(f) Limbic encephalitis might also present with an amnestic syndrome, although these are usually accompanied with confusion and focal neurological signs.

Treatment

TGA has a favorable prognosis.

Acute management: Primarily supportive, ensuring the patient's safety and monitoring for any other neurological symptoms. Intravenous thiamine may be administered.

Long-term management: No specific treatment is typically required. Addressing vascular risk factors and lifestyle modifications may be beneficial. In rare cases of frequent TGA recurrence, metoprolol has been used as a prophylactic [10].

References

1. Arena JE, Rabinstein AA. Transient global amnesia. Mayo clinic proceedings 2015 90 2, pp. 264–272). Elsevier.
2. Torres JR, de Andrade Chemim E, Macari AR, Farneda LP, Iachinski RE. Amnésia Global Transitória: Uma Revisão De Literatura. Revista Thêma et. Scientia. 2016;6(1E)
3. Buratti L, Petrelli C, Potente E, Plutino A, Viticchi G, Falsetti L, Provinciali L, Silvestrini M. Prevalence of obstructive sleep apnea syndrome in a population of patients with transient global amnesia. Sleep Medicine. 2017;32:36–9.
4. Larner AJ. Transient global amnesia: model, mechanism, hypothesis. Cortex. 2022;149:137–47.

5. Döhring J, Schmuck A, Bartsch T. Stress-related factors in the emergence of transient global amnesia with hippocampal lesions. Frontiers in behavioral neuroscience. 2014;8:287.
6. Ogawa K, Suzuki Y, Akimoto T, Shiobara K, Hara M, Morita A, Kamei S, Soma M. Relationship between cytotoxicity in the hippocampus and an abnormal high intensity area on the diffusion-weighted images of three patients with transient global amnesia. Internal Medicine. 2018;57(18):2631–9.
7. Sander D, Winbeck K, Etgen T, Knapp R, Klingelhöfer J, Conrad B. Disturbance of venous flow patterns in patients with transient global amnesia. The Lancet. 2000;356(9246):1982–4.
8. Peer M, Nitzan M, Goldberg I, Katz J, Gomori JM, Ben-Hur T, Arzy S. Reversible functional connectivity disturbances during transient global amnesia. Annals of neurology. 2014;75(5):634–43.
9. Lorch MP. Multiple languages, memory, and regression: an examination of Ribot's Law. Aphasiology. 2009;23(5):643–54.
10. Berlit P. Successful prophylaxis of recurrent transient global amnesia with metoprolol. Neurology. 2000;55(12):1937–8.

49 Headache and Seizures in a Previously Healthy Female: The Skeptical Husband

Grade Easy.

Abstract An adult female with no previous comorbidities presenting with subacute onset headache, followed by seizures.

Story Mario is upset with his wife Suchitra. She has been complaining of a headache for a month now, and he thinks she is making up these complaints because their family doctor did not find anything abnormal when he examined her.

"You have to do something productive with your time," he tells her.

"It is just boredom which is causing this long list of imaginary ailments."

"I'm not making it up!" Suchitra says in tears. "I'm not!"

"Stop watching those depressing soap operas on television, then you'll be fine," he says, leaving her angry and frustrated.

Mario notices Suchitra has become quiet and dull after this incident—she no longer seems interested in his "exciting" stories of life as a used car salesman. He tells himself she is sulking, that she'll get over it soon and gets on with his work and his life.

He is quite shocked and terrified, therefore, when in the midst of a quiet dinner at home, Suchitra falls off the chair with a loud cry and starts convulsing. He weeps quietly during the ambulance ride to the hospital, berating himself for not taking Suchitra's complaints seriously.

You are on duty in the emergency department when they are brought in. You do a quick examination and note that her pupils are 3 mm and sluggishly reactive (fundus examination revealed blurring of the disc margins). There are no lateralizing signs, no neck stiffness. B/L plantar is upgoing.

You start the patient on a levetiracetam infusion and order an urgent MRI brain.

In the meanwhile, you try to find out more from Mario.

"Has she had any past history of fits?"

S. Bhat, *Clinical Conundrums to Practice Diagnostic Reasoning*,
https://doi.org/10.1007/978-981-95-0636-1_49

"No, doctor. She's been having a headache the last month, but I didn't take it that seriously. I did take her to a clinic and got her eyes checked. The doctor there advised a CT scan of the brain. Everything was normal then. The blood pressure was normal. I really didn't neglect her health," he says tearfully.

"I'm sure you didn't," you say reassuringly.

"I need to ask you a couple of questions."

"Yes, doctor?"

"Has she been on any regular medications for diabetes or hypertension or anything?"

"No, she's been very healthy so far. She just takes calcium, vitamins, oral contraceptives."

"Noted. Does she consume alcohol on a regular basis? Or any recreational drugs?"

"No!" says Mario, quite shocked. "Nothing like that."

By then, the radiologist calls with the preliminary MRI report.

Questions What do you think was Suchitra's diagnosis? How would you manage her?

Analysis

The clues are as follows:

(a) Adult female on oral contraceptives.
(b) Subacute headache.
(c) Apathy.
(d) Seizures.
(e) No lateralizing signs on examination.
New onset of headache, followed by seizures in a patient with risk factors for hypercoagulability (viz. oral contraceptives) should prompt one to consider the possibility of cerebral venous thrombosis (CVT).

Cerebral venous thrombosis may be classified into [1].

(a) Acute: Less than 48 h.
(b) Subacute: 48 h to 30 days.
(c) Chronic: Greater than 1 month.

Etiopathogenesis [2, 3]

The risk factors for CVT are indicated in Fig. 49.1.

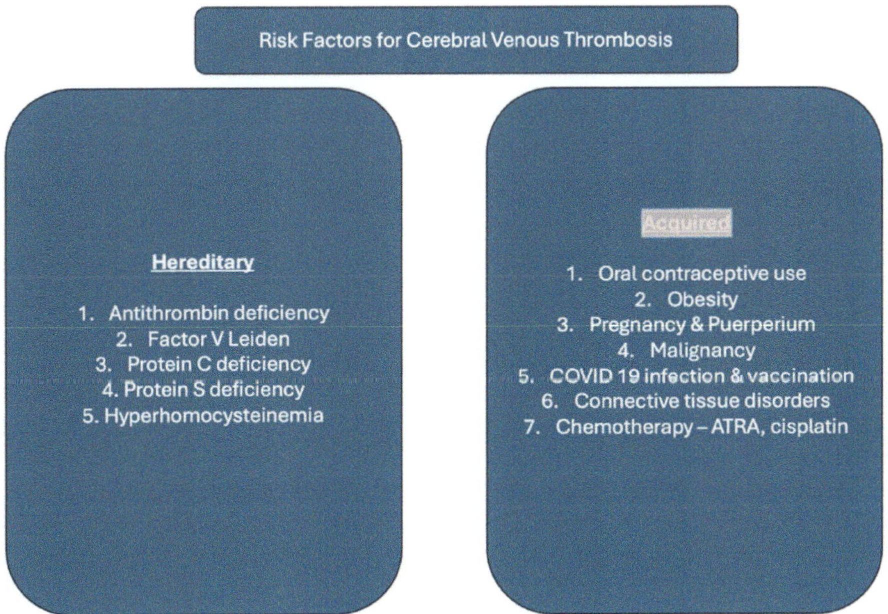

Fig. 49.1 Risk factors for cerebral venous thrombosis

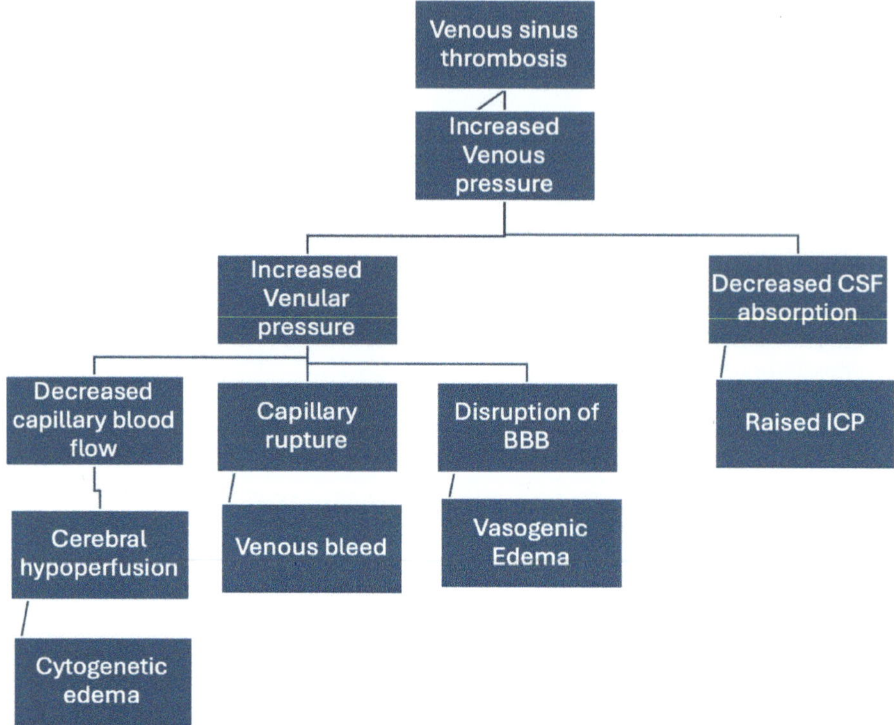

Fig. 49.2 Pathophysiology of CVT

Pathophysiology The cerebral veins lack valves, and crucial to the pathophysiology, the sagittal sinus also drains CSF from the subarachnoid space. The increased venous pressure results in the signs and symptoms of CVT (Fig. 49.2).

Clinical Features

1. Headache: Localized or diffuse, worse while lying down.
2. Blurring of vision.
3. Seizures: Focal or generalized; the patient may present in status epilepticus.
4. Altered responsiveness, apathy, delirium.
5. Motor weakness.
6. Aphasia.

The most common cause of death in CVT is transtentorial herniation [4].

Investigations [5]: The sensitivity of noncontrast CT in the diagnosis of CVT is variable and may be as low as 40% [6]. MRI with MR venography and contrast CT venogram are more sensitive (Fig. 49.3).

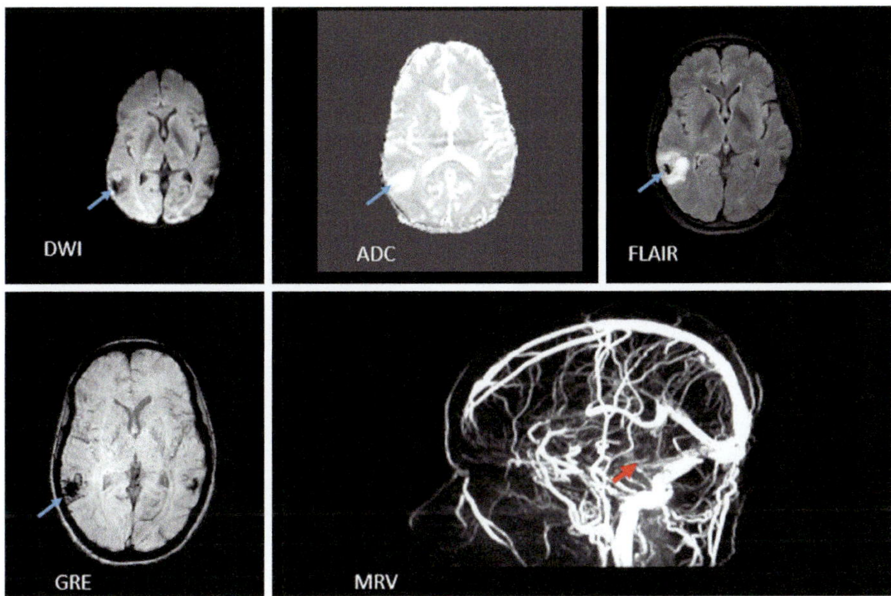

MRI Brain(various sequences as labelled)- Showing a venous infarct in the right temporal lobe (Blue arrow). MRV showing a thrombosed vein of Labbe (Red arrow)

Fig. 49.3 MRI brain showing venous infarct in the right temporal lobe (Image contributed by Dr. Vimala Colaco, neurologist, FMMC)

Thrombophilia workup may be required when no obvious risk factor for CVT is found.

Differential Diagnosis

1. Subarachnoid hemorrhage.
2. Intracerebral hemorrhage.
3. Meningitis and encephalitis.
4. PRES—Posterior reversible encephalopathy syndrome (PRES).
5. RCVS—Reversible cerebral vasoconstriction syndrome.
6. In pregnant women, eclampsia must be considered as a cause for new onset seizures.

Treatment [7]

1. Anticoagulation with either unfractionated or low-molecular-weight heparin initially, followed by warfarin or direct oral anticoagulant for the next 3–12 months.
2. Seizure prophylaxis.

3. Endovascular thrombectomy may be considered if there is evidence of the thrombus propagating, despite adequate anticoagulation.
4. Anti-edema measures: Decompressive surgery including hemicraniectomy may be required as a life-saving procedure.

Key Takeaway

In any patient with or without risk factors presenting with new onset headache with seizures and a focal neurological deficit not coinciding with a vascular territory, consider CVT and order neuroimaging on an emergency basis.

References

1. Idiculla PS, Gurala D, Palanisamy M, Vijayakumar R, Dhandapani S, Nagarajan E. Cerebral venous thrombosis: a comprehensive review. Eur Neurol. 2020;83(4):369–79.
2. Martinelli I, Sacchi E, Landi G, Taioli E, Duca F, Mannucci PM. High risk of cerebral-vein thrombosis in carriers of a prothrombin-gene mutation and in users of oral contraceptives. N Engl J Med. 1998;338(25):1793–7.
3. Ropper AH, Klein JP. Cerebral venous thrombosis. N Engl J Med. 2021;385(1):59–64.
4. Canhão P, Ferro JM, Lindgren AG, Bousser MG, Stam J, Barinagarrementeria F. Causes and predictors of death in cerebral venous thrombosis. Stroke. 2005;36(8):1720–5.
5. Saposnik G, Barinagarrementeria F, Brown RD Jr, Bushnell CD, Cucchiara B, Cushman M, Deveber G, Ferro JM, Tsai FY. Diagnosis and management of cerebral venous thrombosis: a statement for healthcare professionals from the American Heart Association/American Stroke Association. Stroke. 2011;42(4):1158–92.
6. Linn J, Pfefferkorn T, Ivanicova K, Müller-Schunk S, Hartz S, Wiesmann M, Dichgans M, Brückmann H. Noncontrast CT in deep cerebral venous thrombosis and sinus thrombosis: comparison of its diagnostic value for both entities. Am J Neuroradiol. 2009;30(4):728–35.
7. Ferro JM, Aguiar de Sousa D. Cerebral venous thrombosis: an update. Curr Neurol Neurosci Rep. 2019;19:1–9.

50 Complicated Course of an Adult Patient Admitted with Hiccup, Vomiting, and Altered Sensorium: Pass the Salt Please

Grade Easy.

Abstract An elderly male patient admitted with altered sensorium and vomiting, diagnosed to have hyponatremia, perhaps due to SIADH. Hospital stay is prolonged due to complications.

Story Mr George is a 70-year-old male, a known case of hypertension on cilnidipine 10 mg twice a day. He is also on atorvastatin for his dyslipidemia. Citalopram has been prescribed by his psychiatrist 15 days ago. He was apparently well on these drugs until 5 days prior, when his wife noticed that he looked a little switched off, tired, and confused. She passed it off as fatigue due to the summer heat, but George got worse, rather than better, and she brings him to your hospital emergency department.

After obtaining the history from the wife, you proceed with the examination. George vomits twice while you are with him. You note that he is conscious but confused, disoriented to time, place, and person. He is afebrile. The neck is supple, and there are no focal neurological deficits.

- Pulse: 88/min
- BP: 130/80 mm Hg

The tongue is moist, and the cardiovascular, abdomen, and respiratory systems appear normal.

Labs are as follows:

1. Blood sugar: 96 mg%
2. Sodium: 110 mEq/L
3. S. osmolality: 268 mOsm/kg

S. Bhat, *Clinical Conundrums to Practice Diagnostic Reasoning*,
https://doi.org/10.1007/978-981-95-0636-1_50

4. Urine osmolality: 200 mOsm/kg
5. S creatinine, thyroid function, and cortisol: Normal

You diagnose SIADH causing hyponatremia and commence correction as per formula. You are gratified when, later in the day, you call your colleague in the ICU and hear that Mr George is slightly better. Vomiting has ceased, and he is able to recognize and greet his wife.

His labs are better too—the sodium is now 122 mEq/L.

The next day, you visit the ward to check in on George's progress. His wife, sitting by him, looks a little worried.

"How are things?" you enquire.

"I'm a little puzzled, doctor. He has gone down a lot since yesterday."

"Really? in what way?"

"Well, I tried to feed him, and he couldn't swallow—he started coughing. And his speech seems odd."

"Mr George, good morning. How are you?" you ask, gently shaking him.

He looks confused and mumbles something that you cannot comprehend.

You quickly check for neurological deficits and find that there is weakness of all four limbs. Tendon reflexes are exaggerated, and the plantar is upgoing bilaterally.

Questions What do you think happened with George? Why was the initial improvement not maintained?

Analysis

This is a fairly straightforward case of

(a) Hyponatremia—euvolemic, hypo-osmolar—SIADH [1] perhaps secondary to the antidepressants
(b) Too rapid correction of hyponatremia resulting in osmotic demyelination

Osmotic demyelination or central pontine myelinolysis is the consequence of overly rapid correction of hyponatremia on the nervous system [2]

Etiopathogenesis

Brain adaptation to hyponatremia occurs within 48 h, and hyponatremia that occurs over the course of 2–3 days is less likely to cause cerebral edema, tentorial herniation, and seizures [3]

During rapid correction of chronic hyponatremia, water moves extracellularly to maintain similar osmolarities intracellularly and extracellularly. This results in rapid cell shrinkage which in turn causes axonal shear injury, apoptosis of astroglial cells, and disruption of the blood brain barrier [4].

Clinical Features [5]

1. Paraparesis and quadriparesis [6]
2. Dysarthria and dysphagia
3. Ataxia
4. Mutism, agitated delirium, and catatonia [7]
5. Parkinsonism, dystonia, and tremor [8]
6. Encephalopathy "Locked-in" syndrome, coma, and seizures
7. Impairment in short-term memory
8. Deficits in attention span

Risk Factors [9]

- Alcohol abuse
- Malnutrition
- Hypokalemia
- Hypophosphatemia

Investigations

Urgent MRI is the investigation of choice; however, it may take 1–4 weeks for MRI to show findings. Diffusion-weighted imaging is more sensitive.

Approach to Hyponatremia (Fig. 50.1)

Hyponatremia is defined as serum sodium less than 135 mEq/L and is most commonly due to impaired water excretion [10].

History

1. Diuretic use, antidepressants
2. Volume loss—due to vomiting or loose stools
3. CCF
4. Detailed prescription review—diuretics, antidepressants, and anticonvulsants

Physical Examination: Look for [11]

1. Orthostatic hypotension
2. Low jugular venous pressure
3. Decreased skin turgor
4. Signs of fluid overload—pedal edema, ascites
5. Thyroid swelling, bradycardia, nonpitting edema, skin and mucosal hyperpigmentation (suggestive of hypoadrenalism)

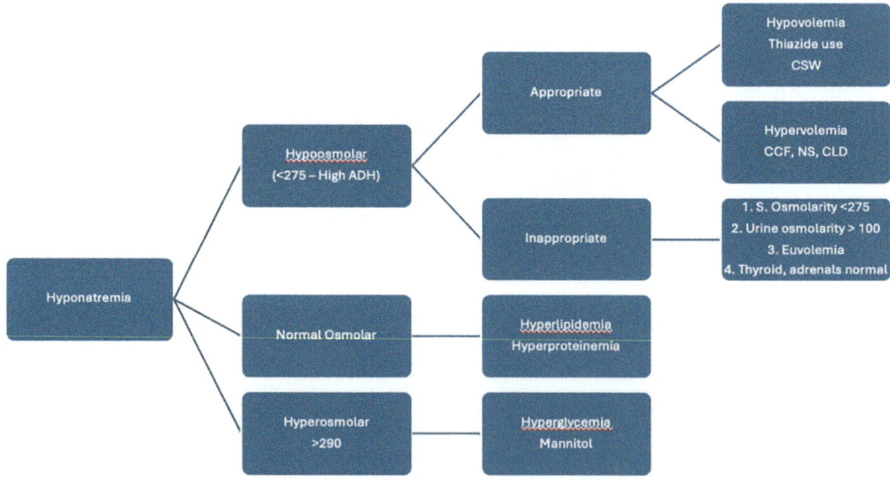

Fig. 50.1 Approach to hyponatremia

Investigations [12]

1. Serum sodium, potassium, blood urea, serum creatinine, and serum osmolarity
2. Urine sodium and urine osmolarity

Management [13]

1. Asymptomatic hyponatremia—If hypovolemic, administer saline.
   If fluid overloaded, restrict fluids.
   If it is a case of stable SIADH and the hyponatremia is asymptomatic, correct initially by fluid restriction.
   (Urine sodium+urine potassium)/serum sodium
   (a) If < 0.5, restrict to 1 L/day
   (b) If 0.5–1—500 mL/day
   (c) If > 1, give high solute load or tolvaptan
2. In symptomatic hyponatremia
   First, calculate the delta Na+ per liter fluid infused
   ◆Delta sodium = (sodium (i) + potassium (i))—Na (s))/TBW +1
   Now, divide the desired rate of correction per hour by the delta sodium.

Correction of Hyponatremia [14]

Though a correction of serum sodium in patients with chronic hyponatremia of 8–12 mEq/L is acceptable, even this amount may result in ODS in patients with the aforementioned risk factors.

It is important to realize that in situations where the stimulus of vasopressin release is removed, there is autocorrection of hyponatremia by secretion of a dilute urine. If exogenous 3% saline is being administered (even at the calculated correct rate), autocorrection plus exogenous saline results in an overly rapid correction of serum sodium and possible ODS.

Autocorrection can occur in the following situations:

(a) Correction of volume deficit
(b) Cessation of drug causing SIADH—SSRIs and carbamazepine
(c) Cessation of thiazide diuretics
(d) Administration of corticosteroids in patients with hypoadrenalism

Key Takeaway

Though hyponatremia may be dangerous, correction of hyponatremia may be more so. Therefore, increase serum sodium levels cautiously, slowly, and with frequent monitoring.

In patients who show a rapidly rising serum sodium, 5% dextrose (6 mL/kg body weight over 2 h) or desmopressin may be administered to mitigate the risk of ODS.

Glossary

ADH Antidiuretic hormone
CCF Congestive cardiac failure
CLD Chronic liver disease
NS Nephrotic syndrome
CSW Cerebral salt wasting

References

1. Adrogué HJ, Madias NE. The syndrome of inappropriate antidiuresis. N Engl J Med. 2023;389(16):1499–509.
2. Sterns RH, Rondon-Berrios H, Adrogue HJ, Berl T, Burst V, Cohen DM, Christ-Crain M, Cuesta M, Decaux G, Emmett M, Garrahy A. Treatment guidelines for hyponatremia: stay the course. Clin J Am Soc Nephrol. 2024;19(1):129–35.
3. Gankam KF. Adaptation of the brain to hyponatremia and its clinical implications. J Clin Med. 2023;12(5):1714.
4. Gankam-Kengne F, Couturier BS, Soupart A, Brion JP, Decaux G. Osmotic stress–induced defective glial proteostasis contributes to brain demyelination after hyponatremia treatment. J Am Soc Nephrol. 2017;28(6):1802.
5. King JD, Rosner MH. Osmotic demyelination syndrome. Am J Med Sci. 2010;339(6):561–7.
6. Fitts W, Vogel AC, Mateen FJ. The changing face of osmotic demyelination syndrome. Neurol Clin Pract. 2021;11(4):304–10.
7. Argitis P, Karampas A, Peyioti M, Goudeli A, Karavia S, Chaviaras Z. Osmotic demyelination syndrome (ODS), and psychiatric manifestations. Eur Psychiatry. 2024;67(S1):S479–80.
8. de Souza A. Movement disorders and the osmotic demyelination syndrome. Parkinsonism Relat Disord. 2013;19(8):709–16.
9. Ambati R, Kho LK, Prentice D, Thompson A. Osmotic demyelination syndrome: novel risk factors and proposed pathophysiology. Intern Med J. 2023;53(7):1154–62.
10. Adrogué HJ, Madias NE. Hyponatremia. N Engl J Med. 2000;342(21):1581–9.
11. Chung HM, Kluge R, Schrier RW, Anderson RJ. Clinical assessment of extracellular fluid volume in hyponatremia. Am J Med. 1987;83(5):905–8.
12. Barhaghi K, Molchanova-Cook O, Rosenberg M, Deal B, Palacios E, Nguyen J, et al. Osmotic demyelination syndrome revisited: review with neuroimaging. J La State Med Soc. 2017;169:89–93.
13. Adrogué HJ, Madias NE. The challenge of hyponatremia. J Am Soc Nephrol. 2012;23(7):1140–8.
14. Adrogué HJ, Madias NE. Diagnosis and treatment of hyponatremia. Am J Kidney Dis. 2014;64(5):681–4.

Part II

Call the Lab

Monitoring Glycemic Status in Patients with End-Stage Renal Disease

51

Abstract A patient with uncontrolled diabetes and renal insufficiency on maintenance hemodialysis has unexpectedly low glycated hemoglobin, though fasting and postprandial sugars are high.

NH, a 65-year-old male is a known case of diabetes and hypertension for 25 years. He was diagnosed to have chronic kidney disease 8 years ago. Maintenance hemodialysis was initiated 2 years ago.

He is referred to your clinic for diabetes management.

His prescription is as follows:

(a) T. Nifedipine retard 10 mg thrice a day
(b) T. Linagliptin 5 mg BD
(c) T. Clonidine 100 microgram thrice a day
(d) Inj. Human insulin 10 units 8th hourly
(e) Inj. Levemir 10 units in the evening
(f) T. Calcium + Vit D3 500 mg twice a day
(g) Inj. Erythropoietin 6000 iu subcutaneously thrice a week

These are his recent lab values:

- FBG: 148 mg %; PPBG: 200 mg %; HbA1C: 6.5

How would you explain the apparent discrepancy between blood glucose levels and HbA1C? How would you address this issue?

Answer Erythropoietin affects HbA1C levels, making them unreliable markers of glycemic status in patients with diabetes [1].

S. Bhat, *Clinical Conundrums to Practice Diagnostic Reasoning*,
https://doi.org/10.1007/978-981-95-0636-1_51

HbA1C is formed by nonenzymatic glycation of hemoglobin. The process of glycation of hemoglobin is irreversible and lasts for the lifespan of the RBC, that is, 120 days. Hence, Hba1C is a marker of glycemic status for the previous 4 months. Erythropoietin stimulates red blood cell production, leading to increased turnover and shortened lifespan [2]. This results in a falsely low HbA1c, potentially misleading the clinician about the glycemic status.

Thus, alternative markers of glycemia such as glycated albumin [3], fructosamine, and continuous glucose monitoring may be used.

References

1. Brown JN, Kemp DW, Brice KR. Class effect of erythropoietin therapy on hemoglobin A1c in a patient with diabetes mellitus and chronic kidney disease not undergoing hemodialysis. Pharmacother: J Human Pharmacol Drug Ther. 2009;29(4):468–72.
2. Jelkmann W. Physiology and pharmacology of erythropoietin. Transfus Med Hemother. 2013;40(5):302–9.
3. Inaba M, Okuno S, Kumeda Y, Yamada S, Imanishi Y, Tabata T, Okamura M, Okada S, Yamakawa T, Ishimura E, Nishizawa Y. Glycated albumin is a better glycemic indicator than glycated hemoglobin values in hemodialysis patients with diabetes: effect of anemia and erythropoietin injection. J Am Soc Nephrol. 2007;18(3):896–903.

High Creatinine and Very High Urea: The Risk of Roadside Munchies

52

Abstract A previously heathy female has impaired renal function with disproportionately elevated urea after an attack of gastroenteritis.

Your secretary peeps into your cabin and says "Doc, are you free for a moment?"
"Sure, Babita. What can I do for you?"

"My friend's mother had a bit of a tummy upset—loose motions and puking—after eating some snacks at a dodgy roadside vendor. She got some blood tests done and she's worried that the results look like kidney failure. Can you have a look at the reports?"

"Certainly."

These are the reports:

- Blood urea: 85 mg/dL (Normal: 7–20 mg/dL)
- Serum creatinine: 2.1 mg/dL (Normal: 0.6–1.2 mg/dL)
- Serum sodium: 148 mg/dL (Normal: 135–145 mg/dL)
- Serum potassium: 5 mg/dL (Normal: 3.5–5.0 mg/dL)
- Serum chloride: 110 mg/dL (Normal: 96–106 mg/dL)
- BUN/creatinine ratio: 40:1

What do these lab results indicate? What is the pathophysiological basis? What management would you advise?

Answer The combination of elevated serum creatinine with disproportionately elevated blood urea in the background of a "tummy upset"—loose stools and vomiting—indicates volume loss.

S. Bhat, *Clinical Conundrums to Practice Diagnostic Reasoning*,
https://doi.org/10.1007/978-981-95-0636-1_52

Pathophysiological Basis

Both urea and creatinine are filtered in the glomerulus, but 40–50% of urea is reabsorbed in the tubule, parallel to the reabsorption of sodium and water [1]. Hence, the normal ratio of blood urea to creatinine (UCR) is up to 10:1. However, in hypovolemia, activation of the Renin Angiotensin System causes avid salt and water reabsorption, and urea is passively reabsorbed. The elevation in urea increases the UCR, sometimes greater than 20:1.

Indicators of Hypovolemia

Clinical

1. Thirst, fatigue, muscle cramps, decreased urine output, and postural symptoms like dizziness
2. Dry tongue, decreased skin turgor, narrow pulse pressure, postural hypotension, and decreased jugular venous pressure

Laboratory

1. Increased UCR
2. Increased hematocrit (unless hypovolemia is due to blood loss)
3. Decreased urinary sodium (< 20 mEq/L) unless hypovolemia is due to diuretic use or if the hypovolemia is accompanied by metabolic alkalosis

Other Causes of Elevated UCR [2]

1. Steroid use (due to increased urea production)
2. GI blood loss (apart from hypovolemia, due to catabolism of blood products in the gut)
3. Low muscle mass—lowers serum creatinine
4. High protein intake

On the other hand, low UCR may be seen in [3]:

1. Low protein intake
2. Decompensated liver disease
3. Rhabdomyolysis

Management

1. Oral fluid replacement.
2. Intravenous fluids may be required in moderate hypovolemia in hospitalized patients. The amount that should be replaced is equal to the GI losses plus urine

output plus the insensible water loss (which is between 25 and 50 mL/h). One regime is to administer 50 mL/h greater than the estimated fluid loss.

Note

1. Elevated UCR (>100) even in the absence of hypovolemia is independently associated with poor outcomes in patients with chronic kidney disease [4].
2. In the clinical setting described above, the elevated creatinine indicates that the hypovolemia was severe enough to decrease the glomerular filtration rate.

References

1. Matsue Y, et al. Blood urea nitrogen-to-creatinine ratio in the general population and in patients with acute heart failure. Google Search [Internet]. [cited 2025 Jan 12].
2. Uchino S, Bellomo R, Goldsmith D. The meaning of the blood urea nitrogen/creatinine ratio in acute kidney injury. Clin Kidney J. 2012;5(2):187–91.
3. Hosten AO. BUN and creatinine. In: Clinical methods: the history, physical, and laboratory examinations. 3rd ed. Boston: Butterworths; 1990.
4. Brookes EM, Power DA. Elevated serum urea-to-creatinine ratio is associated with adverse inpatient clinical outcomes in non-end stage chronic kidney disease. Sci Rep. 2022;12(1):20827.

53 Fatigue and Hiccup in an Elderly Lady: Weakness Is Not a Symptom of Normal Aging!

Abstract An elderly female, hypertensive, presents with hiccup and extreme fatigue.

Mrs. Sumitha Masceranhas is a 78-year-old woman with a long history of hypertension who presents with complaints of progressive weakness, fatigue, and persistent hiccups for the past 7 days. She mentions that she feels "more tired than usual" and has had difficulty completing her daily activities. The hiccups began intermittently but have become more frequent and bothersome, particularly in the evening.

Her past medical history includes hypertension, osteoarthritis, and glaucoma. She is on paracetamol for joint pain and timolol eye drops.

She appears fatigued.

Vitals

- BP: 128/76 mmHg
- HR: 88 bpm
- RR: 16/min
- Temperature: 36.8 °C

Neurological examination reveals mild confusion and slight muscle weakness, more pronounced in the lower extremities.

S. Bhat, *Clinical Conundrums to Practice Diagnostic Reasoning*, https://doi.org/10.1007/978-981-95-0636-1_53

Lab Values

- Hb: 12. 8 gm%; TC: 7200/mL; platelets: 245,000/mL
- Sodium: 118 mEq/L; potassium: 3.2 mEq/l; chloride: mEq/L; bicarbonate: 26 mEq/L
- BUN: 18 mg%; s. creat: 0.9 mg %
- Serum osmolality: 245 mOsm/kg
- Urine osmolarity: 520 mOsm/kg
- Urine sodium: 95 mEq/L

Questions What might be the cause of Mrs. Masceranhas' hyponatremia? Is there any other factor contributing to her weakness?

Answer The labs indicate a hypo-osmolar hyponatremia with inappropriately high urine osmolarity and natriuresis. It appears that Mrs. Masceranhas was on thiazide diuretics for her hypertension and has developed thiazide-induced hyponatremia.

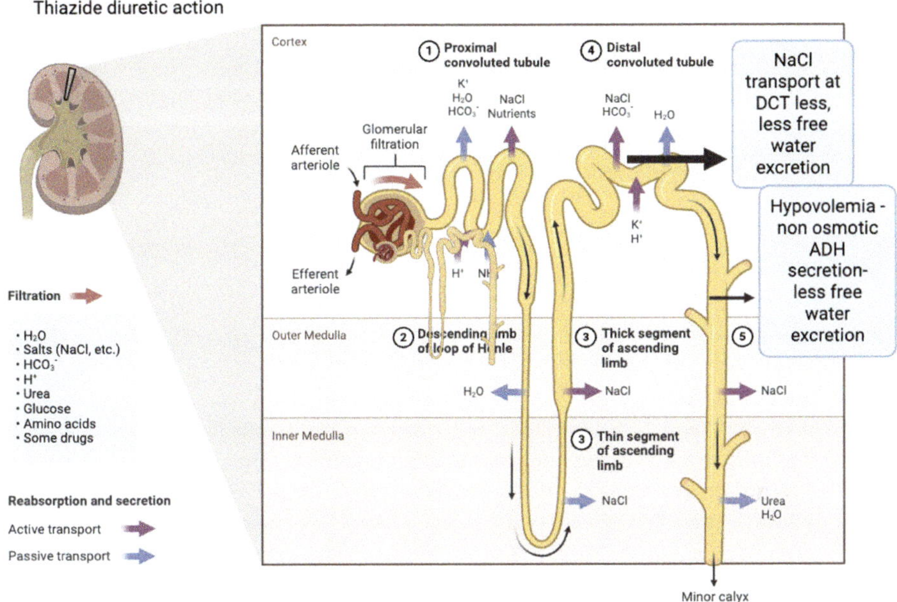

Fig. 53.1 Mechanism of thiazide-induced hyponatremia. (Created in BioRender. Bhat (2025) https://BioRender.com/k551t9v)

Pathophysiology [1] (Fig. 53.1)

1. Impaired diluting capacity: Hydrochlorothiazide inhibits the Na+/Cl– cotransporter in the distal convoluted tubule, reducing the kidney's ability to produce dilute urine. This occurs because:
   - With decreased NaCl reabsorption in the DCT, less free water clearance occurs.
   - The tubular fluid reaching the collecting duct is less dilute than normal.
   - Even with normal ADH suppression, the kidneys cannot excrete maximally dilute urine.
2. Volume depletion and ADH stimulation: Thiazide diuretics cause mild volume depletion, which:
   - Activates baroreceptors.
   - Stimulates ADH release despite hyponatremia.
   - Promotes water reabsorption at the collecting ducts.
   - This nonosmotic ADH release overrides the normal osmotic regulation of ADH.
3. Potential age-related factors:
   - Decreased renal function with aging (her eGFR is at the lower limit of normal)
   - Decreased thirst regulation
   - Higher sensitivity to medication effects

Thiazides increase the risk for hospitalization due to hyponatremia [2].

Risk Factors [3]

(a) Female gender
(b) Frailty
(c) Age
(d) Concomitant use of spironolactone [4].

Management [5]

1. Discontinue hydrochlorothiazide
2. Fluid restriction to 800–1000 mL/day
3. Sodium correction:
   - Given symptomatic hyponatremia (confusion, weakness):
     - Administer 3% hypertonic saline at a controlled rate.
     - Target correction rate of 6–8 mEq/L in the first 24 h to avoid osmotic demyelination.
     - Initial correction of 1–2 mEq/L in first 1–2 h to address neurological symptoms.
     - Frequent monitoring of serum sodium (every 2–4 h initially).
4. Potassium replacement:
   - Potassium chloride supplementation to address hypokalemia.
   - Correcting hypokalemia will help with sodium correction by reducing intracellular sodium shift.

Key Takeaway
It should be noted that elderly females are at a high risk for thiazide-induced hyponatremia, and hence this class of drugs must be prescribed with caution in them.

References

1. Kim GH. Pathophysiology of drug-induced hyponatremia. J Clin Med. 2022;11(19):5810.
2. Mannheimer B, Bergh CF, Falhammar H, Calissendorff J, Skov J, Lindh JD. Association between newly initiated thiazide diuretics and hospitalization due to hyponatremia. Eur J Clin Pharmacol. 2021;77:1049–55.
3. Chow KM, Szeto CC, Wong TH, Leung CB, Li PT. Risk factors for thiazide-induced hyponatraemia. QJM. 2003;96(12):911–7.
4. Kwon S, Kim H, Lee J, Shin J, Kim SH, Hwang JH. Thiazide-associated hyponatremia in arterial hypertension patients: a nationwide population-based cohort study. J Evid Based Med. 2024;17(2):296–306.
5. Adrogué HJ, Tucker BM, Madias NE. Diagnosis and management of hyponatremia: a review. JAMA. 2022;328(3):280–91.

Patient on Regular MHD Presents with Carpopedal Spasm: Post-Holiday Blues

54

Grade Easy.

Abstract An elderly female with diabetes, hypertension, osteoporosis, and chronic kidney disease on maintenance hemodialysis presents with carpopedal spasm.

Story Mrs. Alka, an elderly female, a known case of Type 2 diabetes mellitus, hypertension, osteoporosis, and end-stage renal disease (ESRD) is on regular maintenance hemodialysis (MHD) twice a week at your hospital. You are in the ER when her son brings her to hospital with severe muscle cramps and spasming of the hands and feet 3 days after a family trip.

"I'm afraid I'm a little to blame, doctor. I insisted that Mama accompany me on the trip to Pondicherry. I thought that she could undergo dialysis at a centre there. In fact, I had even arranged for it, but an epidemic of leptospirosis in the area meant that slots were not available. Actually, she has missed dialysis off and on in the past, and there have been no problems at all. "

"Ok, let me examine her. In the meanwhile, can you help me with her present drug chart current medications?"

"Sure doctor, right now she is on

- Insulin glargine
- Amlodipine
- Sevelamer
- Calcitriol 0.25 mcg daily
- Calcium carbonate 1500 mg TID with meals

S. Bhat, *Clinical Conundrums to Practice Diagnostic Reasoning*,
https://doi.org/10.1007/978-981-95-0636-1_54

Also, she received her first dose of denosumab 60 mg subcutaneously for osteoporosis treatment 10 days ago."

"OK, noted."

You examine Mrs. Alka and find that her blood pressure is 160/100 mm Hg, HR 92 bpm, RR 18/min, Temp 36.8 °C. She goes into carpal spasm when the BP is being measured. Chvostek's sign is positive.

Questions What do you think is responsible for Mrs. Alka's symptoms? Does the recent addition of denosumab have anything to do with her presentation?

Analysis

This is a fairly straightforward case of denosumab-induced hypocalcemia in a patient on dialysis.

Diagnosis

Severe hypocalcemia secondary to denosumab administration in a dialysis-dependent patient.

These are Mrs. Alka's lab reports:

1. S. calcium: 6 mg %
2. S. phosphorus: 5.5 mg %
3. S. PTH: 650 pG/mL
4. S. Mg++: 1.2 mg%
5. S. albumin: 3.2 G/L

Pathophysiology

Denosumab is a human monoclonal antibody that binds to RANKL (Receptor Activator of Nuclear Factor κB Ligand), preventing its interaction with RANK on osteoclast precursors [1]. This inhibition blocks osteoclast formation, function, and survival, thereby reducing bone resorption. Hence, the normal osteoclast-induced resorption and release of calcium into the circulation that occurs as a response to hypocalcemia is abolished.

Other factors that are contributing to hypocalcemia [2] in Mrs. Alka are:

1. Baseline-disrupted calcium homeostasis: ESRD patients already have impaired vitamin D activation (due to reduced 1-α-hydroxylase activity in the kidneys), intestinal calcium absorption issues, and secondary hyperparathyroidism.
2. Compromised alternate compensatory pathways: ESRD patients cannot increase renal calcium reabsorption (a normal compensatory mechanism).
3. Precipitous calcium drop: The combination of blocked bone resorption, impaired intestinal absorption, and inability to reabsorb calcium leads to severe hypocalcemia.

Dialysis-dependent patients are vulnerable to denosumab-induced hypocalcemia for several reasons [3]:

1. Absent renal compensation
2. Pre-existing mineral bone disorder
3. Dialysis-related factors:

- Dialysate calcium concentration influences serum calcium.
- Missed dialysis sessions (as in this case) can exacerbate mineral imbalances.
- Dialysis regimens may not fully correct underlying mineral disorders.

4. Medication interactions: Common medications in ESRD (phosphate binders, calcitriol, and cinacalcet) affect calcium metabolism and may interact with denosumab's effects.
5. High-turnover bone disease: Many ESRD patients have high bone turnover due to secondary hyperparathyroidism. Denosumab's sudden blockade of this high-turnover state creates a more dramatic drop in serum calcium than in patients with normal bone turnover.
6. Nutritional factors: Dialysis patients often have poor appetite and dietary restrictions.

Management [4]

1. IV calcium gluconate: 1–2 ampules (10–20 mL of 10% solution) slow IV.
2. Urgent dialysis with high calcium bath: Utilizing dialysate with 3.5 mEq/L calcium concentration.
3. Oral calcium supplementation.
4. Calcitriol adjustment: Increase to 0.5–1 mcg daily to enhance intestinal calcium absorption.
5. Magnesium repletion: If hypomagnesemia is present, as it can impair PTH function and calcium homeostasis.
6. Close monitoring: Check calcium levels every 4–6 h initially until stable.

Safe Retreatment with Denosumab [5]

1. Pretreatment phase (2–4 weeks before administration):
   - Optimize serum calcium (target 9.0–9.5 mg/dL).
   - Ensure 25-OH vitamin D levels >30 ng/Ml.
   - Adjust calcitriol to 0.5–1.0 mcg daily.
   - Initiate prophylactic calcium carbonate 2000–3000 mg elemental calcium daily.
   - Ensure magnesium is in normal range.
2. Administration day:
   - Verify normal calcium, phosphorus, and magnesium levels.
   - Administer denosumab after a dialysis session.
   - Consider reduced dose (30 mg instead of 60 mg) for initial treatment.
   - Schedule next dialysis session within 48 h.
3. Post-administration monitoring:
   - Check calcium levels 3–4 days after administration.
   - Follow-up with twice-weekly calcium monitoring for 2 weeks.

  - Weekly monitoring for the next 2–4 weeks. Biweekly monitoring for 2–3 months.
4. Prophylaxis:
  - Continue high-dose calcium supplementation for 4–6 weeks.
  - Maintain higher calcitriol dose for 1–2 months.
  - Adjust dialysate calcium as needed based on serum levels.

Refractory hypocalcemia may be due to [6]

1. Hypomagnesemia
2. Hungry bone syndrome
3. Medication interactions: like bisphosphonates, anticonvulsants, or proton-pump inhibitors
4. Malnutrition and hypoalbuminemia
5. Citrate toxicity: citrate can bind calcium and worsen hypocalcemia

Key Takeaway

Patients with chronic kidney disease on MHD are more prone to develop hypocalcemia after densumab administration; this risk can be minimized by ensuring that patient is calcium-replete before administering densumab.

References

1. Hanley DA. Denosumab: mechanism of action and clinical outcomes. Int J Clin Pract. 2012. Wiley Online Library [Internet]. [cited 2025 Mar 30]. Available from: https://onlinelibrary.wiley.com/doi/full/10.1111/ijcp.12022.
2. Foley RN, Parfrey PS, Harrnett JD, Kent GM, Hu L, O'Dea R, et al. Hypocalcemia, morbidity, and mortality in end-stage renal disease. Am J Nephrol. 2008;16(5):386–93.
3. Bird ST, Smith ER, Gelperin K, Jung TH, Thompson A, Kambhampati R, et al. Severe Hypocalcemia with denosumab among older female dialysis-dependent patients. JAMA. 2024;331(6):491–9.
4. Pepe J, Colangelo L, Biamonte F, Sonato C, Danese VC, Cecchetti V, et al. Diagnosis and management of hypocalcemia. Endocrine. 2020;69(3):485–95.
5. Diab DL, Watts NB. The use of denosumab in osteoporosis—an update on efficacy and drug safety. Expert Opin Drug Saf. 2024;23(9):1069–77.
6. Humphrey E, Clardy C. A framework for approaching refractory hypocalcemia in children. Pediatr Ann. 2019;48(5):e208–11.

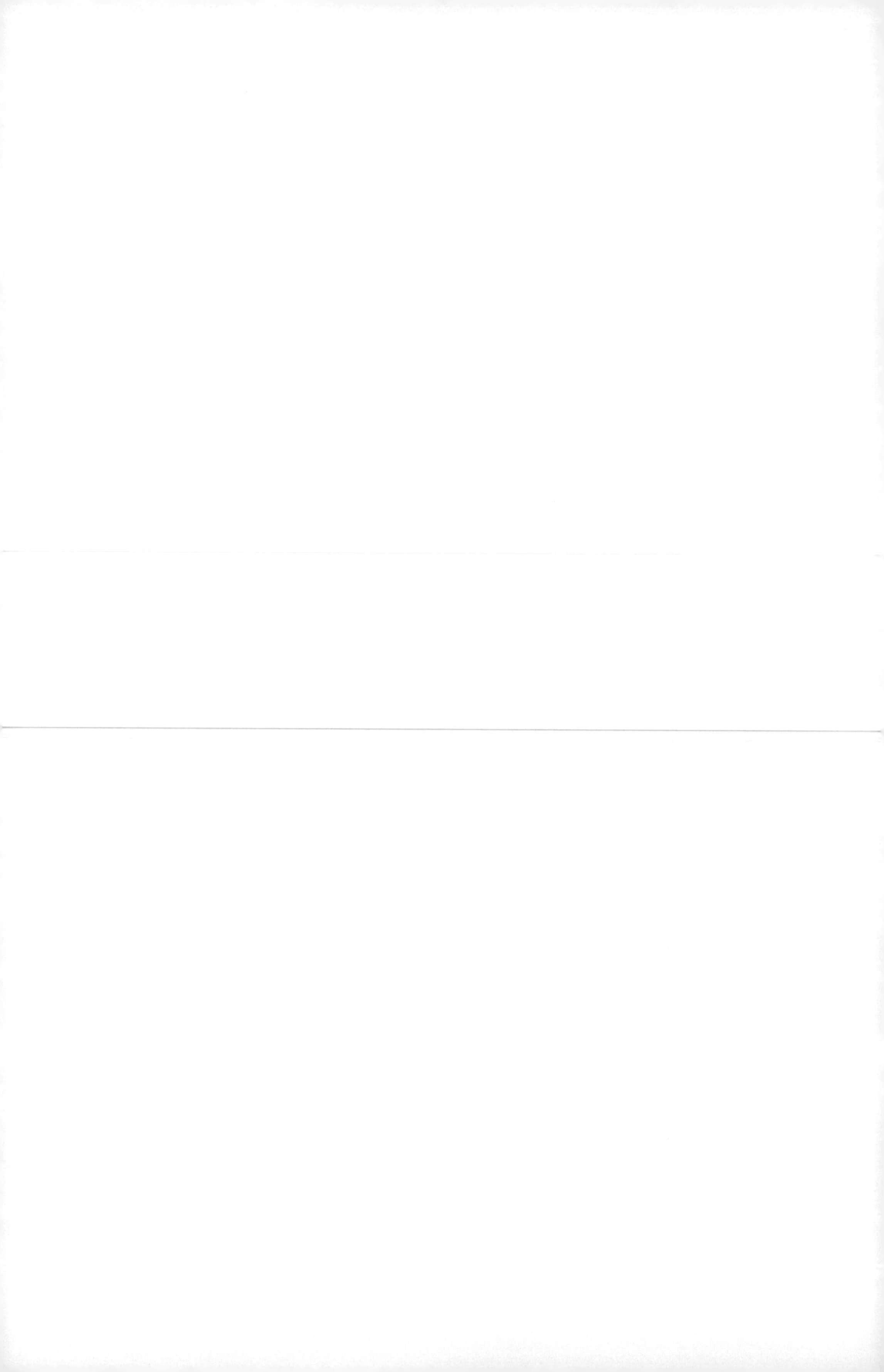

Fever, Body Ache, and Decreased Urine Output: The Flu that Wasn't a Flu

55

Abstract A young male immigrant worker presents with fever and myalgia and is provisionally diagnosed to have flu. However, he does not respond to supportive care.

Wesley, a 28-year-old software engineer from Mumbai, India, arrives in Vienna for a 3-month work assignment. One week after arrival, he develops high fever, severe muscle aches, and headache. He visits a local emergency department where doctors initially suspect influenza. They prescribe antipyretics, rest, and fluids. He returns to hospital after 2 days, looking much worse. He now complains of a decreased urine output, too.

On examination, he is febrile and appears to be in some pain. His conjunctiva are suffused, and there is a suspicion of icterus.

Lab reports are as follows:

Complete Blood Count
- WBC: 15,200/μL (4000–11,000/μL)
  - Neutrophils: 82%
  - Lymphocytes: 12%
  - Monocytes: 6%
- Hemoglobin: 14.2 g/dL (13.5–17.5 g/dL)
- Platelets: 52,000/μL (150,000–450,000/μL)

Renal Function
- Creatinine: 2.8 mg/dL (0.7–1.3 mg/dL)
- BUN: 48 mg/dL (7–20 mg/dL)

S. Bhat, *Clinical Conundrums to Practice Diagnostic Reasoning*, https://doi.org/10.1007/978-981-95-0636-1_55

Liver Function

- Total Bilirubin: 4.8 mg/dL (0.3–1.2 mg/dL)
- Direct Bilirubin: 3.2 mg/dL (0–0.3 mg/dL)
- AST: 82 U/L (5–40 U/L)
- ALT: 76 U/L (7–56 U/L)
- ALP: 185 U/L (45–115 U/L)

Questions

1. What might be wrong with Wesley? What additional laboratory test would you order to support your diagnosis, and what empiric treatment would you initiate while awaiting results?
2. Can you explain why the liver function tests show predominantly elevated bilirubin with only mild elevation of transaminases? How does this pattern differ from viral hepatitis?

Analysis

Lab reports may be summarized as follows:

(a) Thrombocytopenia (52,000/μL) with leucocytosis (15,200/μL)
(b) Renal involvement: Creatinine (2.8 mg/dL)—acute kidney injury
(c) Hepatic involvement: Predominantly conjugated hyperbilirubinemia (direct bilirubin 3.2 mg/dL) with relatively mild transaminitis

This pattern is characteristic of Weil's syndrome, the severe form of leptospirosis. [1]

This pattern occurs because:

- The primary hepatic injury is to the bile canaliculi, affecting bile transport.
- There is relatively less hepatocellular damage (hence lower transaminases).
- The mechanism involves bacterial proteins affecting membrane transport systems.

Diagnostic Confirmation [2]

- Microscopic agglutination test (MAT)—gold standard
- IgM ELISA for leptospirosis
- PCR testing of blood and urine
- Dark-field microscopy of urine
- Blood cultures in special media

Empiric treatment should begin immediately [3]:

- Intravenous penicillin G (4 million units every 6 h) or
- Ceftriaxone 2 g daily or
- Doxycycline 100 mg twice daily

Supportive Care

- Close monitoring of renal function
- Platelet transfusion if bleeding
- Fluid and electrolyte management
- Possible dialysis if severe renal failure

Key Takeaway

The characteristic lab picture of neutrophilic leucocytosis, thrombocytopenia, mild transaminitis, conjugated hyperbilirubinemia, and acute kidney injury in a patient presenting with fever and body ache should prompt one to suspect leptospirosis and commence treatment immediately.

References

1. Abdulkader RC, Seguro AC, Malheiro PS, Burdmann EA, Marcondes M. Peculiar electrolytic and hormonal abnormalities in acute renal failure due to leptospirosis. Am J Trop Med Hyg. 1996;54(1):1–6.
2. Pinto GV, Senthilkumar K, Rai P, Kabekkodu SP, Karunasagar I, Kumar BK. Current methods for the diagnosis of leptospirosis: issues and challenges. J Microbiol Methods. 2022;195:106438.
3. Suputtamongkol Y, Niwattayakul K, Suttinont C, Losuwanaluk K, Limpaiboon R, Chierakul W, Wuthiekanun V, Triengrim S, Chenchittikul M, White NJ. An open, randomized, controlled trial of penicillin, doxycycline, and cefotaxime for patients with severe leptospirosis. Clin Infect Dis. 2004;39(10):1417–24.

Young Lady with Possible Drug Overdose Admitted with High Anion Gap Metabolic Acidosis

56

Abstract A young female admitted with suspected poisoning, initially found to have alkalosis. This is followed after some hours by acidosis.

Case Scenario Devina is a 19-year-old college student studying art in a college. Her room-mate Alice walks in to find Devina lying on the bed looking ill. There is vomitus on the floor and a couple of empty pill bottles lying on the bed. "What have you done?!" asks Alice shaking Devina, but Devina is anxious and confused and unable to answer coherently. Alice calls an ambulance, and Devina is rushed to a nearby hospital.

You are the doctor in the emergency department, and you do a quick assessment of Devina. You note the vitals are as follows: respiratory rate: 28 breaths/min; heart rate: 120 beats/min; BP 130/85 mm Hg; SpO_2: 90% on room air.

The tongue is dry, and the patient appears agitated and diaphoretic. Devina has a bout of vomiting as you examine her, and you note that the vomitus is blood-streaked. Crackles are auscultated bilaterally.

- Glucometer RBS: 75 mg%
- Initial ABG: pH 7.60
- pCO_2: 20 mmHg
- HCO_3: 22 mEq/L
- Na: 135 mEq/L
- K: 5.8 mEq/L
- Cl: 98 mEq/L

6 hours later:

- pH: 7.32
- pCO_2: 32 mmHg
- HCO_3^-: 16 mEq/L

S. Bhat, *Clinical Conundrums to Practice Diagnostic Reasoning*,
https://doi.org/10.1007/978-981-95-0636-1_56

- Na^+: 140 mEq/L
- Cl^-: 98 mEq/L
- pO2: 95 mmHg
- Anion gap: 26

Question What toxicity are these ABGs suggestive of? What is the mechanism?

The combination of early respiratory alkalosis, followed by metabolic acidosis is suggestive of salicylate toxicity [1]:

- Early salicylate toxicity presents with respiratory alkalosis due to stimulation of the medullary respiratory center and tachypnea.
- Later in the course, salicylate toxicity shows predominant metabolic acidosis. Uncoupling of oxidative phosphorylation leads to lactate accumulation, and increased catabolism leads to keto acid accumulation, both together contributing to a high anion gap metabolic acidosis.

Pathogenesis [2] (Fig. 56.1)

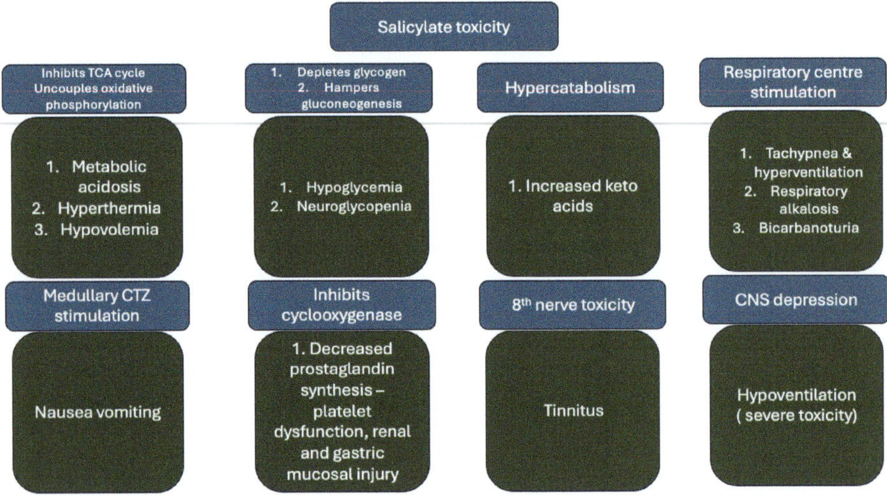

Fig. 56.1 Mechanisms and features of salicylate toxicity

Management

1. Airway, breathing, circulation
2. Decontamination with activated charcoal
3. IV fluids to achieve euvolemia
4. Monitoring of blood glucose and treatment of hypoglycemia
5. Serum and urine alkalinization [3]
6. Hemodialysis [4]

Key Points

1. Avoid endotracheal intubation.
2. Avoid mechanical ventilation unless absolutely necessary—respiratory alkalosis helps compensate for metabolic acidosis.
3. Mortality correlates with central nervous system rather than serum salicylate concentration.

References

1. Palmer BF, Clegg DJ. Salicylate toxicity. N Engl J Med. 2020;382(26):2544–55.
2. Temple AR. Pathophysiology of aspirin overdosage toxicity, with implications for management. Pediatrics. 1978;62(5s):873–6.
3. Flomenbaum N. Salicylates. In: Nelson L, Lewin NA, Howland MA, Hoffman RS, Goldfrank LR, Flomenbaum NE, editors. Goldfrank's toxicologic emergencies. 10th ed. New York: McGraw-Hill Medical Publishing Division; 2015.
4. Fertel BS, Nelson LS, Goldfarb DS. The underutilization of hemodialysis in patients with salicylate poisoning. Kidney Int. 2009;75(12):1349–53.

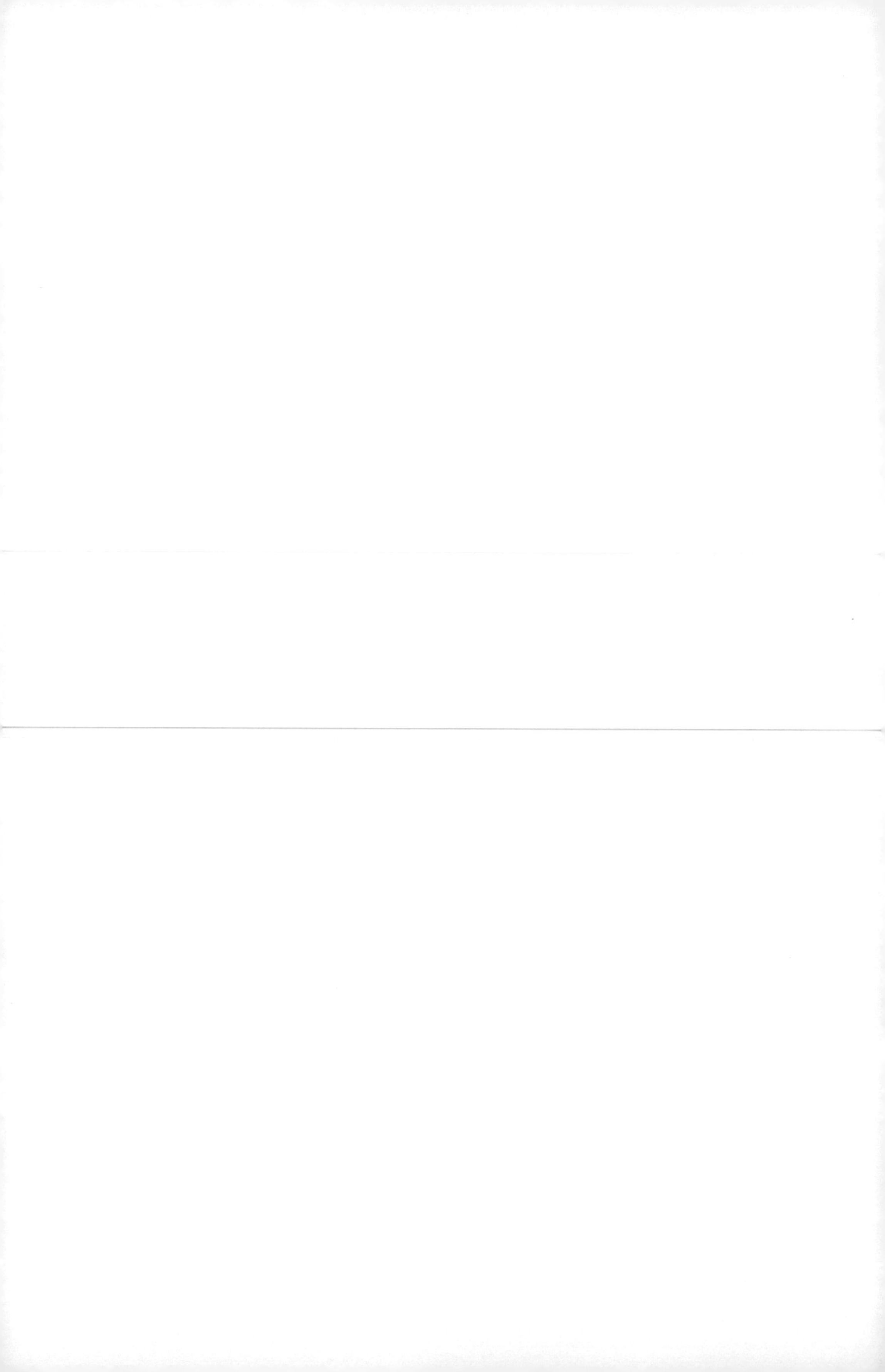

57 Sudden Deterioration in Malnourished Female When Given Nutritious Diet: The Peril of Good Intentions

Abstract A young malnourished female whose nutritional recovery course is complicated by edema and muscle ache.

Raakhee and Ramesh travel to Mumbai from their small village in Karnataka to visit their daughter Manaswini who is studying in a fashion design college. They are shocked when they see her. She looks like a shadow of her former self—she has become skinny and pale, and the dark circles under her eyes look painted on. She confesses that her weight is 30 kg which means that her 1.6 m frame looks like skin stuck on bones. Manaswini's parents insist on bringing her back home to rest and recuperate. Raakhee cooks hot, healthy meals bursting with nutrition and calories, and Ramesh has long talks with Manaswini every evening to find out what went wrong with his strictly brought up daughter that she has become like this.

Things are going ok, but on the third day at home, Manaswini complains of severe muscle ache and weakness. Her mum notes some swelling of her feet, and they take her to a local clinic immediately. There, the nurse practitioner examines her and orders some blood tests.

This is what she finds:

- Weight: 30 kg; height: 160 cm
- Heart rate: 98/min; BP: 100/60 mm Hg
- JVP: elevated;
- Pedal edema: +
- Hb: 9 gm%
- TC: 4000
- RBS: 78 mg%, sodium: 136 mEq/L, potassium: 3 mEq/L, Mg: 1.2 mEq/L, PO4: 2 mEq/L

S. Bhat, *Clinical Conundrums to Practice Diagnostic Reasoning*,
https://doi.org/10.1007/978-981-95-0636-1_57

- SGOT: 55
- SGPT: 58
- Bilirubin: 1.8 mg%

What is the diagnosis? How may it have been prevented?

Answer The characteristic combination of hypophosphatemia and volume overload in a malnourished adult who has been commenced on normal diet/replacement feeds is indicative of refeeding syndrome.

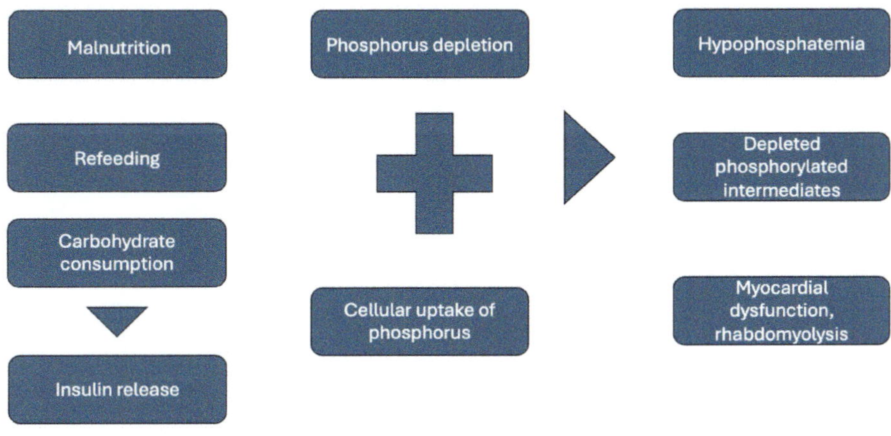

Fig. 57.1 Pathogenesis of refeeding syndrome

Pathogenesis [1] (Fig. 57.1)

Treatment and Prevention [4]

Prevent by avoiding rapid increases in daily caloric intake while replenishing nutrients in a malnourished adult [1, 2].

Treatment: Reduce nutritional support and correct hypomagnesemia, hypophosphatemia, and hypokalemia [3].

References

1. Ponzo V, Pellegrini M, Cioffi I, Scaglione L, Bo S. The refeeding syndrome: a neglected but potentially serious condition for inpatients. A narrative review. Intern Emerg Med. 2021;16:49–60.
2. Bioletto F, Pellegrini M, Ponzo V, Cioffi I, De Francesco A, Ghigo E, et al. Impact of refeeding syndrome on short- and medium-term all-cause mortality: a systematic review and meta-analysis. Am J Med. 2021;134(8):1009–1018.e1.
3. Krutkyte G, Wenk L, Odermatt J, Schuetz P, Stanga Z, Friedli N. Refeeding syndrome: a critical reality in patients with chronic disease. Nutrients. 2022;14(14):2859.
4. da Silva JS, Seres DS, Sabino K, Adams SC, Berdahl GJ, Citty SW, Cober MP, Evans DC, Greaves JR, Gura KM, Michalski A. ASPEN consensus recommendations for refeeding syndrome. Nutr Clin Pract. 2020;35(2):178–95.

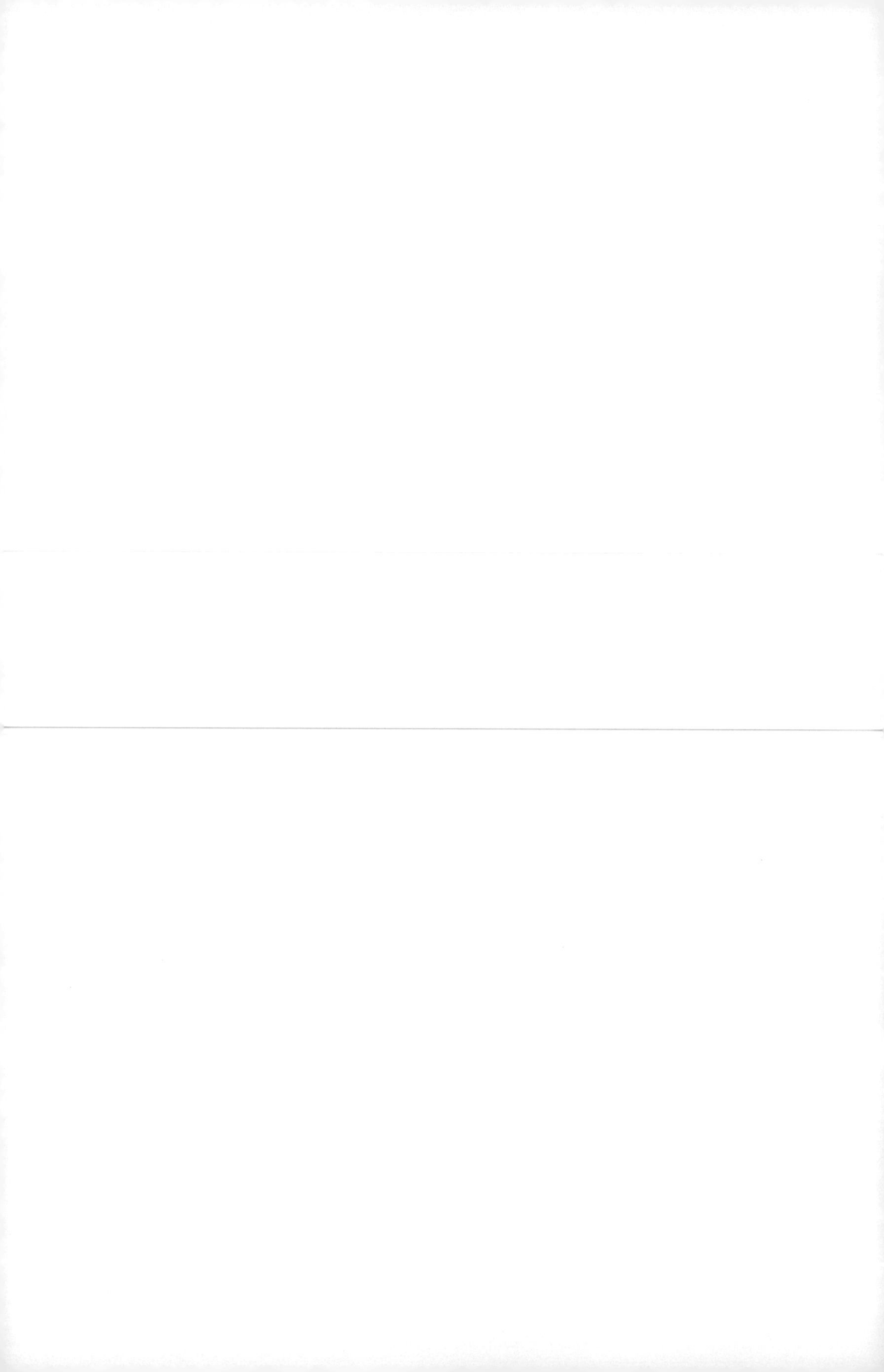

Anemia, Rash, and Jaundice in a Young Woman

58

Abstract A previously healthy young woman is admitted with fever, jaundice, and lower limb petechiae. Labs reveal renal insufficiency.

A 28-year-old woman presents to the emergency department with a 3-day history of fatigue, headache, and mild confusion. Two days prior, she noted dark urine and developed petechiae on her lower extremities. She reports having diarrhea about 1 week ago that resolved without treatment. Her past medical history is unremarkable. She does not take any prescription or over-the-counter medications on a regular basis and denies recent travel. On examination, she appears pale and lethargic with scattered petechiae on her legs and mild jaundice. Her blood pressure is 158/92 mmHg, heart rate is 110 bpm, and she is afebrile.

Her lab reports are as follows:

1. Hemoglobin: 7.2 g/dL (12.0–15.5 g/dL)
2. Hematocrit: 21% (36–46%)
3. Platelet count: 15 × 10^3/μL (150–450 × 10^3/μL)
4. Peripheral blood smear: Numerous schistocytes
5. Reticulocyte count: 4.5% (0.5–2.5%)
6. Lactate dehydrogenase (LDH): 1850 U/L (140–280 U/L)
7. Haptoglobin: <10 mg/dL (30–200 mg/dL)
8. Total bilirubin: 3.2 mg/dL (0.1–1.2 mg/dL); Indirect bilirubin: 2.7 mg/dL (0.1–0.9 mg/dL)
9. Blood urea nitrogen (BUN): 42 mg/dL (7–20 mg/dL)
10. Creatinine: 2.4 mg/dL (0.6–1.2 mg/dL)
11. Prothrombin time (PT): 12.3 s (11–13.5) s
12. Partial thromboplastin time (PTT): 32 s (25–35 s)

S. Bhat, *Clinical Conundrums to Practice Diagnostic Reasoning*,
https://doi.org/10.1007/978-981-95-0636-1_58

13. Fibrinogen: 320 mg/dL (200–400 mg/dL)
14. D-dimer: 2.5 μg/mL (<0.5 μg/mL)
15. Urinalysis: 3+ protein, 2+ blood
16. ADAMTS13 activity: <5% (>70%)

Questions

1. What might the diagnosis be?
2. What is the significance of the low haptoglobin?

Analysis

The hemoglobin is low. The unconjugated hyperbilirubinemia and increased LDH indicate that the etiology of anemia might be hemolysis. The schistocytes and decreased haptoglobin point toward an intravascular rather than extravascular hemolysis. The intravascular hemolysis, thrombocytopenia (15 × 10^3/μL), and AKI (2.4 mg/dL), when taken together, direct us toward the diagnosis of thrombotic microangiopathy—perhaps hemolytic uremic syndrome (considering the preceding history of diarrhea).

Pathophysiology

Widespread microvascular thrombosis that results in microvascular occlusion, platelet consumption, and mechanical destruction of erythrocytes as they travel through partially occluded vessels is a characteristic shared by TTP and HUS.

ADAMTS13, a protease that typically cleaves ultra-large von Willebrand factor (vWF) multimers, is either deficient or inhibited in TTP. Ultra-large vWF multimers build up in the absence of ADAMTS13, leading to spontaneous platelet adhesion and aggregation in the microcirculation [1].

In HUS: Usually brought on by E. coli that produces Shiga toxin (STEC), which leads to tissue factor exposure, complement activation, platelet adhesion, and thrombus formation by damaging endothelial cells. This damage can especially affect the renal microvasculature [2]. The patient demonstrates thrombocytopenia concurrent with hemolytic anemia because of the following:

Platelets are consumed by microvascular thrombi, which result in thrombocytopenia. RBCs are mechanically damaged as they travel through microvessels which are partially occluded with fibrin strands, causing them to fragment (schistocytes). This extravascular mechanical hemolysis explains the elevated LDH (released from damaged RBCs), low haptoglobin (which binds free hemoglobin), and elevated indirect bilirubin. Normal PT, PTT, and fibrinogen are characteristic of TMA and help differentiate it from disseminated intravascular coagulation (DIC) [3]. In TMA:

- Clotting occurs locally in the microcirculation due to platelet aggregation and endothelial damage.
- The systemic coagulation system is not significantly activated.
- Fibrinogen remains normal (unlike in DIC where it is consumed).
- This "microvascular thrombosis without systemic coagulopathy" is a hallmark ofTMA.

Haptoglobin is reduced (<10 mg/dL) as it is a hemoglobin scavenger. The liver produces haptoglobin, a protein whose main function is to bind free hemoglobin that is released during hemolysis. A haptoglobin–hemoglobin complex is created as a result. Thus, one of the most sensitive markers of hemolysis is haptoglobin, which usually drops before other markers start to show abnormalities. As long as hemolysis persists, it stays low. The diagnosis of microangiopathic hemolytic anemia in TTP/HUS is supported by the hallmark laboratory findings of intravascular hemolysis, which include an elevated LDH and undetectable haptoglobin [4]. They are especially helpful when taken in conjunction with elevated indirect bilirubin and the presence of schistocytes on peripheral blood smears. PCR for EHEC genes in stool sample; stool culture for STEC and Shiga toxin testing (positive in typical HUS); ADAMTS13 activity (severely reduced <10% in TTP); ADAMTS13 inhibitor assay (present in acquired TTP); and complement studies (C3, C4, factor H, and factor I) are further tests that would be necessary.

Treatment [5]

1. Plasmapheresis
2. Corticosteroids (methylprednisolone, 1 g/day) if acquired TTP is suspected
3. Supportive care
4. Eculizumab should be considered if atypical HUS is suspected
5. Caplacizumab if available and TTP is likely
6. Continuous monitoring of platelet count, hemoglobin, LDH, and creatinine to assess response

References

1. Hassan S, Westwood JP, Ellis D, Laing C, Mc Guckin S, Benjamin S, Scully M. The utility of ADAMTS 13 in differentiating TTP from other acute thrombotic microangiopathies: results from the UK TTP registry. Br J Haematol. 2015;171(5):830–5.
2. Fakhouri F, Zuber J, Frémeaux-Bacchi V, Loirat C. Haemolytic uraemic syndrome. Lancet. 2017;390(10095):681–96
3. Page EE, Kremer Hovinga JA, Terrell DR, Vesely SK, George JN. Thrombotic thrombocytopenic purpura: diagnostic criteria, clinical features, and long-term outcomes from 1995 through 2015. Blood Adv. 2017;1(10):590–600.
4. George JN, Nester CM. Syndromes of thrombotic microangiopathy. N Engl J Med. 2014;371(7):654–66.
5. Cuker A, Cataland SR, Coppo P, de La Rubia J, Friedman KD, George JN, Knoebl PN, Kremer Hovinga JA, Lämmle B, Matsumoto M, Pavenski K. Redefining outcomes in immune TTP: an international working group consensus report. Blood J Am Soc Hematol. 2021;137(14):1855–61.

Patient Admitted with Exacerbation of Bronchial Asthma Does Not Improve: Lab Report Trends Are More Important Than Numbers

59

Abstract An adult female admitted with exacerbation of asthma is not responding to treatment.

"Why is it"—you grumble to your friend Dr. Maitreyee during your coffee break—"why is it that my family members eschew modern allopathic medicine and put their faith in local practitioners and quacks when I'm a fairly well known and successful physician and I'm only too ready to volunteer my expertise?"

"The mystique of a healer whose methods and medicines are not available on a Google search." your friend mutters. "I've had my fair share of these cases too. In fact, I'm dealing with a particularly troublesome patient at the moment."

"What's the story?"

"Well, it's a middle-aged female named Poornima—she's a fairly straightforward case of obstructive airway disease.

For the last 2 years, her daughter—a staunch follower of native medicine—has got her off inhaled corticosteroids and has put her on some native concoction. Apparently, she recovered miraculously with this treatment. She had a bit of cough and fever for the last couple of days, the breathlessness got worse and that is why Poornima insisted on coming here, but her daughter thinks that this is a bad decision."

"What's your diagnosis?"

"Acute infective exacerbation of bronchial asthma, but the problem is, she is not getting better. In fact, it looks like she is getting worse., The daughter is trying very hard not to say, 'I told you so', but I can see it in her face. Would you mind having a look? I could do with a second opinion."

"Sure. I'll pop round in the afternoon."

When you go to the ward later that day, you see that Mrs. Poornima is sitting up in her bed in some discomfort. Her SpO_2 is 92% on venturi 40%, the respiratory rate is 24 cycles per minute, and accessory muscles are in use. There is an extensive bilateral polyphonic wheeze.

S. Bhat, *Clinical Conundrums to Practice Diagnostic Reasoning*,
https://doi.org/10.1007/978-981-95-0636-1_59

"I'm not feeling that great"—Poornima says with difficulty—"in fact I am feeling worse. Maybe I should do what my daughter suggested and get back to native medicine."

"Give me a moment. Let me have a look at your labs."

These are the labs:

Hb: 10 gm%, TC: 12500 N85 L10 M10%

- Sodium: 133 mEq/L (Normal: 135–145 mEq/L)
- Potassium: 5.4 mEq/L (Normal: 3.5–5.0 mEq/L)
- Chloride: 98 mEq/L (Normal: 98–107 mEq/L)
- Bicarbonate: 24 mEq/L (Normal: 22–29 mEq/L)
- BUN: 18 mg/dL (Normal: 7–20 mg/dL)
- Creatinine: 0.9 mg/dL (Normal: 0.6–1.1 mg/dL)
- Glucose: 68 mg/dL (Normal: 70–100 mg/dL)

You look for the drug chart and find that it is a textbook prescription. Antibiotics, bronchodilators, mucolytics, and oxygen.

Why do you think Mrs. Poornima is not getting better in spite of the treatment?

Analysis

Though none of the individual lab values is strikingly out of range, when viewed as whole, the results are suggestive.

The low normal blood sugar and sodium, and the high normal potassium, in the context of native medicine intake, followed by abrupt withdrawal, point toward a subacute Addison's, perhaps due to steroid withdrawal. The most likely diagnosis for this patient is adrenal insufficiency secondary to exogenous steroid use. Specifically, this represents a case of hypothalamic–pituitary–adrenal (HPA) axis suppression from undisclosed steroid content in the "natural herbal remedies" the patient has been taking.

These undisclosed steroids explain the excellent control of her asthma symptoms over the past 6 months but also explain her current presentation. Recent interruption or reduction in steroid intake has led to symptoms of adrenal insufficiency because of the following:

1. Long-term exogenous steroid use suppresses the HPA axis.
2. The adrenal glands atrophy and lose their ability to produce cortisol.
3. When exogenous steroids are reduced or discontinued, the suppressed adrenal glands cannot immediately resume normal function.
4. This results in relative adrenal insufficiency despite elevated ACTH levels.

The system of ayurveda and other native medicines are major players in the healthcare system of India. While licensed practitioners do a lot of good, it is unfortunately true that many times, steroids are prescribed under the guise of "natural remedies" [1]. Hence, when a patient is switched to allopathic treatment for various reasons, including disease exacerbation, on hospital admission, there is an unexplained deterioration in the patient's condition which is due to a subacute Addison's disease or a worsening of the underlying illness [3]. A high index of suspicion, confirmation of diagnosis by documenting low serum cortisol, followed by reintroduction of steroids and gradual tapering would improve Mrs. Poornima's condition.

Additional Tests to Confirm Diagnosis [2]

1. ACTH stimulation test (cosyntropin stimulation test): This is the gold standard for diagnosing adrenal insufficiency. Synthetic ACTH is administered, and cortisol levels are measured at baseline, 30 min, and 60 min. A subnormal response confirms adrenal insufficiency.
2. CRH stimulation test: Can help differentiate between primary, secondary, and tertiary adrenal insufficiency.

Immediate Treatment Recommendations

1. Corticosteroid replacement therapy
2. Patient education
3. Electrolyte correction if symptomatic from hyponatremia or hyperkalemia

Key Takeaway
1. Always consider undisclosed steroid use in patients with good symptom control using "alternative" or "natural" remedies for inflammatory conditions [4].
2. The combination of hyponatremia, hyperkalemia, and hypoglycemia should raise suspicion of adrenal insufficiency.
3. Recovery of the HPA axis after exogenous steroid use can take months to years, depending on the duration and dose of steroid exposure [5].

References

1. Gupta SK, Kaleekal T, Joshi S. Misuse of corticosteroids in some of the drugs dispensed as preparations from alternative systems of medicine in India. Pharmacoepidemiol Drug Saf. 2000;9(7):599–602.
2. Nicholas MN, Li SK, Dytoc M. An approach to minimising risk of adrenal insufficiency when discontinuing oral glucocorticoids. J Cutan Med Surg. 2018;22(2):175–81.
3. Chen YT, Chang CJ, Yao WJ, Wang PW, Wang JD. One year follow-up study of the recovery of adrenal insufficiency induced by formulated herb drugs. J Formosan Med Assoc Taiwan yi zhi. 1993;92:S250–7.
4. Kempegowda P, Quinn L, Shepherd L, Kauser S, Johnson B, Lawson A, Bates A. Adrenal insufficiency from steroid-containing complementary therapy: importance of detailed history. Endocrinol Diabetes Metab Case Rep. 2019;2019(1):1–4.
5. Younes AK, Younes NK. Recovery of steroid induced adrenal insufficiency. Transl Pediatr. 2017;6(4):269.

Lung Cancer with Bone Metastasis: Unexpected Normal Calcium Values

60

Abstract Mr. Momin is a 65-year-old male admitted to the orthopedic ward with severe back pain. Examination by the orthopedist reveals something more sinister, and Momin is referred to you for further evaluation and management.

Mr. Momin has a 30 pack year history. Apart from the backache which has been troubling him for a month now, he has been having a sharp pain in the right side of the chest and loss of weight of 9 kg over the last 2 months.

Figure 60.1 shows the patient.

Figure 60.2 shows the chest X-ray.

Relevant labs are as follows:

- Hb: 10 gm%, TC: 5000/mm^3.
- RBS: 94 mg%, Ca++: 9 mg/dL
- Serum albumin: 2 g/dL
- Blood urea: 40 mg%, serum creatinine: 1.1 mg/dL

Is there anything surprising in the labs? What might the explanation be, and how do you adjust for it?

Answer Considering the likely diagnosis, that is, carcinoma bronchus with vertebral metastasis, one would have expected the serum calcium to be elevated. However, it is surprisingly within range.

The key here is the hypoalbuminemia which causes a falsely low calcium.

Corrected calcium may be corrected by the formula

$$\text{Corrected calcium}\left(\text{mg / dL}\right) = \text{measured total Ca}\left(\text{mg / dL}\right) \\ +0.8\left(4.0 - \text{serum albumin}\left[\text{g / dL}\right]\right)$$

S. Bhat, *Clinical Conundrums to Practice Diagnostic Reasoning*, https://doi.org/10.1007/978-981-95-0636-1_60

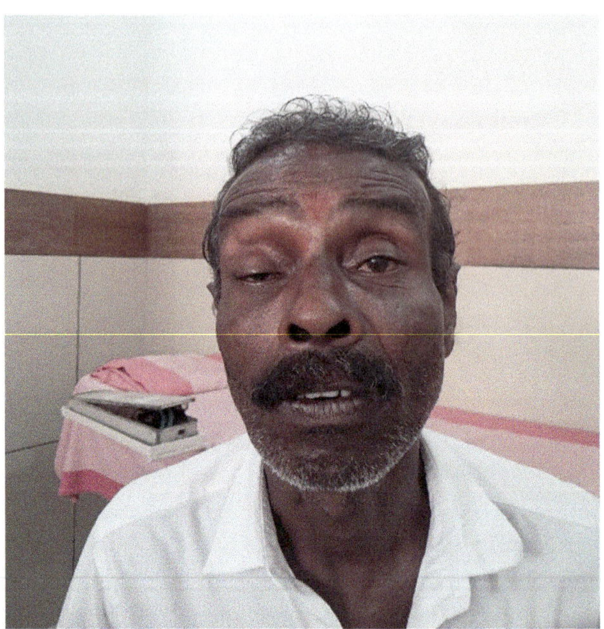

Fig. 60.1 Ptosis of right eye, suggestive of Horner's syndrome. (Patient consent obtained)

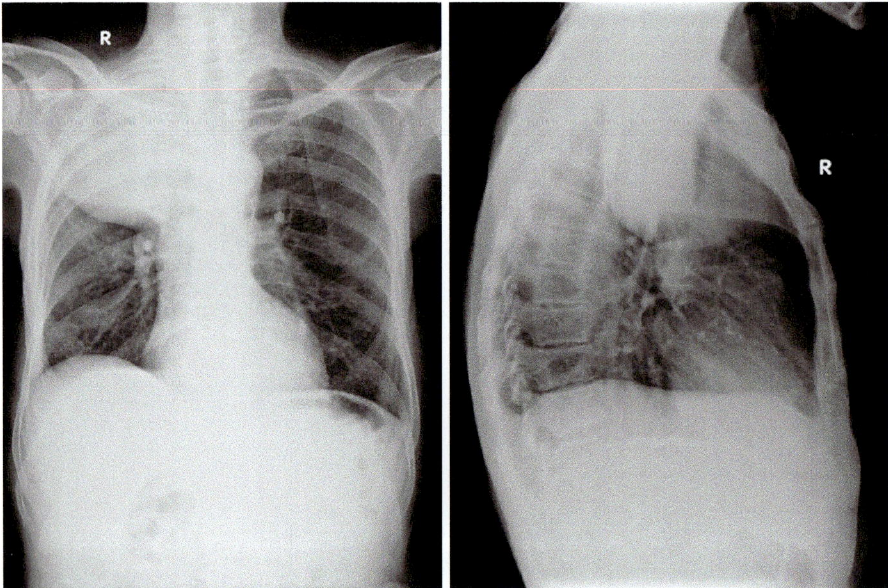

Fig. 60.2 Chest X-ray. (Image contributed by Dr. Srishankar Bairy, pulmonologist, FMMC)

$$9\,\mathrm{mg\%} + 0.8(4.0 - 2)$$

$$9 + 0.8 \times 2$$

$$9 + 1.6 = 10.16\,\mathrm{mg\%}$$

It should be noted that not all clinicians consider it necessary or useful to correct serum calcium for the level of albumin [1].

Humoral hypercalcemia of malignancy is due to the production of parathormone-related peptide (PTHrP), which mimics the action of parathormone [2]. This leads to increased bone resorption, release of calcium into the bloodstream, and hypercalcemia. It is especially common in squamous cell carcinoma [3].

Severe hypercalcemia defined as a corrected calcium more than 14 mg % must be treated emergently with [4]

1. Intravenous fluids
2. Salmon calcitonin
3. Zoledronic acid
4. Denosumab

References

1. Smith, J. D., Wilson, S., & Schneider, H. G. (2018). Misclassification of Calcium Status Based on Albumin-Adjusted Calcium: Studies in a Tertiary Hospital Setting. Clinical chemistry, 64(12), 1713–1722. https://doi.org/10.1373/clinchem.2018.291377.
2. Stewart AF. Hypercalcemia associated with cancer. N Engl J Med. 2005;352(4):373–9.
3. Carroll MF, Schade DS. A practical approach to hypercalcemia. Am Fam Physician. 2003;67(9):1959–66.
4. Guise TA, Wysolmerski JJ. Cancer-associated hypercalcemia. N Engl J Med. 2022;386(15):1443–51.

Part III

Short Puzzles

61 Fluctuating Somatic and Psychological Complaints in a New Mother: The Worried Grandmum

Grade Moderate.

Abstract Mother of a newborn baby having a difficult postpartum period, followed by mood changes.

The Story Mrs. Rukmini is at her wits end. She has come to help her daughter Priya through her first delivery and postpartum period, but she is quite unable to figure out how to deal with Priya's labile mood and irritability. The delivery in itself was uneventful, and Mrs. Rukmini falls in love with her tiny doll of a granddaughter, Rani, at first sight. Priya seems happy too, initially—singing funny ditties of her own composition to the little baby. But things change when Rani turns a month old. Everything seems to make Priya angry.

"Maybe it's because she is sleep-deprived," Rukmini tells her husband Krishna as they drink their morning tea. "I hear her pace up and down in the middle of the night—no wonder she is so short-tempered."

"Yes, but I wish she wouldn't be so snappy with poor baby Rani."

"I know! And she turns on the fan so fast that the wee mite must be trembling with cold."

"Yes, what's wrong with her that she needs the fan on in December?!"

"She says it is to muffle the noise of the street outside."

"Let her wear ear plugs! By the way, speaking of trembling, have you noticed that Priya's hands tremble when she is really angry?"

"Yes! I told you we should have sent her for the meditation classes when she was tense before the exam."

"No point in blaming me at this point. Do you think we should take her to a counsellor now?"

"No, no—she will be furious if we make that suggestion."

"Ok. I just really wish she would quieten down a bit. It is like having a caged tiger at home," Rukmini says.

S. Bhat, *Clinical Conundrums to Practice Diagnostic Reasoning*, https://doi.org/10.1007/978-981-95-0636-1_61

She is soon to regret that wish, however. In another couple of months, Priya swings to the opposite extreme. She now sits at the window like a slug, trying to bask in the weak light of the winter sun. This sedentary lifestyle—not surprisingly—reflects on the weighing scale, and Priya resorts to buying larger and even larger clothes online. She wakes up so late that Mrs. Rukmini has to resort, much against her wishes, to plying baby Rani with formula feeds to tide her over until her mother wakes up.

She gently broaches the topic of meeting a counsellor to Priya who drearily responds

"I'm ok! Just tired. Don't you remember being a new mother? It's not as easy as being a grandmom."

Stung at the injustice of this statement, Rukmini spends an hour in her garden to find solace among the winter blooms.

Questions What do you think is happening here? A straightforward case of the postpartum blues? Or something else?

Analysis

Minus all the conversations and drama, it boils down to this.

A postpartum lady who is irritable, has insomnia (pacing up and down in the middle of the night), and heat intolerance (fan turned on full speed even in winter).

This is followed by weight gain (larger clothes), cold intolerance (needs to bask in the sun all the time), and lethargy (wakes up late, inactive as a slug even upon waking).

This characteristic picture of hyperthyroid followed by hypothyroid features after delivery is typical of postpartum thyroiditis (PPT).

Postpartum thyroiditis tends to occur in women with a past history or a family history of autoimmune diseases. It has a prevalence of around 5% [1] and occurs in the first year following delivery. It occurs postpartum, until a year after delivery, since this period coincides with the end of the immune tolerance induced by pregnancy.

Natural History of the Disease

PPT presents with symptoms of thyrotoxicosis (irritability, fatigue, and heat tolerance) due to the release of preformed hormones by the thyroid gland [2]. This is followed by symptoms of hypothyroidism (dry skin, drowsiness, and constipation). The disease normally remits within a year, and the patient becomes euthyroid again; hypothyroidism, however, persists in approximately half the patients and tends to recur following subsequent pregnancies as well.

Postpartum thyroiditis must be differentiated from Grave's disease in the thyrotoxic phase (Table 61.1). Since the symptoms of postpartum depression overlap with the hypothyroid phase of PPT, a high index of suspicion is required for diagnosis, and *all postpartum women presenting with low mood, fatigue, and weight gain must have a thyroid function assessment.*

Management

Antithyroid drugs are not required as the symptoms are due to the release of preformed hormones. Symptoms of thyrotoxicosis may be managed with beta-blockers which are safe during lactation, like metoprolol [3]. Thyroid function must be

Table 61.1 Grave's disease and postpartum thyroiditis

	Graves	PPT
TRAb	Positive	Positive
Anti-TPO	Positive	–
T3:T4 ratio	20: 1	
Presentation	6–12 months postpartum	1–4 months postpartum

assessed 6–8 weeks after the resolution of the symptoms in the thyrotoxic phase. Thyroxine may be required in the hypothyroid phase. This phase normally lasts for a year, and thyroxine may be tapered and stopped after that. Since PPT tends to recur, annual monitoring of TSH is recommended.

References

1. Nicholson WK, Robinson KA, Smallridge RC, Ladenson PW, Powe NR. Prevalence of postpartum thyroid dysfunction: a quantitative review. Thyroid. 2006;16(6):573–82.
2. Stagnaro-Green A. Approach to the patient with postpartum thyroiditis. J Clin Endocrinol Metabol. 2012;97(2):334–42.
3. Dickens LT, Cifu AS, Cohen RN. Diagnosis and management of thyroid disease during pregnancy and the postpartum period. JAMA. 2019;321(19):1928–9.

62 Hypoglycemia Not Reverting with Sugar: The Unexplained Hypos

Grade Easy.

Abstract A patient with T2DM presents with signs and symptoms of hypoglycemia. These symptoms did not revert after self-administration of sugar.

Story Mr. Ashok, a 55-year-old male with diabetes, comes to you with a history of diabetes detected recently during a routine health check. He lives in Mangalore but commutes to Udupi, an hour away, where he works as a clerk in a factory.

You note that he is not a smoker, does not consume ethanol, and has a BMI of 30. You counsel him about diet management and foot care and plan a Target Organ Damage evaluation at the next visit.

You start him on a combination of oral antidiabetic drugs that includes sulfonylurea. In view of this, you educate him about the symptoms of hypoglycemia and advise him to carry juice or a sweet snack with him and to consume them if he develops any of the described symptoms.

Mr. Ashok, an educated, committed patient, follows your instructions religiously. Unfortunately, one morning, his bus journey is unavoidably prolonged as an accident on the highway has blocked the road.

When he next visits your clinic, it is with the history that he had developed seizures, and when taken to a hospital Emergency Department, his random blood sugar tested by a glucometer was found to be 50 mg%. Surprisingly, his colleague and co-passenger claim that when stuck in the traffic jam, Mr. Ashok complained of weakness and sweating and immediately consumed four pieces of candy.

1. Questions: Why did Mr. Ashok develop hypoglycemia in spite of consuming the candy? (No, it was not sugar-free candy).
2. How would you modify your advice (not the prescription)?

S. Bhat, *Clinical Conundrums to Practice Diagnostic Reasoning*,
https://doi.org/10.1007/978-981-95-0636-1_62

Answer

The key here is "combination of oral antidiabetic drugs that includes a sulfonylurea". Considering the fact that the hypoglycemia did not respond to the sugar in chocolate, it is likely that the OAD prescribed along with sulfonylurea was an alpha-glucosidase inhibitor (acarbose)

Ans 1. The hypoglycemia caused by sulfonylurea could not be treated with sucrose, as acarbose inhibits 1 alpha-glucosidase (an enzyme that is located in the brush border of epithelial cells, mainly in the upper half of the small intestine) which degrades disaccharides such as sucrose to glucose and fructose. The alpha-glucosidase inhibitors bind reversibly in a dose-dependent manner to the oligosaccharide-binding site of these enzymes and delay the degradation of polysaccharides and starch to glucose. Since the patient consumed sucrose which could not be converted to glucose, his hypoglycemia did not revert.

Ans 2. Ask patient to carry glucose powder instead of chocolates. Vide infra, the package insert information for acarbose

"Use glucose tablets or liquid glucose to help manage a hypoglycemic event while you're taking acarbose. Cane sugar (sucrose) won't work to treat hypoglycemia while you're taking acarbose. Use oral glucose (dextrose) products instead."

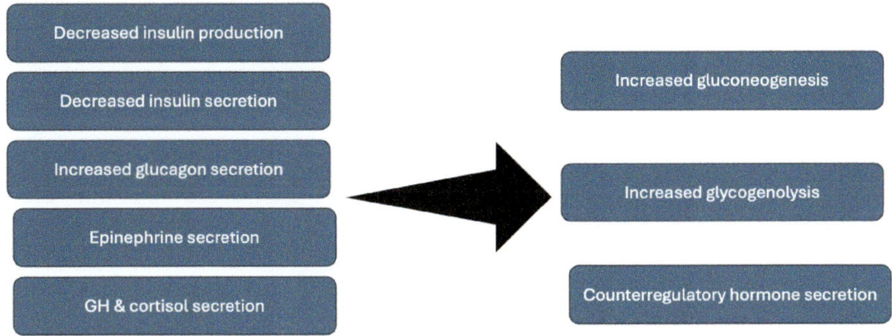

Fig. 62.1 Low serum glucose leads to counter-regulatory hormone secretion and sympatho- adrenal activation, resulting in the characteristic symptoms of hypoglycemia.

Hypoglycemia

Definition Blood glucose less than 70 mg%

Etiopathogenesis (Fig. 62.1)

In patients on treatment for diabetes, hypoglycemia may be a possible side effect of the following drugs:

A. Insulin
B. Sulfonylureas
C. Meglitinides

Clinical Features

(a) Tremors
(b) Palpitations
(c) Sweating
(d) Anxiety

If hypoglycemia is not corrected promptly, neuroglycopenia ensues: fatigue, dizziness, headache, abnormal behavior, drowsiness, seizures, and loss of consciousness.

It is important to note that in long-standing diabetes, with recurrent attacks of hypoglycemia, the counter-regulatory hormone response may be blunted, resulting in **hypoglycemia unawareness**.

Severe untreated hypoglycemia may be fatal.

Diagnosis

Whipple's triad of hypoglycemia:

1. Symptoms of hypoglycemia
2. Low blood glucose
3. Symptoms relieved by administration of glucose

Treatment [1]

1. If the patient is conscious, give oral carbohydrate immediately—either juice, candy, or biscuits. The 15–15 rule should be followed—15 g carbohydrate (e.g., half a cup of juice, one tablespoon of sugar), followed by checking blood sugar 15 min later.
2. If the patient has lost consciousness, 50 mL of 50% dextrose, followed by 5% dextrose infusion to maintain blood glucose >100 mg% may be given.

Unfortunately, setting tight glycemic goals to prevent the complications of diabetes is a double-edged sword and comes with an increased risk of hypoglycemia [2]. Endocrine Society guidelines include strong recommendations for education of patients with diabetes about the causes, consequences, and management of hypoglycemia. Repeated attacks of hypoglycemia cause fear of hypoglycemia in patients with diabetes, which might lead to them adjusting medication doses downward and result in inadequate glycemic control. Attacks of severe hypoglycemia may precipitate cardiac event [3].

Key Takeaway

All patients with diabetes on medicines which might cause hypoglycemia *must* have immediate access to glucose, especially when outside their home or traveling. Additionally, their family members must be instructed to recognize and treat hypoglycemia at an early stage. It is also advisable to have Glucagon IM or intranasal at hand for the management of severe hypoglycemia.

References

1. Nakhleh A, Shehadeh N. Hypoglycemia in diabetes: an update on pathophysiology, treatment, and prevention. World J Diabetes. 2021;12(12):2036.
2. Diabetes Control and Complications Trial Research Group. Hypoglycemia in the diabetes control and complications trial. Diabetes. 1997;46(2):271–86.
3. Przezak A, Bielka W, Molęda P. Fear of hypoglycemia—an underestimated problem. Brain Behav. 2022;12(7):e2633.

63 Ascending Weakness with No Sensory Signs in a 5-Year-Old Girl: Holiday Blues

Grade Easy.

Abstract A young girl returns from holiday and shortly thereafter develops fatigue and malaise, followed by ascending paralysis.

Story You are on the Saturday night shift in the ER when a young lady walks in with a small girl in her arms.

"Doctor, please help us. This is my daughter Riya—she's not well at all."

"Can you put her on the examination couch, please?"

Riya is maybe 5 or 6 years old. She compliantly lies down on the couch and looks at you with wide eyes.

"What exactly is the problem?" you ask the mother.

"We returned from a holiday in Florida 5 days ago. Riya was looking dull and out of sorts since we got back. This morning, she seemed to be a little unsteady while walking.

I thought it was tiredness after the trip, but by this afternoon, I noticed she wasn't moving her arms much. What terrified me was this: I tried to feed her this evening, and I guess she wasn't able to swallow, doctor, because she started coughing and brought out the soup that she had just eaten."

"That must have been scary for you," you say sympathetically. "Can I ask you a couple of questions while I have a quick look at her?"

"Sure."

"Has she been ok prior this? No hospital admissions or doctor visits?"

"Only for routine vaccinations."

"And did anything unusual happen on your trip to Florida? I ask only because the problem started soon after your holiday."

"No, doctor. We spent most of our time outdoors—did a fair bit of walking in the woods. And she absolutely loved it."

"Was there fever at any point of time?"

S. Bhat, *Clinical Conundrums to Practice Diagnostic Reasoning*, https://doi.org/10.1007/978-981-95-0636-1_63

"No."

You hand Riya a lollipop and say "I'm going to quickly examine you, ok? Your mom will be right here, and you will feel no pain."

"Ok" she says, but her speech seems a little slurred.

You become increasingly concerned as you examine Riya. She is afebrile; there is no rash. She is conscious and is able to answer simple questions correctly.

However, the power is 3 in both lower limbs and 4 in upper limbs. There is hypotonia in all limbs, and deep tendon reflexes are absent. There is left LMN facial palsy. The sensory examination is normal. The child does not understand the instructions to perform a single breath test, but her shallow rapid respiration worries you, and you decide to shift her to the pediatric ICU.

Basic blood investigations are noncontributory. Serum electrolytes are normal. Toxicology screen is negative. You ask for a nerve conduction study and MRI.

You are discussing the case with the pediatric intensivist who will soon be in charge of the patient. You inform him of the travel history and the signs and symptoms. He walks to the patient and examines her from head to toe. He finds something, does something, and the next day the patient (who you thought would need to be intubated and mechanically ventilated) is sitting up and asking when she can go home.

Questions What is the diagnosis in this case? What do you think the pediatrician found? And what did he do?

Analysis

This is a case of acute neuromuscular paralysis (ANMP)—flaccid, ascending, pure motor weakness with facial palsy.

Some causes of ANMP are [1] as follows:

(a) GBS (Guillain Barre syndrome)
(b) Porphyria
(c) Diphtheria
(d) Lyme neuroborreliosis
(e) Toxins like organophosphate and heavy metals
(f) Critical illness neuropathy
(g) Tick paralysis
(h) Snake bite
(i) Botulism
(j) Periodic paralysis

The first differential diagnosis that leaps to mind, of course, is Guillain Barre syndrome. Botulism can also cause weakness of all limbs, but it is descending rather than ascending [2]. Myasthenia, polio, and organophosphorus consumption do have certain features in common with this case, but this particular presentation is unlikely to be any of them. Hypokalemia is a possibility, but serum potassium is normal.

Looking at the etiology again—why would a 5-year-old girl who has recently travelled to Florida present with ascending weakness with no sensory involvement?

This is a case of tick paralysis. In fact, some experts say that a meticulous search for ticks must be made in patients with relevant travel history before entertaining a diagnosis of Guillain Barre Syndrome.

Tick paralysis is a toxin-mediated ascending paralysis seen in Australia, the United States, and Canada [3].

Etiopathogenesis Tick paralysis may occur after the bite of a female tick. In Florida, the American dog tick or *Dermacentor variabilis* is commonly seen (Fig. 63.1).

The female tick injects toxin while feeding on its blood meal. The toxin inhibits sodium flux across channels, thus impairing nerve transmission [4].

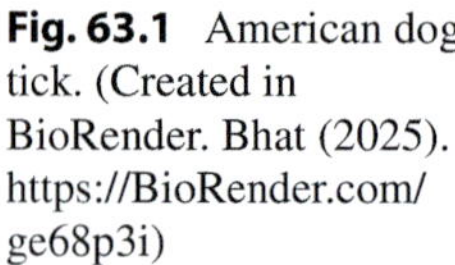

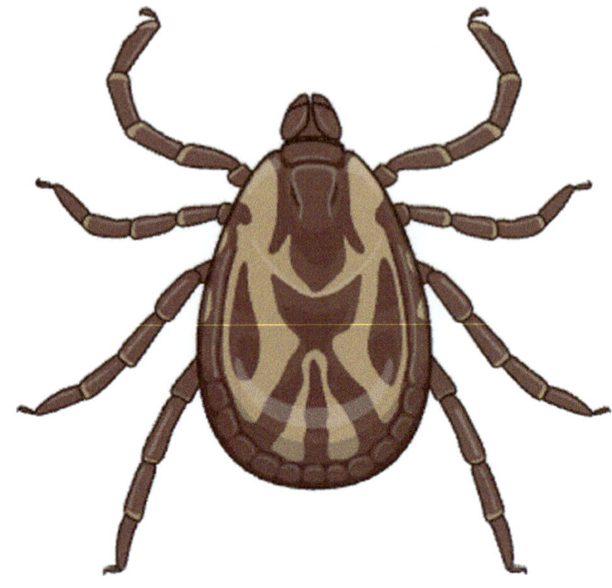

Fig. 63.1 American dog tick. (Created in BioRender. Bhat (2025). https://BioRender.com/ge68p3i)

Clinical Features

(a) Weakness of lower limbs ascending to involve upper limbs and cranial nerves.
(b) Sometimes, ophthalmoplegia may be seen [5].
(c) Pupillary dilatation may be seen in some cases, especially in Australia [6].

It is seen more often in children because the dose of tick toxin per kg body weight is more in them. It is also more frequent in girls whose long hair may mask the tick.

Treatment Removal of the tick.

Key Takeaway
In areas where tick paralysis is known, in all cases presenting with paraparesis/quadriparesis with no sensory involvement, a meticulous search for ticks must be made before considering the diagnosis of Guillain Barre syndrome [7].

Behind the ear, between the scalp and the ear, is a common spot where ticks hide.

References

1. Nayak R. Practical approach to the patient with acute neuromuscular weakness. World J Clin Cases. 2017;5(7):270–9.
2. Kobaidze K, Wiley Z. Botulism in the 21st century: a scoping review. Brown J Hosp Med. 2023;2(2):72707.
3. Edlow JA, McGillicuddy DC. Tick paralysis. Infect Dis Clin N Am. 2008;22(3):397–413. vii
4. Krishnan AV, Lin CS, Reddel SW, Mcgrath R, Kiernan MC. Conduction block and impaired axonal function in tick paralysis. Muscle Nerve. 2009;40(3):358–62.
5. Edlow JA. Tick paralysis. Curr Treat Options Neurol. 2010;12(3):167–77.
6. Hall-Mendelin S, Craig SB, Hall RA, O'Donoghue P, Atwell RB, Tulsiani SM, et al. Tick paralysis in Australia caused by Ixodes holocyclus Neumann. Ann Trop Med Parasitol. 2011;105(2):95–106.
7. Salman F, Atlantawi A, Maraqa N. Tick paralysis: a thorough examination may prevent unnecessary harm. Cureus [Internet]. 2023 [cited 2025 Mar 30]; Available from: https://www.cureus.com/articles/144415-tick-paralysis-a-thorough-examination-may-prevent-unnecessary-harm

Middle Aged Male Meets with an Accident While Driving on a Straight Well-Lit Empty Road: The Improbable Accident

64

Grade Moderate.

Abstract A middle-aged male patient admitted to a hospital with rib fractures after a road traffic accident is referred for neurological evaluation as there is no apparent cause for the accident.

Story You visit the orthopedics ward to see a consult. Mr. Ratnakar is a 45-year-old man, a known hypertensive on treatment, who was apparently well when he started driving from his home to his office at 10 am in the morning. His car crashed into a tree around half an hour later. Ratnakar called an ambulance and was brought to the hospital where you work. The road where his car crashed is straight, well lit, and extremely safe; neither Ratnakar nor the orthopedist treating him can figure out what caused the crash. The orthopedist suspects seizures and refers the patient to you for further evaluation.

You speak to Ratnakar and find that he has been a hypertensive for the last 3 years, on treatment with telmisartan 40 mg once a day. He remembers driving on the road and also calling for help soon after the accident. There is no past history of seizures, head trauma, fever, or ethanol use. In fact, apart from the fact that he wakes up four or five times every night to pass urine, the history is not contributory. Examination reveals a BMI of 32 and blood pressure of 150/100 mm Hg. There are no focal neurological deficits. The fundus is normal, and the lungs are clear. Labs reveal normal blood sugar, electrolytes, and thyroid function. Echocardiogram and ECG are normal apart from left ventricular hypertrophy. The 24-h Holter monitoring is normal. An MRI that had been done on the day of the accident to rule out cerebral trauma is normal.

Questions What would be your next step? Would you order an EEG? Or something else? What might have caused Ratnakar's accident?

S. Bhat, *Clinical Conundrums to Practice Diagnostic Reasoning*, https://doi.org/10.1007/978-981-95-0636-1_64

Analysis

It is clear from the story that the cause of the accident is not due to anything on the road but something to do with Ratnakar himself. The normal MRI rules out a structural central nervous system lesion, and the fact that he was oriented enough to ask for assistance immediately after the accident makes a seizure less likely.

Similarly, the practically normal Holter and echocardiogram suggest that there is no cardiovascular cause for a possible loss of consciousness and loss of control of the vehicle, which resulted in the accident.

The clues in the story are the fact that his BMI and blood pressure are elevated, and an additional hint is the history of nocturia. Taken together, it seems to be a case of sleep apnoea syndrome resulting in Ratnakar falling asleep at the wheel and crashing his car.

Sleep Apnoea Syndrome (SAS) is characterized by frequent episodes of apnea and hypopnea during sleep, leading to symptoms such as excessive daytime sleepiness and increased cardiovascular morbidity [1]. Obstructive Sleep Apnea (OSA), a common type of SAS, involves the dynamic collapse of upper airway tissues during sleep, resulting in apnea and hypopnea and both short and long term physiological consequences [2].

SAS encompasses a spectrum of sleep-disordered breathing, including central, mixed, and obstructive apneas and hypopneas. It is a common disorder, affecting a significant portion of the adult population. The prevalence varies depending on the definition used but is estimated to be approximately 15–30% in males and 5–15% in females when OSA is defined as an apnea–hypopnea index (AHI) greater than five events per hour of sleep.

The primary classification is based on the underlying mechanism:

(a) Obstructive sleep apnea (OSA): Results from upper airway collapse despite ongoing respiratory effort.
(b) Central sleep apnea (CSA): Occurs due to a lack of respiratory drive from the brain.
(c) Mixed sleep apnea: A combination of both obstructive and central components.
(d) Treatment-emergent central sleep apnea: Emergence or persistence of central apneas with the use of positive airway pressure (PAP).

Etiopathogenesis

The etiology of OSA is multifactorial, involving a combination of anatomical and physiological factors.

Risk factors include:

1. Obesity: Excess weight contributes to increased soft tissue in the upper airway (Fig. 64.1).
2. Craniofacial abnormalities that narrow the upper airway.

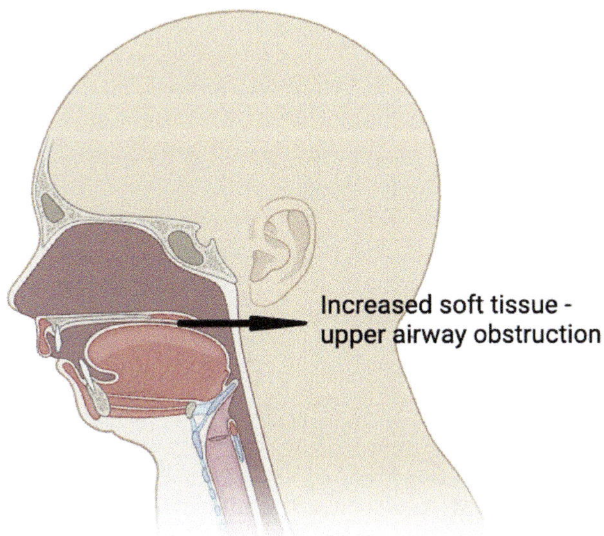

Fig. 64.1 OSA—increased soft tissue due to obesity. (Created in BioRender. Bhat (2025). https://BioRender.com/ge68p3i)

3. Nasal obstruction: Such as septal deviation or nasal polyps.
4. Family history: A genetic predisposition may increase the risk of OSA.

Pathogenesis

The pathogenesis of OSA involves repetitive collapse of the upper airway during sleep, leading to intermittent hypoxia and sleep fragmentation. This process triggers a cascade of physiological consequences, including:

(a) Increased sympathetic nervous system activity
(b) Endothelial dysfunction
(c) Systemic inflammation
(d) Increased cardiovascular morbidity [3].

Clinical Features [4]

Patients with OSA often present with a constellation of symptoms, including

(a) Loud, disruptive snoring—because of narrowing of airways
(b) Witnessed apneas during sleep
(c) Excessive daytime sleepiness
(d) Nonrestorative sleep
(e) Morning headaches
(f) Nocturia—due to hypoxia which stimulates ANP

Investigations [5]

(a) Polysomnography (PSG): The gold standard for diagnosing OSA, PSG involves overnight monitoring of various physiological parameters, including brain activity, eye movements, muscle activity, heart rate, and respiratory effort.
(b) Home sleep apnoea testing (HSAT): Portable monitoring devices can be used to diagnose OSA in the home setting, particularly in patients with a high pretest probability of moderate to severe OSA.
(c) Epworth sleepiness scale (ESS): This questionnaire helps quantify daytime sleepiness, with a score > 9 indicating abnormal sleepiness.

Diagnosis

OSA is diagnosed based on the presence of characteristic symptoms and objective evidence of sleep-disordered breathing on sleep testing. Diagnostic criteria include an AHI of ≥5 events per hour, accompanied by symptoms such as sleepiness, fatigue, insomnia, or other symptoms that impair sleep-related quality of life.

Treatment: The management of OSA aims to alleviate symptoms, improve sleep quality, and reduce the risk of long-term complications.

Treatment options include the following:

(a) Continuous positive airway pressure (CPAP): CPAP therapy involves delivering pressurized air through a mask to keep the upper airway open during sleep.
(b) Oral appliances: Mandibular advancement devices (MADs) can be used to reposition the lower jaw and tongue, thereby increasing the size of the upper airway [5].
(c) Weight loss: Weight reduction can improve OSA severity in overweight or obese patients.
(d) Positional therapy: Avoiding sleeping in the supine position can reduce the frequency of apneas in patients with positional OSA.
(e) Surgery: In selected cases, surgical procedures such as uvulopalatopharyngoplasty (UPPP) or maxillomandibular advancement (MMA) may be considered.
(f) Hypoglossal nerve stimulation: This involves implanting a device that stimulates the hypoglossal nerve to maintain upper airway patency.

References

1. Sforza E, Bacon W, Weiss T, Thibault A, Petiau C, Krieger J. Upper airway collapsibility and cephalometric variables in patients with obstructive sleep apnea. Am J Respir Crit Care Med. 2000;161(2):347–52.
2. Sunwoo JS, Hwangbo Y, Kim WJ, Chu MK, Yun CH, Yang KI. Prevalence, sleep characteristics, and comorbidities in a population at high risk for obstructive sleep apnea: a nationwide questionnaire study in South Korea. PLoS One. 2018;13(2):e0193549.

3. Peppard PE, Young T, Palta M, Skatrud J. Prospective study of the association between sleep-disordered breathing and hypertension. N Engl J Med. 2000;342(19):1378–84.
4. Donovan LM, Kapur VK. Prevalence and characteristics of central compared to obstructive sleep apnea: analyses from the sleep heart health study cohort. Sleep. 2016;39(7):1353–9.
5. Quinnell TG, Bennett M, Jordan J, Clutterbuck-James AL, Davies MG, Smith IE, Oscroft N, Pittman MA, Cameron M, Chadwick R, Morrell MJ. A crossover randomised controlled trial of oral mandibular advancement devices for obstructive sleep apnoea-hypopnoea (TOMADO). Thorax. 2014;69(10):938–45.

Middle-Aged Male Concerned About Verruca: Just a Wart?

65

Abstract A known case of diabetes and hypertension presents to a physician concerned about warts on his body.

Mr. NH has been your patient for many years, following up once in a while for his diabetes and hypertension. You ask the routine questions, do a brief examination, and find that his blood pressure and blood sugar are under control.

"Hey doc, can you refer me to a skin doctor?"

"Sure, what's up?" you ask.

"There are these sudden funny warty growths I've got on my ear, on my palms, and on my groin. They itch quite a bit. My wife says I have to get it looked into," he says.

The lesions that he shows you are as in Figs. 65.1a and b.

Question What do you think NH has. Does he need a referral to a dermatologist or someone else?

Answer The lesions are seborrheic keratoses, and this is the "sign of Leser Trelat." Panel 1 shows a background of acanthosis nigricans. Mr. NH must be referred immediately to an oncologist.

S. Bhat, *Clinical Conundrums to Practice Diagnostic Reasoning*, https://doi.org/10.1007/978-981-95-0636-1_65

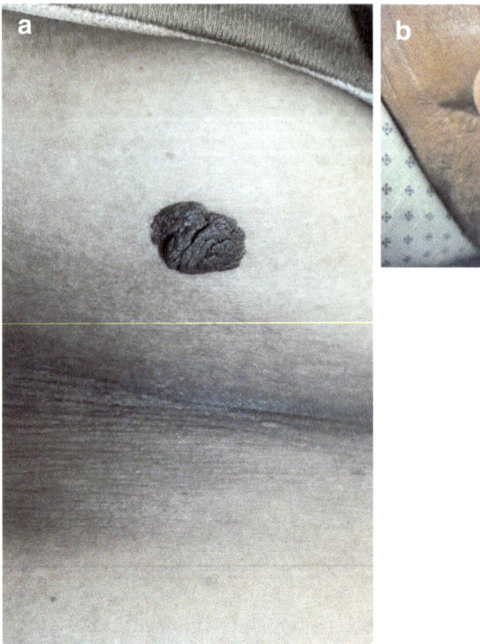

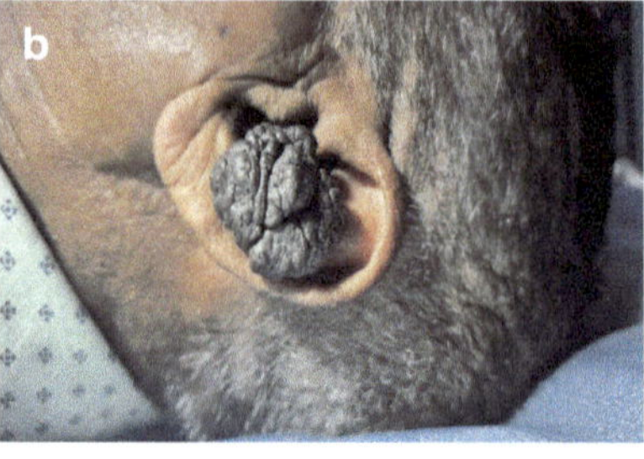

Figs. 65.1 (**a** and **b**) Images contributed by Dr. Michelle, Department of Dermatology, FMMC

Disease Description

The sign of Leser Trelat is one of the dermatological manifestations of malignancy—seborrheic keratoses, sometimes on a background of acnathosis nigricans. It most commonly seen in gastric adenocarcinoma [1]. It can also be seen in colon, lung, and breast cancer [2]. However, it must be noted that seborrheic keratoses are fairly common and are often not associated with malignancy. It is the **sudden explosive increase in the number and size** which must give rise to a suspicion of malignancy [3]. This increase is due to cytokines and growth factors—epidermal growth factor and alpha-transforming growth factor—secreted by the malignancy.

Other cutaneous lesions associated with malignancy are tripe palms, malignant acanthosis nigricans, and florid cutaneous papillomatosis. It is important to note that seborrheic keratoses might also be a side effect of cyclophosphamide.

Curth's postulates [4] which increase the probability of dermatosis being associated with a malignancy.

1. Concurrent onset: Dermatosis and malignancy occur concurrently.
2. Parallel course: Treatment of malignancy results in the remission of dermatosis.

3. Uniformity: Specific malignancy associated with specific dermatosis.
4. Statistical significance: Statistically significant association between malignancy and dermatosis.
5. Genetic basis: Genetic association between dermatosis and malignancy.

The sign of Leser Trelat, if associated with malignancy, has sinister prognostic significance since it is associated with more malignant tumors. However, recent published literature questions the association of seborrheic keratosis with malignancy [5].

Key Takeaway
The importance of the sign of Leser Trelat is that it may occur prior to the development of malignancy and is an indicator that the patient must be screened for malignancy.

References

1. Sign of leser-Trélat – ScienceDirect [Internet]. [cited 2025 Mar 2]. Available from: https://www.sciencedirect.com/science/article/abs/pii/0738081X9390111O
2. Sign of Leser-Trelat Differential Diagnoses [Internet]. [cited 2025 Mar 2]. Available from: https://emedicine.medscape.com/article/1097299-differential
3. Ponti G, Luppi G, Losi L, Giannetti A, Seidenari S. Leser-Trélat syndrome in patients affected by six multiple metachronous primitive cancers. J Hematol Oncol. 2010;3(1):2.
4. Thiers BH, Sahn RE, Callen JP. Cutaneous manifestations of internal malignancy. CA Cancer J Clin. 2009;59(2):73–98.
5. Bräuer J, Happle R, Gieler U, Effendy I. The sign of Leser-Trélat: fact or myth? J Eur Acad Dermatol Venereol. 1992;1(1):77–80.

66 Transfusion-Dependent Adolescent Presents with Rhinorrhea and Epistaxis: The Troubled Teen

Grade Easy.

Abstract An adolescent who has received multiple transfusions presents with epistaxis and rhinorrhea.

Story Your neighbor approaches you as you arrive home in the evening. You greet her.

"Hi, Mrs Mehra."

"Hello, Doctor. I'm so sorry to trouble you when you are just reaching home."

"No problem. You look very upset, what's the matter?"

"You know my nephew Kripal, who stays with me? He is not keeping very well."

"Yes, I've heard you discussing this with my mother."

"He went to hospital last Saturday for his routine blood transfusion. He was ok then. Then he started having a bit of a cold and headache. He suddenly started feeling worse, he started having some eye pain, and this morning, he started bleeding from the left nostril. He's looking really sick today and I'm wondering whether to call my sister—his mum—from their home in the village. Would you mind having a look at him?"

"Certainly, Mrs Mehra. Let me just pop into my house, freshen up, and I will be at your place in 15 minutes."

After a while, you go to Mrs. Mehra's house.

"Hi, Kripal," you say as you see the 15-year-old boy lying in bed looking miserable. "Your aunt asked me to have a quick look at you. Would that be ok?"

"Yes, doctor," Kripal says wearily.

"How are you feeling right now?"

S. Bhat, *Clinical Conundrums to Practice Diagnostic Reasoning*,
https://doi.org/10.1007/978-981-95-0636-1_66

"Not that good, doctor. I'm feeling pretty sick and I couldn't keep my lunch down. My face hurts too—the left side."

You observe that there is rhinorrhea, and the left side of the face looks swollen and a little red. The left eye looks a little red too.

Questions What do you think is happening to Kripal? Is it a simple sinusitis, or something more dangerous?

Analysis

We have a young boy who is receiving regular blood transfusions. This means that Kripal might have either beta-thalassemia or sickle cell disease or aplastic anemia. Regardless of the reason for transfusions, a consequence of repeated blood transfusion is iron overload [1]. One of the drugs used to manage iron overload is deferoxamine [2]. Deferoxamine increases the risk for invasive fungal infections like mucormycosis [3].

Thus, the rhinorrhea, epistaxis, swelling, and redness of one side of the face indicate that Kripal may have developed mucormycosis.

Iron chelation is used to remove excess iron, detoxify non-transferrin-bound iron and prevent iron accumulation in patients who have iron overload secondary to repeated blood transfusions [4].

Indications for iron chelation include [5] the following:

After 10–20 RBC transfusions, at least 100 mL of RBCs per kg have been administered along with either

- Ferritin level of 1000 ng/mL on two consecutive tests obtained when well
- Liver iron concentration ≥5 mg/g dry weight or
- Cardiac T2* magnetic resonance imaging (MRI) <20 milliseconds

Deferoxamine It is an efficient iron chelator; however, it must be infused subcutaneously overnight for 5–7 days a week, which increases noncompliance [6].

Mucormycosis Mucor is ubiquitous, and the rarity of human infection is because of the intact immune system [7]. It follows that patients who develop mucormycosis have a predisposing factor, possibly one which results in immunocompromise.

The following are the risk factors for mucormycosis [8]:

(a) Diabetic ketoacidosis
(b) Glucocorticoids
(c) Hematologic malignancies
(d) Hematopoietic stem cell transplantation
(e) Solid organ transplantation
(f) Deferoxamine
(g) Recent COVID-19
(h) Malnutrition

Key to the pathogenesis of mucorales is its ability for [9]

(a) Utilizing excess free iron
(b) Angioinvasion

Clinical Features [10]

Patients present initially as acute sinusitis with headache, fever, and nasal discharge. The infection then escalates into a pansinusitis, following which contiguous structures are involved as well.

Spread of infection beyond sinuses is indicated by

(a) Palatal necrosis and eschars
(b) Turbinate destruction
(c) Facial swelling and erythema
(d) Black eschar due to tissue necrosis secondary to vascular invasion
(e) Periorbital edema, proptosis, and blindness
(f) Loss of facial sensation
(g) Obtundation

Treatment [11]

1. Surgical debridement
2. Liposomal amphotericin
3. De-escalation to posaconazole or isavuconazole

Key Takeaway

In a patient with the risk factors for mucormycosis who presents with features of sinusitis but looks disproportionally ill, consider mucormycosis.

References

1. Shander A, Cappellini MD, Goodnough LT. Iron overload and toxicity: the hidden risk of multiple blood transfusions. Vox Sang. 2009;97(3):185–97.
2. Brittenham GM, Griffith PM, Nienhuis AW, McLaren CE, Young NS, Tucker EE, et al. Efficacy of deferoxamine in preventing complications of iron overload in patients with thalassemia major. N Engl J Med. 1994;331(9):567–73.
3. Daly AL. Mucormycosis: association with deferoxamine therapy. Am J Med. 1989;87(4):468–71.
4. Faa G, Crisponi G. Iron chelating agents in clinical practice. Coord Chem Rev. 1999;184(1):291–310.
5. Poggiali E, Cassinerio E, Zanaboni L, Cappellini MD. An update on iron chelation therapy. Blood Transfus. 2012;10(4):411–22.
6. Porter JB. Practical management of iron overload. Br J Haematol. 2001;115(2):239–52.
7. Mallis A, Mastronikolis SN, Naxakis SS, Papadas AT. Rhinocerebral mucormycosis: an update. Eur Rev Med Pharmacol Sci. 2010;14(11):987–92.

8. Gamaletsou MN, Sipsas NV, Roilides E, Walsh TJ. Rhino-orbital-cerebral mucormycosis. Curr Infect Dis Rep. 2012;14(4):423–34.
9. Challa S. Mucormycosis: pathogenesis and pathology. Curr Fungal Infect Rep. 2019;13(1):11–20.
10. Abdollahi A, Shokohi T, Amirrajab N, Poormosa R, Kasiri A, Motahari S, et al. Clinical features, diagnosis, and outcomes of rhino-orbito-cerebral mucormycosis- a retrospective analysis. Curr Med Mycol. 2016;2(4):15–23.
11. Palejwala SK, Zangeneh TT, Goldstein SA, Lemole GM. An aggressive multidisciplinary approach reduces mortality in rhinocerebral mucormycosis. Surg Neurol Int. 2016;7:61.

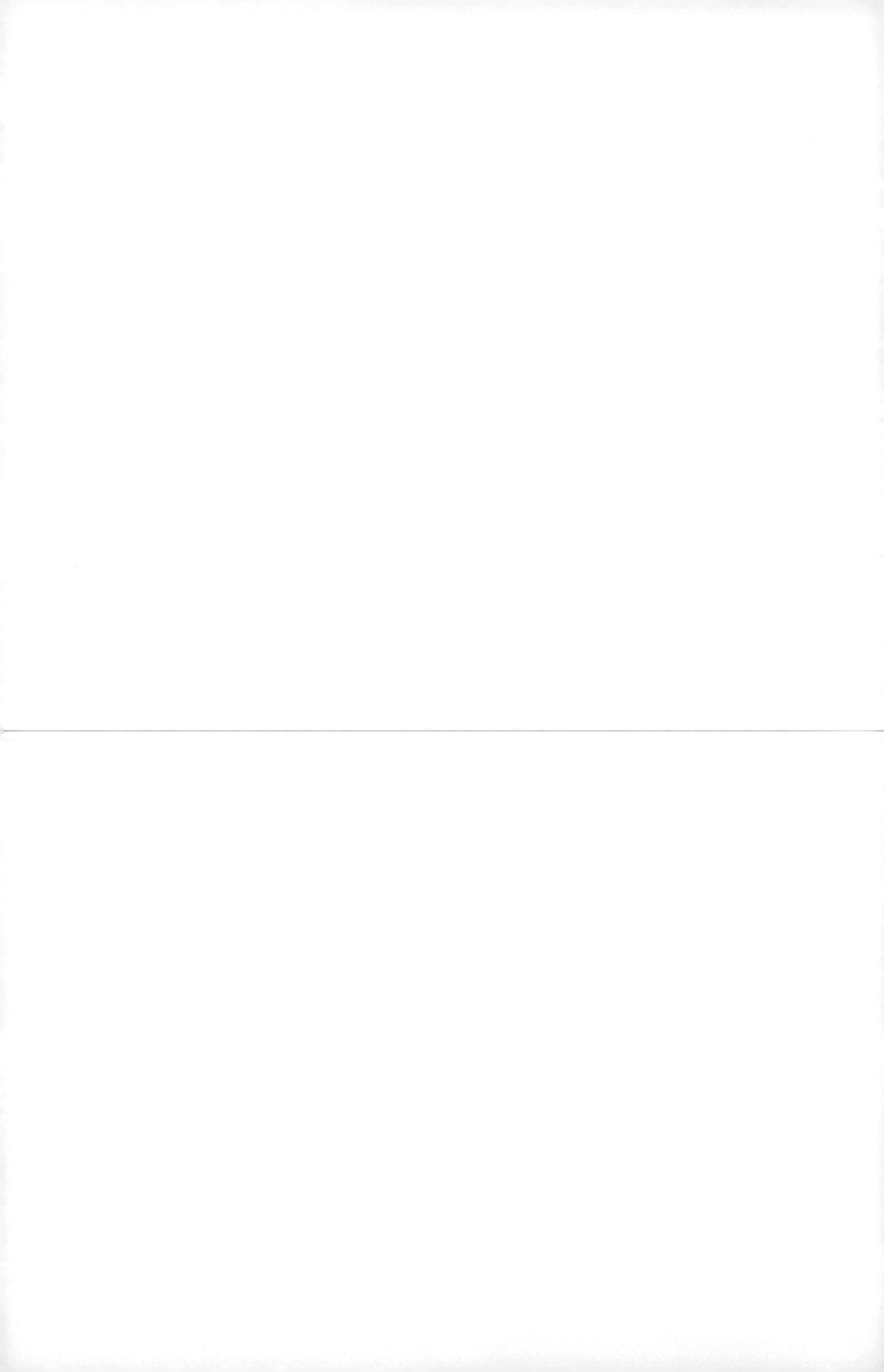

67 Weakness of Limbs and Difficulty in Swallowing After an Attack of Gastroenteritis: Supercilious Sanjay

Grade Easy.

Abstract A haughty uncle admitted to a hospital with sudden illness after an attack of gastroenteritis.

Story You are at your customary monthly dinner with your favorite cousin Anju—you generally spend a pleasant couple of hours discussing work, travel, and music. This evening, however, Anju seems a little upset and moody.

"Ok, spill. What's up with you today?"

"Sorry I'm so glum, Ritu. It's just that I visited Uncle Sanjay this evening, and I really got bugged. I did it as a matter of politeness and because my dad asked me to. It's not like I enjoy meeting him."

"What did he do to piss you off?"

"Well, he asked me how work was going at the gallery. I got a little carried away talking about this painter who I'm convinced is going to make it big very soon."

"Ok..."

"And he sat there all the while, listening to me with this sneer on his face as if he couldn't be less interested in what I was saying."

"That must have been irritating."

"Yes, but what's worse, he then sat there with his eyes half closed like I was boring him to a coma. I'm talking about my gallery—my life's work!"

"Yes, I do understand, but listen, you really shouldn't let our relatives aggravate you like this, you know what they're like."

"That's true," Anju says and asks for another martini.

It is probably 2 weeks later that you are sitting in a very busy outpatient clinic when your aunt—Sanjay's wife—Sunaina calls you.

S. Bhat, *Clinical Conundrums to Practice Diagnostic Reasoning*,
https://doi.org/10.1007/978-981-95-0636-1_67

"Just a quick question, Ritu. Your uncle had loose stools and a tummy upset after eating at that new chaat place. I went to the neighborhood clinic and the doctor prescribed racecodotril and ciprofloxacin. Can he take these?"

"Yes, yes sure," you say absently as the clinic nurse peers in to give you a stern look and say "Many patients are waiting, doctor."

A couple of days later, Sunaina calls again, this time in a panic.

"Ritu, I've just admitted Sanjay to the hospital. Since yesterday, he had severe weakness in his arms and legs and could barely keep his eyes open. I'm really frightened," she says and starts weeping.

"I'll be there as soon as I can," you tell her.

Questions What is happening with Sanjay? Is it just an intercurrent infection in a haughty man? Or is something else at play here?

Analysis

These points must be noted:

(a) The initial history of a sneering look and half-shut eyes
(b) The weakness of limbs and eyes after taking ciprofloxacin

This looks like an undiagnosed case of myasthenia gravis with sudden worsening due to the fluoroquinolone prescription.

Myasthenia gravis (MG) is an autoimmune neuromuscular disorder characterized by weakness of ocular, bulbar, limb, and respiratory muscles. The intensity of weakness varies, depending on exertion and rest [1].

It occurs due to antibodies against acetylcholine receptors (AChR) in the post-synaptic membrane, which prevent sodium ingress and depolarization [2]. This results in muscle weakness. The global prevalence is 150–200 cases per 1,000,000 population [3].

Classification

Based on involvement:

(a) Ocular myasthenia
(b) Generalized myasthenia where ocular, bulbar, limb, and respiratory muscles are involved [2]

Based on severity, MG may be classified as follows [4]:

- Class I—Isolated ocular muscle weakness
- Class II—Mild weakness involving non-ocular muscles
- Class III—Moderate weakness involving non-ocular muscles
- Class IV—Severe weakness involving non-ocular muscles
- Class V—Intubation due to respiratory muscle weakness

Pathogenesis

Myasthenia gravis is an autoimmune disease. The following have been implicated in the pathogenesis:

(a) Autoantibodies are formed against ACh receptors. Initially, the receptors are cross-linked and internalized, preventing the action of ACh on them. However, later in the course of the disease, there is complement-mediated destruction of the receptors [5] (Fig. 67.1).

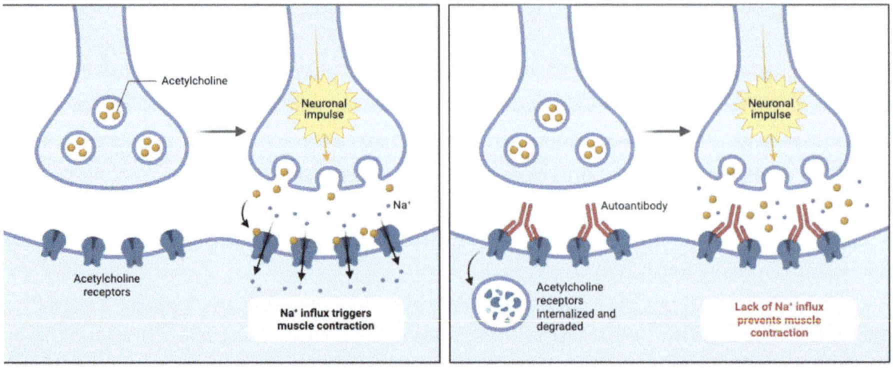

Fig. 67.1 Normal neuromuscular transmission (Panel 1); Ach receptors preventing Ach binding to receptors in MG (Panel 2). (Created in BioRender. Bhat, S. (2025) https://BioRender.com/8pqtizu)

(b) MuSK—Some patients have antibodies against the muscle-specific kinase which is a transmembrane protein in the postsynaptic area of the neuromuscular junction [6].
(c) More than 90% of patients with MG have thymic abnormalities [7]. Thymic hyperplasia or malignancy may be the source of the antigen that drives autoimmunity.
(d) There may be a genetic component as well, as the following haplotypes have been found to be more common in patients with myasthenia—HLA-B8, DRw3, and DQw2 [8].

Clinical Features [9]

1. Fatiguable proximal muscle weakness—decreased strength of contraction with sustained activity.
2. Ptosis, diplopia—pupillary involvement is not seen and goes against a diagnosis of MG [10].
3. Myasthenic sneer when the patient tries to smile—the corners of the mouth do not move, only the middle part of the lip moves, causing the characteristic sneer [11].
4. Dysarthria, dysphagia, and difficulty in chewing hard foods [12].

Diagnosis

(a) Ice pack test [13]
(b) Presence of autoantibodies against AChR and MuSK

(c) Electrodiagnosis: nerve conduction studies with repetitive nerve stimulation tests
(d) Single fiber electromyogram

Treatment

1. General measures: Patient education—all patients must be provided with a list of drugs that exacerbate myasthenia (in this case, fluoroquinolones were the culprit) [14].
2. Vaccination—seasonal flu and pneumococcal vaccinations; however, live attenuated vaccines must be avoided in patients on immunosuppression.
3. Chronic immunotherapy—oral glucocorticoids [15].
4. Symptomatic therapy—acetylcholinesterase inhibitor pyridostigmine [16].
5. Thymectomy in patients who are unresponsive to ACh inhibitors [17].

Myasthenic Crisis [18]

Myasthenic crisis is a life-threatening exacerbation of myasthenia gravis causing respiratory failure.

Management
Plasmapheresis
Intravenous immunoglobulins
Pulsed glucocorticoids
Biologicals like efgartigimod alfa

References

1. Conti-Fine BM, Milani M, Kaminski HJ. Myasthenia gravis: past, present, and future. J Clin Invest. 2006;116(11):2843–54.
2. Drachman DB, Adams RN, Josifek LF, Self SG. Functional activities of autoantibodies to acetylcholine receptors and the clinical severity of myasthenia gravis. N Engl J Med. 1982;307(13):769–75.
3. Dresser L, Wlodarski R, Rezania K, Soliven B. Myasthenia gravis: epidemiology, pathophysiology and clinical manifestations. J Clin Med. 2021;10(11):2235.
4. Jaretzki A, Barohn RJ, Ernstoff RM, Kaminski HJ, Keesey JC, Penn AS, et al. Myasthenia gravis: recommendations for clinical research standards. Task Force of the Medical Scientific Advisory Board of the Myasthenia Gravis Foundation of America. Neurology. 2000;55(1):16–23.
5. Antibodies in Myasthenia Gravis and Related Disorders – VINCENT – 2003 – Annals of the New York Academy of Sciences – Wiley Online Library [Internet]. [cited 2025 Mar 28]. Available from: https://nyaspubs.onlinelibrary.wiley.com/doi/abs/10.1196/annals.1254.036.

6. Cartaud A, Strochlic L, Guerra M, Blanchard B, Lambergeon M, Krejci E, et al. MuSK is required for anchoring acetylcholinesterase at the neuromuscular junction. J Cell Biol. 2004;165(4):505–15.
7. Utsugisawa K, Nagane Y. Thymic abnormalities in patients with myasthenia gravis. Brain Nerve Shinkei Kenkyu No Shinpo. 2011;63(7):685–94.
8. Carlsson B, Wallin J, Pirskanen R, Matell G, Smith CI. Different HLA DR-DQ associations in subgroups of idiopathic myasthenia gravis. Immunogenetics. 1990;31(5–6):285–90.
9. Cortés-Vicente E, Álvarez-Velasco R, Segovia S, Paradas C, Casasnovas C, Guerrero-Sola A, et al. Clinical and therapeutic features of myasthenia gravis in adults based on age at onset. Neurology. 2020;94(11):e1171–80.
10. Kaminski HJ, Maas E, Spiegel P, Ruff RL. Why are eye muscles frequently involved in myasthenia gravis? Neurology. 1990;40(11):1663–9.
11. Keesey JC. Clinical evaluation and management of myasthenia gravis. Muscle Nerve. 2004;29(4):484–505.
12. Pal S, Sanyal D. Jaw muscle weakness: a differential indicator of neuromuscular weakness—preliminary observations. Muscle Nerve. 2011;43(6):807–11.
13. Chatzistefanou KI, Kouris T, Iliakis E, Piaditis G, Tagaris G, Katsikeris N, et al. The ice pack test in the differential diagnosis of myasthenic diplopia. Ophthalmology. 2009;116(11):2236–43.
14. Jones SC, Sorbello A, Boucher RM. Fluoroquinolone-associated myasthenia gravis exacerbation: evaluation of postmarketing reports from the US FDA adverse event reporting system and a literature review. Drug Saf. 2011;34(10):839–47.
15. Sanders DB, Wolfe GI, Benatar M, Evoli A, Gilhus NE, Illa I, et al. International consensus guidance for management of myasthenia gravis: executive summary. Neurology. 2016;87(4):419–25.
16. Mehndiratta MM, Pandey S, Kuntzer T. Acetylcholinesterase inhibitor treatment for myasthenia gravis. Cochrane Database Syst Rev. 2014;2014(10):CD006986.
17. Aydin Y, Ulas AB, Mutlu V, Colak A, Eroglu A. Thymectomy in myasthenia gravis. Eurasian J Med. 2017;49(1):48–52.
18. Myasthenic crisis demanding mechanical ventilation | Neurology [Internet]. [cited 2025 Mar 28]. Available from: https://www.neurology.org/doi/10.1212/WNL.0000000000008688.

68 Cardiovascular Deterioration After Sexual Intercourse: The Happy Couple

Grade Very easy.

Abstract Man found dead in bed on honeymoon.

Story Glen is happier than he ever thought he would be. His business is booming, he is newly married, and he is in beautiful Bali for his honeymoon along with his gorgeous wife Sharol (Fig. 68.1). Here in the sun, sipping on mimosas with Sharol—the real world seems very far away. His niggling health issues—his blood pressure which never came down, his cholesterol level which seemed to be rising at every clinic visit, his chronic acidity—they all seem imaginary. He feels ready to take on the world. Why, didn't he accomplish a spectacular win at the badminton court this morning? Of course, his opponent was a resort employee who was probably playing to lose, but still.

He stretches luxuriously and tells Sharol to get ready and join him at the dock so they can take a ride on a speedboat.

That night, after a scrumptious meal in the moonlight, Glen and Sharol decide to go to bed. Glen showers and surreptitiously swallows a pill that his friend had given him—winking and saying—"You have to keep that young bride of yours happy!" In fact, while stocking up on medicines prior to travel, Glen had requested his physician for some help in this regard, but the good doctor categorically refused, saying that it would have adverse effects on his health.

Glen and his bride turn in and turn the lights off. The next morning, Sharol opens her eyes to the terrifying realization that her new husband is very dead. She screams, calls for help, and has the traumatic experience of spending the last day of her honeymoon arranging to repatriate her husband's remains.

Questions Was Glen's death a consequence of overeating, badminton, and honeymoon high jinks? Or was there another factor contributing?

S. Bhat, *Clinical Conundrums to Practice Diagnostic Reasoning*, https://doi.org/10.1007/978-981-95-0636-1_68

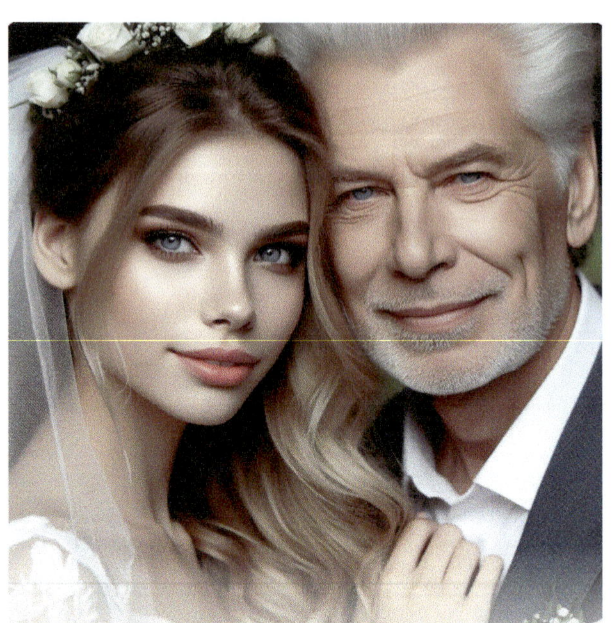

Fig. 68.1 Glen and Sharol

Analysis

This is most likely a case of Sexual Activity-related Sudden Death (SArSD). The common causes of SArSD are [1]

(a) Coronary artery disease
(b) Subarachnoid hemorrhage with ruptured berry aneurysm

Of these, considering his risk factors of hypertension and dyslipidemia, coronary artery disease is likely. However, one must also take in to account the fact that he took a tablet to enhance his performance. This, in all likelihood, was one of the phosphodiesterase inhibitors like sildenafil. If Glen was already on nitrates for ischemic heart disease (again very likely), the two would have interacted to cause hypotension.

Sildenafil [2]

It acts by inhibiting phosphodiesterase. The end effect is increased cGMP causing dilatation of penile arteries, causing increased blood flow to the penis and erection (Fig. 68.2).

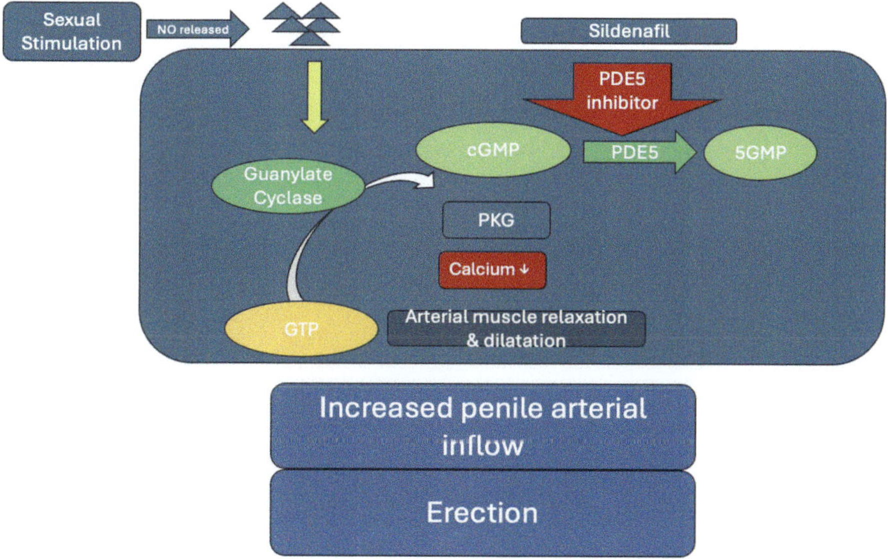

Fig. 68.2 Effect of sildenafil on penile blood flow. *cGMP* cyclic GMP, *PDE5* phosphodiesterase 5, *PKG* phosphokinase

As can be seen from the figure, nitrates also have the effect of combining with guanyl cyclase to increase the formation of cGMP, which causes a generalized arterial dilatation. Hence, nitrates potentiate the action of sildenafil and tend to cause a precipitous fall in blood pressure which may precipitate cardiac death.

Risk factors for SArSD include [3]:

(a) Obesity
(b) Use of cocaine
(c) Medications for erectile dysfunction

Key Takeaway
Patients should avoid taking PDE-5 inhibitors within 24–48 h of nitrate use.

References

1. Lopez-Garcia P, de Leon MSS, Hernandez-Guerra A, Fernandez-Liste A, Lucena J, Morentin B. Sudden death related to sexual activity: a multicenter study based on forensic autopsies (2010–2021). Forensic Sci Int. 2024;354:111908.
2. Smith BP, Babos M. Sildenafil. In: StatPearls [Internet]. Treasure Island (FL): StatPearls Publishing; 2025 [cited 2025 Mar 27]. Available from: http://www.ncbi.nlm.nih.gov/books/NBK558978/.
3. Lee S, Chae J, Cho Y. Causes of sudden death related to sexual activity: results of a medicolegal postmortem study from 2001 to 2005. J Korean Med Sci. 2006;21(6):995–9.

69 Middle-Aged Male with Varicocele—The Bag of Worms

Grade Easy.

Abstract A middle-aged male with loss of weight and fever.

Story Mr. Jijo, a 40-year-old male, is under the care of your surgery colleague for a left scrotal varicocele. He is referred to you for evaluation of fever and loss of weight. You speak to him and elicit a history of fever, night sweats, loss of appetite, and weight. There is no history of contact with tuberculosis. No history of cough, headache, loose stools, or burning micturition, though Jijo says he has passed clots of blood in his urine a week ago.

You examine him and note that his BMI is 17. He is pale. His lungs are clear, abdomen is soft, and nervous system examination is normal. You examine the scrotal varicocele that your colleague has documented—it is quite large and does not drain when the patient is recumbent.

Questions What might be the cause of Jijo's loss of weight and fever? How would you like to proceed with investigations and treatment?

S. Bhat, *Clinical Conundrums to Practice Diagnostic Reasoning*,
https://doi.org/10.1007/978-981-95-0636-1_69

Analysis

The points worth noting here are as follows:

(a) The scrotal varicocele that does not drain on recumbency is itself a red flag.
(b) The passing of clots in the urine is very suggestive of renal cell carcinoma.

With the high clinical suspicion of renal cell carcinoma, Mr. Jijo requires an abdominal CT scan.

Renal cell carcinomas (RCC) originate in the renal cortex and unfortunately are usually asymptomatic until the disease is advanced. It is more common in males than females and are usually seen between the age of 60 and 80 [1].

Etiopathogenesis [2]

The risk factors of RCC are

(a) Smoking
(b) Analgesic abuse
(c) Hypertension
(d) Obesity
(e) Genetic predisposition
(f) Exposure to asbestos and cadmium
(g) Cytotoxic chemotherapy
(h) Acquired cystic disease of the kidney

Clinical Features [3]

1. Fever, loss of weight, and loss of appetite
2. Hematuria, history of passing blood clots in the urine
3. Abdominal mass
4. Varicocele—which does not empty on recumbency since the mass obstructs the gonadal vein at the point of renal vein entry
5. Cachexia
6. Anemia, sometimes erythrocytosis, and thrombocytosis
7. Hypercalcemia

Investigations

CT abdomen
MRI abdomen
Biomarkers

Treatment

Nephrectomy
Adjuvant therapy with pembrolizumab [4]

For metastatic RCC: sorafenib, sunitinib, bevacizumab, pazopanib and axitinib, and everolimus and temsirolimus [5].

References

1. Bukavina L, Bensalah K, Bray F, Carlo M, Challacombe B, Karam JA, Kassouf W, Mitchell T, Montironi R, O'Brien T, Panebianco V. Epidemiology of renal cell carcinoma: 2022 update. Eur Urol. 2022;82(5):529–42.
2. Makino T, Kadomoto S, Izumi K, Mizokami A. Epidemiology and prevention of renal cell carcinoma. Cancers. 2022;14(16):4059.
3. Kirkali Z, Öbek C. Clinical aspects of renal cell carcinoma. EAU Update Ser. 2003;1(4):189–96.
4. Choueiri TK, Tomczak P, Park SH, Venugopal B, Ferguson T, Symeonides SN, Hajek J, Chang YH, Lee JL, Sarwar N, Haas NB. Overall survival with adjuvant pembrolizumab in renal-cell carcinoma. N Engl J Med. 2024;390(15):1359–71.
5. Hsieh JJ, Purdue MP, Signoretti S, Swanton C, Albiges L, Schmidinger M, Heng DY, Larkin J, Ficarra V. Renal cell carcinoma. Nat Rev Dis Primers. 2017;3(1):1–9.

Altered Behavior and Agitation in a Postoperative Patient: The Bike Accident

70

Grade Very easy.

Abstract A patient admitted to a hospital after a fracture sustained in a road traffic accident becomes violent and agitated.

Story Jidin and his friends were getting back home after a party when Jidin's bike crashed, and he sustained a fall and unfortunately fractured his left tibia. The department of orthopedics admits him and advises intramedullary nailing.

The patient is posted for surgery the next morning. The surgery is successful, and Jidin is shifted to the ward for physiotherapy and postoperative care. Jidin is recovering well apart from two episodes of loose stools and a slight headache on postoperative days 1 and 2. However, he takes a turn for the worse on day 4, and a medicine consult is sent.

You go to the orthopedic ward to assess Jidin, and when you near his bed, you are greeted by a stream of colorful invective. You resist the temptation to tell Jidin to go wash his mouth out with soap and proceed to examine him.

You note:
Heart rate: 110/min
BP: 150/70 mm Hg
Respiratory rate: 28 breaths/min

S. Bhat, *Clinical Conundrums to Practice Diagnostic Reasoning*,
https://doi.org/10.1007/978-981-95-0636-1_70

The patient is febrile, diaphoretic, and extremely agitated.
Tongue is dry.
No focal neurological deficits.
No neck stiffness.

Questions Why do you think Jidin is so agitated? Is it the frustration of being cooped up and inactive? Or is something else happening? How do you proceed with investigations and management?

Analysis

This is a very easy puzzle.

Clues: The fact that the patient is returning from a party and has an accident is a clue to the possibility of alcohol intoxication. The headache and GI upset on days 1 and 2 are the first symptoms of minor withdrawal. The extreme agitation, hypertension, tachycardia, and diaphoresis are typical of delirium tremens which can occur between 4 and 8 days after the last drink.

Other causes of agitation/confusion in a patient with alcohol dependence syndrome are

(a) Intoxication
(b) Withdrawal
(c) Wernicke's encephalopathy/Korsakoff's psychosis
(d) Hypoglycemia
(e) Subdural hematoma
(f) Hepatic encephalopathy

The effect of sudden cessation of alcohol in an individual who is habituated to its consumption may have different clinical manifestations:

(a) Withdrawal—anxiety, headache, and gastrointestinal symptoms
(b) Alcohol withdrawal seizures
(c) Alcoholic hallucinosis: visual or auditory hallucinations
(d) Delirium tremens

Etiopathogenesis [1, 2] (Fig. 70.1)

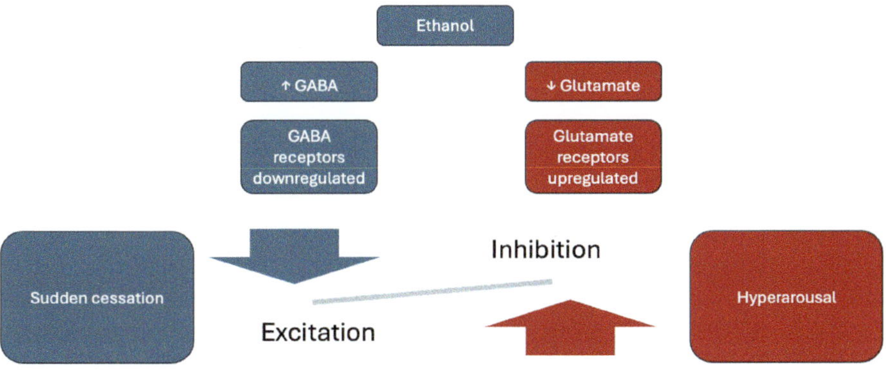

Fig. 70.1 Eetipathogenesis of alcohol withdrawal syndrome

Investigations

1. Blood glucose
2. Serum electrolytes
3. Liver function test
4. Neuroimaging to rule out subdural hematoma as the cause of seizures

Treatment [2, 3]

1. Hydration.
2. Correct hypokalemia, hypomagnesemia, and hypophosphatemia if present.
3. Sedation.
4. Administration of thiamine.
5. Chlordiazepoxide.
6. Treatment of seizures: benzodiazepines and phenobarbital are the preferred agents [4].

Key Takeaway
Always consider alcohol withdrawal as a cause for unexplained agitation and autonomic hyperactivity in a hospitalized patient.

References

1. Bayard M, Mcintyre J, Hill KR, Woodside J. Alcohol withdrawal syndrome. Am Family Phys. 2004;69(6):1443–50.
2. Littleton J. Neurochemical mechanisms underlying alcohol withdrawal. Alcohol Health Res World. 1998;22(1):13.
3. Kosten TR, O'Connor PG. Management of drug and alcohol withdrawal. N Engl J Med. 2003;348(18):1786–95.
4. Gupta A, Khan H, Kaur A, Singh TG. Novel targets explored in the treatment of alcohol withdrawal syndrome. CNS Neurol Disord Drug Targets (Formerly Current Drug Targets-CNS & Neurological Disorders). 2021;20(2):158–73.

Refractory Shock After Trauma—The Bloody Biker

71

Grade Easy.

Abstract A young man presents after a bike accident with shock unresponsive to volume replacement.

Story N is an 18-year-old boy, the proud possessor of a KTM bike. Drunk on cheap whiskey and speed, he not unexpectedly comes a cropper and is brought to a hospital by terrified friends.

You are on duty in the ER when he is brought in—and you do a quick survey. You note that his blood pressure is 90/70 mm Hg, he looks pale, he is conscious, and he is in obvious pain and distress. There are multiple abrasions all over his body; some wounds are bleeding heavily. There are no petechiae on the chest. You send him in for X-rays, start him on iv fluids, send for blood grouping and typing, and administer pain relief.

You have rushed 2 pints of fluids, packed RBC transfusion is on flow, and you are a little worried that the BP is not picking up. There is no fracture of the lower limbs, and the ultrasonogram abdomen shows no signs of splenic/hepatic injury. IVC collapsibility index is normal. You have a look at the chest X-ray (Fig. 71.1) and ECG (Fig. 71.2).

Questions What do you think is the cause of the hypotension? How would you manage Mr. N? What are the other signs that might be seen?

S. Bhat, *Clinical Conundrums to Practice Diagnostic Reasoning*,
https://doi.org/10.1007/978-981-95-0636-1_71

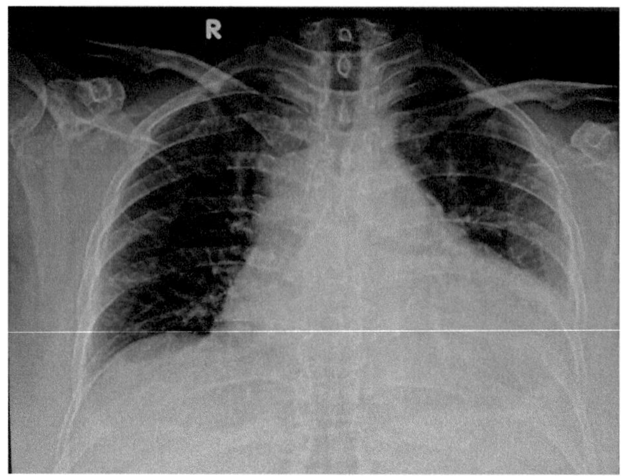

Fig. 71.1 Chest X-ray. (Image from author's collection)

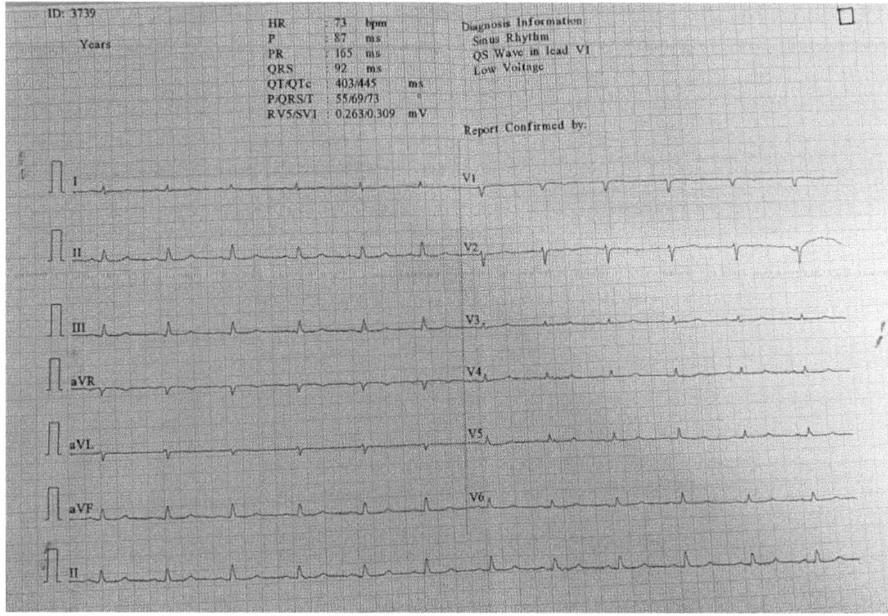

Fig. 71.2 ECG. (Image from author's collection)

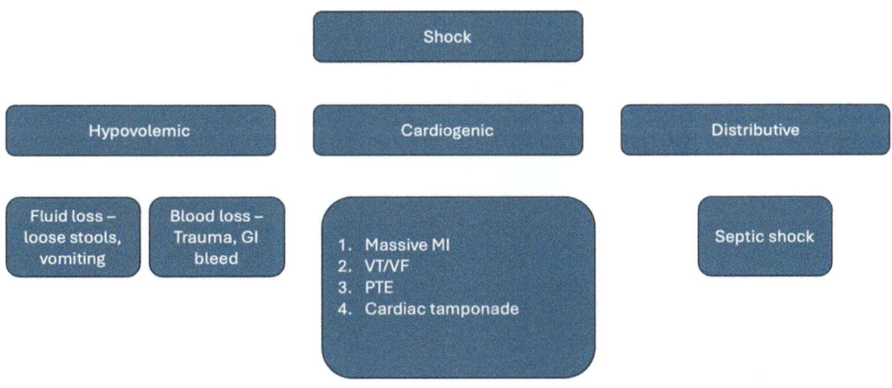

Fig. 71.3 Approach to shock

Analysis

The causes of hypotension are as follows (Fig. 71.3).

Hypovolemia is unlikely since fluid has been replaced and IVC is normal. The timeline of this scenario does not go in favor of septic shock. The patient characteristics are not suggestive of massive MI, and ECG does not show arrhythmia. In a road traffic accident, fat embolism [1] is a possibility; however, there is no fracture femur in this case. Cardiac tamponade is likely, given the chest X-ray demonstrating cardiomegaly and the ECG showing low-voltage complexes.

Cardiac tamponade is due to a pressurized pericardial effusion compressing the ventricles, diminishing venous return and impairing cardiac output.

Common Causes [2]

- Blunt or penetrating trauma to the chest
- Complications from cardiac catheterization or pacemaker insertion
- Postcardiac surgery
- Aortic dissection
- Myocardial infarction

Pathogenesis (Fig. 71.4)

(a) Pressurized pericardial effusion—decreased venous return to right ventricle: Blue arrow
(b) Interventricular septum bulging into left ventricle because of increased interdependence of ventricles: Yellow arrow
(c) Decreased left ventricular volume: Black arrow

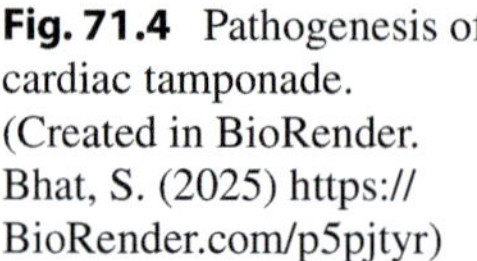

Fig. 71.4 Pathogenesis of cardiac tamponade. (Created in BioRender. Bhat, S. (2025) https://BioRender.com/p5pjtyr)

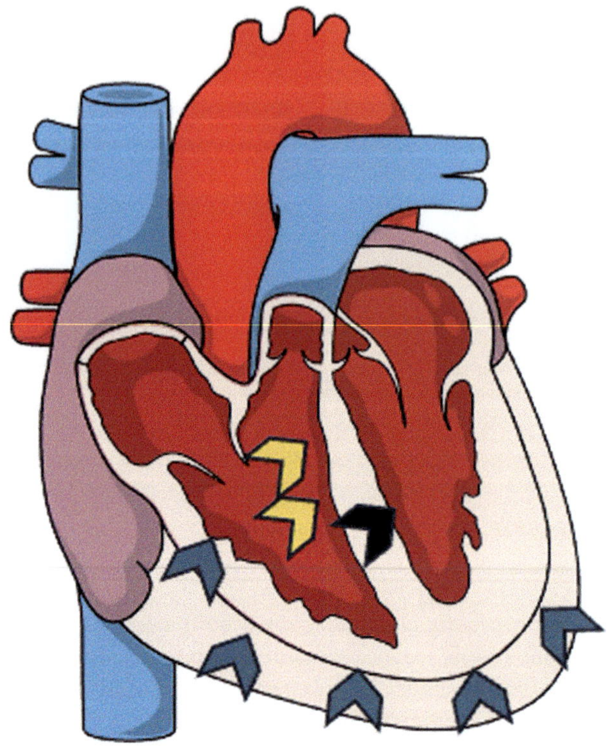

Clinical Features

1. Becks triad [3]
   - Falling arterial pressure
   - Rising venous pressure
   - Muffled heart sounds
2. Prominent x descent and absent y descent [4]
3. Paradoxical pulse: Inspiratory fall in systolic blood pressure >10 mm Hg [5]

Treatment

Emergent pericardiocentesis [6]

References

1. Kwiatt ME, Seamon MJ. Fat embolism syndrome. Int J Crit Illn Inj Sci. 2013;3(1):64–8.
2. Sánchez-Enrique C, Nuñez-Gil IJ, Viana-Tejedor A, De Agustín A, Vivas D, Palacios-Rubio J, et al. Cause and long-term outcome of cardiac tamponade. Am J Cardiol. 2016;117(4):664–9.
3. Cardiac tamponade | Nature Reviews Disease Primers [Internet]. [cited 2025 Mar 30]. Available from: https://www.nature.com/articles/s41572-023-00446-1.
4. Ranganathan N, Sivaciyan V. Jugular venous pulse descent patterns: recognition and clinical relevance. CJC Open. 2022;5(3):200–7.
5. Hamzaoui O, Monnet X, Teboul JL. Pulsus paradoxus. Eur Respir J. 2013;42(6):1696–705.
6. Imazio M, De Ferrari GM. Cardiac tamponade: an educational review. Eur Heart J Acute Cardiovasc Care. 2021;10(1):102–9.